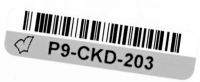

THEORY AND PRACTICE OF BRIEF THERAPY

Theory and Practice of Brief Therapy

SIMON H. BUDMAN
Harvard Community Health Plan
and Harvard Medical School

ALAN S. GURMAN
University of Wisconsin Medical School

Foreword by Paul L. Wachtel

THE GUILFORD PRESS
New York   London

© 1988 The Guilford Press
A Division of Guilford Publications, Inc.
72 Spring Street, New York, New York, 10012

Printed in the United States of America

Last digit is print number: 9 8 7 6 5 4 3

Library of Congress Cataloging in Publication Data

Budman, Simon H.
    Theory and practice of brief therapy
Simon H. Budman & Alan S. Gurman.
        p.   cm.
    Bibliography: p.
    Includes index.
    ISBN 0-89862-716-8
    1. Psychotherapy, Brief. I. Gurman, Alan S. II. Title.
    [DNLM: 1. Psychotherapy, Brief—methods. WM 420 B927t]
RC480.55.B83 1988
616.89'14—dc 19   87-24847
                                                                        CIP

To Drs. Gene Lindsey and John Collins, for saving my life.
                                                                —S.H.B.

To Gerri, Jesse, and Ted, for enriching mine.
                                                                —A.S.G.

Foreword

This excellent book conveys vividly an approach to brief therapy that is comprehensive and based on sound and well thought-out principles. It demonstrates as well as anything I have read how the findings of empirical research can be brought to bear in devising effective therapeutic strategies, and exposes as shallow and uninformed the claim that research has yielded nothing of value to the clinician. Particularly noteworthy is that the research that nourishes this work is not just therapy outcome research but research on basic processes as well. Budman and Gurman's applications of the research findings on bereavement and loss, for example, are extremely impressive.

I found particularly valuable their strong emphases on building on the patient's strengths and on the importance of social support systems throughout the life cycle. Budman and Gurman's approach appreciates the degree to which people's lives are lived in a social context, and it does so without sacrificing attention to the supposedly "deeper" issues which have served as the excuse for many therapists to substantially ignore the world around us. Especially significant is their addressing of the importance of events outside the consulting room in bringing about therapeutic change. All too many therapeutic approaches seem to assume that little outside the few hours a week that the patient spends with the therapist really has an impact. Here, as in other places, this book exposes the false dichotomy between what happens in the session and what happens in daily life. As Budman and Gurman show very well, the impact of the time spent with the therapist is very largely in helping the patient to change his or her daily interactions, which contribute so centrally to the maintenance of the problem. The authors do this without minimizing or ignoring the processes going on in the session itself or between patient and therapist. Their appreciation of the importance of the corrective emotional experience—or perhaps more accurately, their explicit and unhedged appreciation; it is often brought in through the back door of authors' discussions—is salutary and unusual in an era in which that concept is still inappropriately stigmatized.

The book is commendable for its honesty. It confronts the complexity of the real world rather than attempting to fit all observations into the mold of their theories. For example, though the book is about *brief* therapy—and demonstrates very effectively how much more can be accomplished in a brief time than is usually assumed by dynamically oriented therapists—in the case of Shelley the authors present an instance in which therapy over many years was required; albeit in the spirit of the approach described throughout the book, rather than as a kind of Woody Allen continuous immersion in therapy month after month (except August) and year after year. It is a case, moreover, in which even all of this did not stem her decline when contact with the therapist was interrupted. Such confrontation with the actual complexity of what happens in the lives of people who have been in therapy gives the reader much greater confidence in what the authors are presenting and advocating.

The book will be of value to practitioners of long-term therapy as well as those who explicitly think of themselves as brief therapists. It presents a fresh and exciting approach that would be extremely worthwhile for the clinician to learn even if insurance companies wanted to do nothing more than to pay for full scale analyses. Much of what the book advocates is what long-term therapists' common sense has been telling them for years, and the points it articulates account for why therapists do all those things they'd never tell their supervisors (who also secretly do them, without letting on to their supervisees).

The book is beautifully written. It is clear; it is literate; and it is the only book I have read that dares to explore the world historical dialectic between Sophocles and Yogi Berra (see Chapter 11). In addition to its main arguments, the book is filled with insightful asides. Some made me notice in a fresh way what should have been obvious all along; for example, that the research on psychotherapy outcome seems to focus almost exclusively on brief therapy, even if not always presented as doing so. Other points made in passing stimulated further thought and provoked me to generate my own hypotheses. Their early discussion of premature termination, for example, made me wonder if the reason so many "long-term" therapies end with the patient having attended fewer sessions than in the typical brief therapy is that the open-endedness of long-term therapy, its seeming prospect of endlessness, is disturbing to some patients. In effect, they have to leave after 5 to 10 sessions when the prospect looms of hundreds, but can stick it out for 20 or 40 when they know that the plan is quite explicit and that 20 or 40 is all there will be.

All in all, this is one of those rare books that combines clarity with profundity, depicting an approach that, in equally rare fashion, combines flexibility with rigor. The theoretical discussions are consistently sensible, complex, and clarifying, and the clinical vignettes are useful and to the point. Budman and Gurman present a humane and comprehensive approach that should have a powerful influence on how therapy is practiced for many years to come.

Paul L. Wachtel

Preface

To many observers, it appears that interest in brief therapy has greatly increased over the past decade. Psychoanalytic, cognitive, interpersonal, and behavioral clinicians, seemingly persuaded by theoretical factors, research findings and/or the hard realities of third-party reimbursement pressures, have examined ways in which treatment can be made maximally effective in the shortest period of time. Such efforts have spawned the variety of new short-term approaches described in the many psychotherapy "treatment manuals" currently available.

In fact, most therapy is, and has for decades been, brief by any of several criteria. While "brief therapy" has come on the scene in more "acceptable" forms over the past decade, this has often been through the "miniaturization" of "established," psychoanalytic long-term models. We are convinced, however, that most therapists who do brief therapy (whom, we believe, are *most* therapists) are rarely theoretical or technical purists. Rather, they are pragmatic and eclectic, if not integrative, in method and technique.

Furthermore, we are of the belief that most of the actual day-to-day brief therapy that occurs emphasizes current developmental issues (often more neutrally referred to as "situational") and the interpersonal and systemic context of problems. Such a perspective seems to us to be not only practically wise, but also to offer a much more optimistic view of the human condition—hence, the likelihood of change—than many conventional short- or long-term psychotherapeutic models. In like fashion, we see most of this brief therapy as being more comprehensively "systemic," in the sense of paying simultaneous attention to affect, cognition, and behavior and to "the" patient's interactions with others in everyday life.

Thus, in a certain sense, the model of therapy presented here is not particularly unique, but reflects what we see as the essential and common elements in effective brief therapy-as-most-often-practiced. It is a distillation of what we believe to be the central features of any effective brief therapy, even those aspects of the treatment that may not be completely articulated by the therapist.

Our own involvement with brief therapy grew, to a great degree, out of our work settings. As practicing clinicians at health maintenance organizations (HMOs), we were faced with the task of treating large and varied populations of patients without the luxury of extended evaluations or unlimited treatment resources. At the same time, we found that some of the models of brief therapy presented in the literature were difficult or impossible to implement in a general practice setting, or were seemingly developed with very specific types of "ideal patients."

It became clear to us that, for some patients, 10 or 12 consecutive, weekly visits were far too many, while for others change could evolve only by very small incremental steps over many months or years. We also noticed that even our most successful cases often failed to "really" terminate. The longer that we worked at our respective clinical settings, the more apparent it became that a patient would frequently return to us at various points in his or her life with issues related to current developmental hurdles or milestones. Even if such issues were variations on earlier concerns, the likelihood of having been able to anticipate and preventatively treat the "new" problem in an earlier course of therapy was usually not great.

What evolved for us over time was a model of brief treatment that came to appear much more like a primary care or family practice paradigm for internal medicine, than traditional therapeutic models of mental health treatment. Often, we see not only the designated patient, but also significant others, family, friends and so on, as it appears useful. Also, we may treat patients for many intermittent courses of therapy over their life times and, as appropriate, use different techniques and types of interventions. We do not feel constrained by any narrow theoretical orientation and, therefore, feel free to choose from what we see as the most beneficial aspects of many different psychotherapy perspectives.

It is our hope that _Theory and Practice of Brief Therapy_ can serve as a helpful reference for those interested in a practical, flexible, and comprehensive model of brief psychotherapy. There are clearly elements of what we describe that will require future study and examination. For the present, however, we believe that this approach can be applied in a multiplicity of settings, with diverse populations and varied clinical demands.

We are very grateful to Dr. Paul Wachtel for his helpful comments on an earlier draft of this manuscript. Drs. Gerald Klerman and Nick Cummings provided sage advice and insightful critiques. Ms. Tamar Springer was another reader who must be singled out for her invaluable input regarding many aspects of this project.

Special thanks are due to Dr. Howard Frazier, The Institute for Health Research, and The Harvard Community Health Plan Foundation for providing Dr. Budman with the time and resources to carry out this undertaking.

We are indebted to Seymour Weingarten, Editor-in-Chief at The Guilford Press, with whom it has been our great pleasure to work on this and other books.

Our deepest thanks go to our patients, who have shared their stories with us. It is from them that we have learned the most about psychotherapy.

Simon H. Budman
Alan S. Gurman

Contents

1

The Practice of Brief Therapy:
An Introduction

THE HISTORICAL CONTEXT

In the earliest days of the psychoanalytic movement, the psychotherapeutic process was seen as being of relatively brief duration (Marmor, 1979). Many of Freud's treatments and training analyses were completed in a span of weeks or months rather than years. Indeed, the famous analyst Sandor Ferenczi was himself analyzed by Freud in 6 weeks, 3 in 1914 and 3 in 1916 (Jones, 1955). At that time, the prevailing mood among psychoanalytic thinkers was that therapeutic intervention could be brief, concise, and effective. Examples abound of therapies being successfully completed after several visits. In one instance, Freud referred a case to Wilhelm Reich with the notation: "impotence, three months" (Reich, 1967, p. 59). Even in 1930, treatment at the Berlin Psychoanalytic Institute averaged about 1 year in length (Roazen, 1974, p. 130).

It was only as analytic thinking became more complex, as the problems dealt with by analysts became more difficult, and as the goals of analysis became increasingly ambitious that treatment became longer and longer. Freud's personal developmental issues in later years also appear to have had an impact on the length of his analyses. As Roazen (1971) writes:

> By the end of his life, Freud was seeing patients for longer periods—in some instances six years. In part this was due to his ill health; as he grew old he became less attracted to meeting new people, and if he found a patient who could afford his fees and was interesting but not too troublesome, it was easier for him not to interrupt treatment. In addition, Freud was disappointed by the results of some of his early cases, which at the time had appeared to be successful; perhaps lengthier analyses might be more reliable. . . . But questions of how long analysis should last were not really important to Freud. Uppermost in his mind was the advancement of science. (p. 131).

Sections of this chapter are adapted from "The Practice of Brief Therapy" by S. H. Budman and A. S. Gurman, 1983, *Professional Psychology: Research and Practice, 14*, 277–292. Copyright 1983 by *American Psychological Association*. Adapted by permission. And from "Advances in Brief Psychotherapy" by S. H. Budman and J. Stone, 1984, *Hospital and Community Psychiatry, 34*, 939–946. Copyright 1984 by American Psychiatric Association. Adapted by permission.

Although many within analytic circles were distressed by the trend toward more extended treatment, their protests were viewed with great antagonism, especially by Freud himself (Roazen, 1974). One by one, great innovators such as Ferenczi, Rank, Adler, and Strebel, who expressed concern about the development of more efficient modes of analysis, were rejected from Freud's inner circle. These men, all prominent analysts and original thinkers, clashed with Freud on a variety of issues, some related to brevity of therapy and the activity of the analyst. It also appears that Freud's feelings about input from others often made him disinclined to accept innovative positions on the parts of his followers.

> Although he admired originality and talent, he had difficulty tolerating anyone with ideas of his own. As he freely admitted, "I have no use for other people's ideas when they are presented to me at an inopportune moment." Thus Freud repeatedly drove away his best pupils. . . . [H]e enjoyed quoting Heine's saying, "One must forgive one's enemies—but not before they have been hanged." (Roazen, 1971, p. 181).

The tone thus set within the analytic movement was one of orthodoxy and close adherence to the positions recommended by Freud. Although some psychoanalysts continued to raise the issue of more efficient analysis (Ferenczi & Rank, 1925), it was not until years after Freud's death in 1939 that brevity of treatment again emerged as a prominent issue.

By the mid-1940s, when Alexander and French published their seminal volume on brief treatment, *Psychoanalytic Therapy* (1946/1974), the *Zeitgeist* had changed dramatically. Thousands of veterans were returning from World War II in need of mental health services and with an entitlement to such benefits through the Veterans Administration. Many practicing psychiatrists had had experiences as Army physicians with the short-term treatment of "war neuroses" or "battle fatigue" (Grinker & Spiegel, 1944). Furthermore, the prevailing mood in the country of optimism and egalitarianism ran counter to the somber elitism of long-term psychoanalysis, for which few people were candidates and which even fewer could afford.

In their book, Alexander and French directly confronted many of the pivotal analytic dogmas current at that time:

> (1) that the depth of therapy is *necessarily* proportionate to the length of treatment and the frequency of the interviews;
> (2) that therapeutic results achieved by a relatively small number of interviews are *necessarily* superficial and temporary, while therapeutic results achieved by prolonged treatment are necessarily more stable and more profound; and
> (3) that the prolongation of an analysis is justified on the grounds that the patient's resistance will *eventually* be overcome and the desired therapeutic results achieved. (Alexander & French, 1946/1974, p. vi)

The authors went on to call for flexibility on the part of the therapist in regard to frequency of visits and manipulation of the transference in order for the patient to achieve a "corrective emotional experience." What Alexander and French meant by such an experience is that the therapist helps the patient to be re-exposed to some of those emotional situations that were unbearable in the past, but under more favorable circumstances that allow the situation to be handled in a new and more effective way. As a case example of a naturally occurring corrective emotional experience, Alexander and French cited Jean Valjean from Victor Hugo's classic, *Les Miserables* (1862/1938). Valjean, a hardened criminal, is treated with great kindness and compassion by a bishop whom he has tried to rob. The criminal is stunned by this behavior. Shortly after this incident, Valjean is walking on a road and almost automatically attempts to steal two francs from a young boy who has dropped the money. When he suddenly realizes what he is doing, he runs after the crying boy to return the coin. Jean Valjean at that moment has been transformed by the bishop's warmth and forgiveness. This humane "brief treatment" leads him to abandon his former criminality completely.

At nearly the same time that Alexander and French were developing their model in Chicago, Erich Lindemann, in Boston, initiated studies in the area of crisis intervention. Working mainly with relatives and friends of victims of the tragic Cocoanut Grove nightclub fire, Lindemann (1944) mapped the course of "normal" and "morbid" grief reactions. He also described brief psychiatric interventions (8–10 sessions) that could be used with such survivors. Thus, the mid-1940s saw a resurgence of the long-dormant interest in brief therapies.

Nonetheless, it was not until the 1960s that the short-term movement really began to flourish. The Community Mental Health Centers Act, passed during the Kennedy administration, led to the universal availability of psychotherapeutic services. Thus, with great patient demand and chronic staffing shortages came extended waiting times. The sociopolitical climate fueled the brief therapy movement, as did theoretical developments in family therapy and behavioral treatments. In quick succession, Malan (1963), Sifneos (1972), and Mann (1973) published important books on brief treatment from an analytic perspective, while from a more iconoclastic position Haley (1973) published his book on the innovative work of Milton Erickson.

Since the late 1960s, but in particular during the 1980s, the sociopolitical climate has continued to favor the development of short-term therapy models. Insurers of health care have responded to spiraling costs and mandated mental health benefits by placing strict caps on the amount of money provided for such coverage. Newly emerging health care delivery systems, such as health maintenance organizations (HMOs) and independent practice associations (IPAs), have strictly limited the number of mental health visits provided to members (Budman, 1985). In addition, an informed public that is no longer as ready to accept medical recommendations unquestioningly and that seeks faster, less costly, and more efficient therapies is an important factor contributing to the increasing prominence of brief treatment.

The most recent "wave" of short-term therapies has come from clinician/researchers. These individuals, such as Beck, Rush, Shaw, and Emery (1979), Klerman, Rounsaville, Chevron, and Weissman (1984), Luborsky (1984), and Strupp and Binder (1984), have all attempted systematic codifications of their models of brief treatment. Most of these models are the products of extensive research and have often been tested as part of comparative clinical trials. In general (with the exception of the Strupp and Binder model, which is currently being tested), these brief treatments have been found to be highly effective when compared to chemotherapy (Elkin, 1986), or to nonprofessional counseling (Woody *et al.*, 1983). However, it is not at all clear that any one of these models is any more effective than any other. These findings are also consistent with those of large meta-analyses (Smith, Glass, & Miller, 1980). Although occasionally one type of brief treatment is shown to be superior to another, it appears to us that the "winner" in such situations is often the therapy with the "home-court advantage." That is, an experimenter testing his or her own brand of brief therapy against an alternative model imported for the trial probably will find superior results for the local brand (e.g., S. M. Johnson & Greenberg, 1985).

We have found no compelling evidence yet that any specific modes of brief therapy are better than other modes under identical circumstances. Rather, it is probably true that there are a number of ways to approach the same problem, many of which may have comparable benefits. In explaining this phenomenon, G. L. Klerman (personal communication, 1983) uses a medical analogy. He says that in the case of hypertension, for example, a physician may choose to treat this problem in a variety of ways. He or she may use a diuretic, a beta-blocker, a reduction in weight, and/or an increase in exercise as ways of helping the patient control blood pressure. It is our impression that the prevailing trend in current medical practice is to combine a number of these approaches in a successful antihypertensive program. In much the same way, it is our impression that a psychotherapeutic program that flexibly applies a number of strategies and techniques will probably be more successful than will a very rigid and doctrinaire approach.

DEFINING BRIEF THERAPY: HOW LONG IS "SHORT," AND TO WHOM?

The description we have just given of the development of brief psychotherapy seems clear and straightforward. Therapy was once short-term, but for a variety of reasons, it became longer and more protracted. In recent years the pendulum has swung back, with the goal being shorter and more efficient treatment.

In reality, however, the picture is much more hazy and less clear. Although it appears that for many mental health clinicians the ideal image of therapy entails relatively long-term treatment, most therapy as it is actually practiced has been and remains quite short. For example, Garfield (1978) reviewed the data for 1948 to 1970 on average length of psychotherapy in a variety of clinical settings, and found that most patients discontinued treatment well before 20 visits, with the median number in most settings being 5–6 sessions. These typical treatment durations are thus more in line with common patient expectations of the length of therapy (usually less than 3 months; Garfield, 1971) than with the expectations of many psychotherapists.

Also of interest is a survey by Langsley (1978) of psychiatric practice in both private and public settings. He found that across all diagnoses psychiatrists in private practice settings saw patients for 12.8 visits, while the average for community mental health practitioners was 10.3 visits. Similarly, when Koss (1979) examined the length of treatment in a private clinic staffed by psychologists and generally attended by middle-class, reasonably well-educated patients, she found the median duration to be 8 sessions, with nearly 80% of the patients discontinuing treatment prior to their 20th visit.

These surveys contribute to a definitional dilemma in discussing short-term therapy. It must be, after all, "short-term" when compared to some other therapies. As noted earlier, however, available data imply that most major, planned brief treatment approaches are *longer* than the usual length of psychotherapy in either clinic or private settings. Indeed, prominent short-term therapists such as Malan (1976) and Sifneos (1972) have reported cases of up to 40 sessions and 1 year, respectively, although some consensus among clinicians would probably set 25 sessions as the upper limit of brief treatment (Butcher & Koss, 1978).

The problem of definition becomes even more complex when one also takes into account the question of how time is being allocated to treatment. Thus, although Butcher and Koss (1978), in their review of short-term therapy approaches, define 25 sessions as the upper limit of such treatment, they address neither the problem of what constitutes a session nor the question of over what duration of time these 25 sessions must occur in order to be considered "brief." Are fifty 30-minute sessions still "short-term"? Is 1 year or more of monthly sessions—as practiced, for example, in the therapy of Selvini-Palazzoli, Boscolo, Cecchin, and Prata (1978)—to be judged "brief"? Thus, merely tabulating hours spent in clinical contact does not offer an adequate index of whether a therapy is brief. The temporal density of brief therapies allows for varied allocation of therapeutic time for different, although equally compelling, clinical and conceptual reasons.

In our experience as practitioners of brief therapy, we have concluded that (to paraphrase James Thurber) "there is no length in number." *What is, in fact, being examined in any discussion of brief treatment is therapy in which the time allotted to treatment is rationed.* The therapist hopes to help the patient achieve maximum benefit with the lowest investment of therapist time and patient cost, both financial and psychological. "Brief," or "short-term" therapy as it is presented in this book might be more accurately described as "time-sensitive," "time-effective," or "cost-effective" therapy. For the sake of conventionality and convenience, however, we continue to use the more standard and common terminology.

Thus, while brief therapies have received most of their attention only in the last decade or less, the recurrent fact that the typical psychotherapy outpatient receives fewer than 10 sessions has been noted and emphasized for several decades (e.g., Matarazzo, 1965; Rubenstein & Lorr, 1956). By the temporal ideals of most traditionally trained psychotherapists, then, brief therapy is hardly new, and was not ushered in by the recent emergence of HMOs, governmental cost-containing agencies, and the like. The recent explosion of interest in brief psychotherapy has been an explosion of interest in *planned* brief therapy—that is, brief therapy "by design," as opposed to the commonly occurring unplanned brief therapy "by default" (Gurman, 1981, p. 417). This distinction is absolutely essential to keep in mind when we turn to consider the empirical status of brief psychotherapy.

THE EFFECTIVENESS OF BRIEF THERAPY—BY DESIGN AND BY DEFAULT

Given this design–default distinction, it becomes difficult to decide which body of existing research on psychotherapy should be attended to in considering the question of the efficacy of "brief" psychotherapy. Certainly, studies of planned time-limited treatments whose duration is undeniably shorter than traditionally valued therapies (e.g., up to 25 sessions) would qualify. But what about treatments of similar duration in which time limits are not established near the beginning of therapy by therapist–patient agreement? As we have said before, therapeutic brevity is in the mind of the beholder, and we believe that very large numbers of psychotherapists view the latter type of treatment experiences as "brief." Therefore, it follows that outcome research on treatment courses of this latter type—brief therapy by default, that is—deserves to be included in considering the efficacy of brief therapy.

Brief Therapy by Default

While very little research on psychotherapy outcomes has focused on time-limited treatment per se (see below), the overwhelming majority of outcome research has involved therapy that has lasted for very brief periods by the standards of psychoanalysis and traditional psychoanalytic psychotherapy. In our view, the enormous body of research on the outcomes of various individual psychotherapies (psychodynamic, humanistic, eclectic, cognitive-behavioral) (Bergin & Garfield, 1971; Garfield & Bergin, 1978, 1986), taken collectively, constitutes research on time-unlimited brief therapy.

Thus, virtually every major review of the efficacy of various individual therapies (e.g., Bergin, 1971; Bergin & Lambert, 1978; Lambert, Shapiro, & Bergin, 1986; Luborsky, Chandler, Auerbach, Cohen, & Bachrach, 1971; Orlinsky & Howard, 1986) has been an unacknowledged review of time-unlimited brief therapy. For example, the two most influential and widely cited recent meta-analyses of individual psychotherapy outcome studies were based on data from treatments lasting from about 7 (Shapiro & Shapiro, 1982) to about 17 (Smith *et al.*, 1980) sessions. Meta-analysis is a statistical procedure for standardizing and making replicable the practices and criteria for reviewing large bodies of data, in order to establish more dependable generalizations and to assess systematically the impact of numerous potentially important variables (e.g., treatment length) on treatment outcome. Meta-analysis also assesses the size or magnitude of a treatment effect, rather than simply assessing the probability of whether the effects found in given studies were due to chance. Smith *et al.* (1980) found that the average "effect size" in 475 studies that compared treatment and untreated groups was .85, meaning that the mythical, statistically "average person" who received treatment was better off than about 80% of people with similar problems who did not receive treatment.

Although both data-analytic procedures and study samples have varied among the now numerous meta-analyses of individual therapy outcome, "the average [across meta-analyses] effect [size] associated with psychological treatment approaches one standard deviation" (Lambert *et al.*, 1986, p. 159). Translation of such effect sizes into estimates of improvement rates (see Lambert *et al.*, 1986) shows that these reviews reliably find between two-thirds and three-quarters of treated patients to be better off than untreated subjects. Moreover, these results have been obtained from patients with mild and/or limited symptoms *and* from patients with more severe and/or more global symptoms and impairment. Finally, the improvements assessed on a wide range of clinical criteria tend to be quite stable over time (Andrews & Harvey, 1981; Landman & Dawes, 1982; Nicholson & Berman, 1983).

We consider these sorts of data to be solid and impressive evidence of the general effectiveness of time-unlimited brief individual psychotherapy. Moreover, the research literature on the effectiveness of marital and family therapy has shown similar results (Gurman & Kniskern, 1978b; Gurman, Kniskern, & Pinsolf, 1986). Indeed, most of the positive results of the varied forms of marital and family therapy that have received empirical scrutiny have been achieved in treatments lasting fewer than 20 sessions. By traditional time standards, family treatment methods that are both brief and demonstrably helpful have been developed for a range of clinical problems—for example, marital discord, conduct disorders of children, juvenile delinquency, adolescent psychosomatic disorders, adult anxiety disorders, alcohol and other substance abuse, and schizophrenia (Gurman *et al.*, 1986).

The More the Better, or Diminishing Returns?

The kinds of data considered thus far would appear to fly in the face of the generally accepted lore among clinicians that "the more psychotherapy the better." In fact, recent analyses of the relationship between the "dose" (number of sessions) of psychotherapy and its effects (Howard, Kopta, Krause, & Orlinsky, 1986; Orlinsky & Howard, 1986) show that, with an important qualification, this clinical lore has an empirical foundation. Howard *et al.* (1986) conducted a probit analysis of the data from 15 previously published studies of individual therapy outcome. The 2,431 patients from these studies were mostly in the "neurotic" range of disturbance (e.g., depression, anxiety) and were diverse in terms of age and social class. Each of the major mental health disciplines were represented among the therapists, whose orientations were typically psychodynamic or interpersonal, and the studies had been done in various service settings (e.g., private practice, university psychiatry clinic, community mental health centers, and university counseling centers).

Howard *et al.*'s analysis showed that by the 8th session, approximately 50% of patients had shown measurable improvement, and that by the 26th session, almost 75% had improved. Following clinical lore, this trend continued: By the 52nd session, 83% of the patients had improved. (Interestingly, about 15% of the patients improved before the first session!)

These findings might seem to argue against brief (by traditional standards) psychotherapy. That is, these data indicate that "patients who have more therapy get more benefit from it . . . improvement is a linear function of the [logarithm of the] number of sessions" (Orlinsky and Howard, 1986, p. 361). This "the more the better" view of such findings has received tentative support in other reviews of individual psychotherapy outcome research (D. H. Johnson & Gelso, 1980; Luborsky *et al.*, 1971) as well. But the "important qualification" that we have alluded to above is this: "[I]mprovement is proportionately greater in earlier sessions . . . and increases more slowly as the number of sessions grows. . . .This analysis also suggests a course of diminishing returns with more and more effort required to achieve just noticeable difference in patient improvement" (Orlinsky & Howard, 1986, p. 361). The major meta-analysis of outcome research referred to earlier (Smith *et al.*, 1980) similarly found the major positive impact of individual psychotherapy to occur in the first 6–8 sessions, followed by continuing but decreasing positive impact for approximately the next 10 sessions. It is interesting to note that the largest proportion of positive change in individual psychotherapy appears to occur in a time frame (6–8 sessions) that roughly parallels the amount of time most patients expect to stay in treatment (about 6–10 sessions; Garfield, 1971, 1978) and actually do stay in treatment (6–8 sessions; Garfield, 1978, 1986). The reasons for discontinuation of treatment are numerous; they range from interpersonal ones, such as dissatisfaction or conflict with therapists, to mundane and practical ones, such as the ending of insurance benefits (Koss, 1979). Another reason for such "early" termination for many patients is that they have gotten what they came for, or at least a good deal of it.

Brief Therapy by Design

Compared to the enormous amount of research that exists on unplanned, time-unlimited brief psychotherapy, outcome studies of planned, time-limited brief therapy are few. Perhaps this fact accounts for the unanimous view among those who have carefully reviewed the research on time-limited therapy (Butcher & Koss, 1978; Luborsky, Singer, & Luborsky, 1975; Koss & Butcher, 1986; Orlinsky & Howard, 1986) that the existing comparative studies of time-limited versus time-unlimited individual therapy show no reliable differences in effectiveness between the two. A parallel picture can be drawn from the existing studies of time-limited versus time-unlimited marital and family therapy (Gurman & Kniskern, 1978b).

An ironic footnote to all these data is that patients in time-limited therapy (e.g., up to 20–25 sessions) at times receive more treatment than do patients in time-unlimited therapy! This certainly accords with our view, elaborated in the next section, that the essence of brief psychotherapy lies not in its numerical time characteristics, but in the therapeutic values, attitudes, and aims of the therapist. Still, there is a very important message to be derived (and repeated regularly) from the collective body of research on brief therapy both by design *and* by default. This message is that, contrary to the romanticized beliefs about "long-term" therapy and the negative views of brief therapy that exist among many psychotherapists, (1) there is very little research on the efficacy of "long-term" therapy, and hardly enough to justify the claims of its advocates; and (2) a great many consumers of psychotherapy benefit substantially from therapy experiences that last "only" between 2 and 5 months, even when the termination date of these therapies is not set at the start of treatment, and even when there typically is no explicit plan by the therapist for his or her use of the available treatment time. It is the planned, focused use of time in psychotherapy to which we now turn.

ATTITUDINAL AND SYSTEMS LIMITATION FACTORS
IN BRIEF THERAPY

Since we cannot reliably or meaningfully define "brief therapy" in terms of either number of visits or time elapsed since therapy was initiated, we must consider other criteria for defining the nature of brief treatment. In part, brief therapy is a state of mind of the therapist and of the patient; in part, brief therapy involves a set of limitations on service delivery system resources. The techniques of brief therapy are derived from these attitudinal and systems limitation factors.

In this section, we discuss those attitudinal and systems factors that seem to characterize the practice of brief therapy as it occurs modally. Not all the elements we identify here are found in each of the currently influential models of brief therapy (e.g., Beck *et al.*, 1979; Davanloo, 1980; Malan, 1976; Mann, 1973; Sifneos, 1972). Yet we believe that in the long run, brief therapeutic methods will be more effective if the most potent components that transcend specific schools or brief treatment orientations are isolated and refined. We also believe that despite numerous professional workshops, books, and journal articles on brief therapy, few practitioners of brief therapy faithfully use a single model or approach. Indeed, we think that most brief therapists and even most adherents of psychodynamically oriented short-term methods are pragmatically eclectic.

Attitudinally, planned brief therapy requires that the therapist and the patient agree to accept a set of values (to be described below) as to what therapy can and cannot do. Furthermore, these values almost always develop and gain credibility because of system demands, such as low barriers to mental health care (e.g., low-cost care) and a large population of treatment utilizers (Budman, 1985); increased waiting times (Mann, 1973); an enormous influx of psychiatric casualties during wartime (Alexander & French, 1946/1974); or limited mental health insurance benefits, high cost of therapy, and difficult economic times. When such system constraints are not operating, therapy (depending on the patient population) will be either long and continuous (for a small but wealthy or well-insured minority) or brief (because of a high dropout rate) and unplanned. Because of systems pressures on all mental health professionals at this time, we may have to think increasingly "small," realistically, and efficiently.

The Value Systems of the Long-Term and the
Short-Term Therapist

Practitioners of all psychotherapies have spoken and unspoken values regarding the ideal manner in which their specific therapy is practiced. Here we contrast the major divergences in the value systems of the long-term and the short-term therapist. We recognize, of course, that numerous therapists practice both long-term and short-term therapy and that few pure examples of either species actually exist. Moreover, we recognize that these divergencies may not be as extreme or dichotomous as we paint them here; as in a well-painted watercolor caricature, though, something of the essence of the subject is captured and conveyed.

We identify eight major differences in the values of short-term and long-term psychotherapists. These differences are summarized in Table 1-1.

Value Ideals of the Long-Term Therapist

1. First and foremost, the long-term psychoanalytically oriented therapist almost always seeks major character change, and may view such change as synonymous with cure. That is, after successful therapy, the patient should have a modified character structure. Much of this quest derives from Freud's dictum, "where Id was, there Ego shall be." The long-term therapist is unlikely to be looking for mere home improvements, but is much more likely to be striving to rebuild the house from the ground up. Freud addressed this issue of the necessity of character change in the following

Table 1-1. Comparative Dominant Values of the Long-Term and the Short-Term Therapist

Long-term therapist	Short-term therapist
1. Seeks change in basic character.	Prefers pragmatism, parsimony, and least radical intervention, and does not believe in notion of "cure."
2. Believes that significant psychological change is unlikely in everyday life.	Maintains an adult developmental perspective from which significant psychological change is viewed as inevitable.
3. Sees presenting problems as reflecting more basic pathology.	Emphasizes patient's strengths and resources; presenting problems are taken seriously (although not necessarily at face value).
4. Wants to "be there" as patient makes significant changes.	Accepts that many changes will occur "after therapy" and will not be observable to the therapist.
5. Sees therapy as having a "timeless" quality and is patient and willing to wait for change.	Does not accept the timelessness of some models of therapy.
6. Unconsciously recognizes the fiscal convenience of maintaining long-term patients.	Fiscal issues often muted, either by the nature of the therapist's practice or by the organizational structure for reimbursement.
7. Views psychotherapy as almost always benign and useful.	Views psychotherapy as being sometimes useful and sometimes harmful.
8. Sees patient's being in therapy as the most important part of patient's life.	Sees being in the world as more important than being in therapy.

analogy: "If the fire brigade, called to deal with a house that had been set on fire by an overturned oil-lamp, contented themselves with removing the lamp from the room in which the blaze had started . . . a comfortable shortening of the brigade's activities would be effected by this means" (1937/1964, pp. 216–217). Thus, a therapist may rapidly deal with the symptomatic manifestations of the problem, but basically, to use Freud's metaphor, may still leave the house on fire.

Even behavior therapists may strive for "therapeutic perfectionism" (Malan, 1963) by seeking to help the patient deal with each and every aspect of each and every problem about which the patient expresses concern. We believe that the selective overattention and overemphasis placed upon characterological issues by long-term-oriented therapists may set up an endless quest for "fundamental changes" or "core changes," and an unwillingness to be satisfied with what are viewed as "superficial changes" or "flights into health." In the National Institute of Mental Health (NIMH) Collaborative Psychotherapy Study of Depression, one of the major problems in training experienced therapists to do brief interpersonal therapy has centered around their frequent tendencies to overemphasize characterological problems and therefore to have great difficulty in adhering to a problem-oriented focus (G. L. Klerman, personal communication, 1984).

2. The long-term therapist is likely to endorse the idea that only a significant and continuing therapeutic relationship with a mental health professional can begin to "chip away" at the patient's encrusted and unyielding psychological pathology. A corollary to this viewpoint is that adults usually change only in therapy under the watchful eyes of the clinician; otherwise, their personalities are largely static and immutable.

3. A common belief of long-term therapists is that the particular problem the patient presents as a reason for seeking help is only a representation of more deeply entrenched and embedded pathology. Although few long-term therapists currently discuss symptom substitution (Gordon & Zax, 1981), there is a sense that symptomatic improvements are usually not genuine or significant in and of themselves.

4. The long-term therapist has a wish (often unstated, of course) to get *naches* from the patient. Loosely translated from the Yiddish, this means that the therapist wishes to see changes in the patient and receives personal satisfaction from these changes.

5. Therapist and patient are likely to experience an indefiniteness of time. The "timeless" quality that Mann (1981) discusses is often conveyed by an implicit or explicit message from the therapist: "I will be here as long as you need me." Appelbaum (1981) warns that under such circumstances, "Parkinson's law" takes effect, and the work of treatment may expand to fill the time available for it.

6. Also present, but never expressed overtly, may be a desire on the therapist's part to keep a given "slot" of paid time filled on a continual basis.

This is a task that is most effectively accomplished with a regular long-term patient, preferably on a more-than-once-a-week basis. Informal evaluation (but repeated experience) suggests that when our rate of referrals is low, our patients "need" more treatment; when our referrals increase, we find many more patients "ready" to terminate. It is undoubtedly the rare therapist who consciously "strings along" a patient for his or her own financial gain (Hoyt, 1985). Therapists, however, *are* in the business of selling time, and business and clinical issues certainly interact, even for therapists who have been psychoanalyzed.

7. Psychotherapy, in the hands of a "good enough" practitioner, is viewed as almost *always* benign and helpful (as well as possibly useful for problems such as poverty and unemployment). Minimal changes or deterioration following therapy are generally attributed to a lack of patient motivation or to insufficient dosage (i.e., "more treatment is needed"). Usually, the long-term therapist does not attend to research findings indicating that, as Frances and Clarkin (1981) note, "the psychotherapies, like drugs, can produce addiction, side effects, complications and overdosage if prescribed in an unselective fashion" (p. 542).

8. A common overriding value of the long-term therapist is that the patient should *be* in therapy with him or her. "To be in therapy" has all of the existential implications of a total commitment of self to the process and to the therapeutic relationship. The more a therapist adheres to a long-term model, the more he or she wishes the patient to forego money, time, vacations, and so forth in order to be in therapy. Indeed, in describing long-term group therapy, Yalom (1975) writes: "The more important the members consider the group, the more effective the group becomes. I believe that the ideal therapeutic posture for patients is for their therapy group experience to be considered *the most important event in their lives*" (p. 119, emphasis added). This sentiment has been echoed frequently by psychoanalysts and is conveyed most clearly in the analytic rule of abstinence (Freud, 1919/1949).

Value Ideals of the Brief Therapist

1. The brief therapist begins treatment by using the least radical procedure; that is, therapy begins with the least costly, least complicated, and least invasive treatment. Moreover, the brief therapist believes that changes in one area of psychological functioning may have important "ripple effects" in other areas. Thus, parsimony of intervention is a core value for the brief therapist. As we describe later in this book, our view is that under some circumstances even those with severe character pathology can be helped by a relatively circumscribed brief intervention.

2. The brief therapist views cure as inconceivable. The human condition is such that anxieties, doubts, losses, changes, and conflicts are perva-

sive. Even the most thoroughly analyzed individual is faced with these experiences. The brief therapist knows that he or she cannot change the client into someone who is *always* sensitive, assertive, friendly, insightful, patient, orgasmic, attractive, giving, taking, responsible, fun-loving, courteous, kind, obedient, thrifty, brave, clean, and reverent.

3. Brief therapists view people as malleable and as constantly changing and developing. Rather than becoming enamored of a patient's hardened and encrusted character structure (which, for the most part, is fully developed by 6 years of age), the brief therapist maintains an adult developmental perspective. This perspective assumes a degree of continuing personality change throughout life (Gilligan, 1982; Neugarten, 1979; Vaillant, 1977). In assuming such a perspective, the therapist may aid the patient in negotiating some of life's requisite tasks. Since it is understood that change will be inevitable for most people, the therapist can judiciously allocate his or her time to help the patient maximize the trajectory of that change.

4. The brief therapist, while maintaining an appreciation for the role of psychiatric diagnosis, has a health rather than an illness orientation. The brief therapist wishes to help the patient build on his or her existing strengths, skills, and capacities. For the brief therapist, it is very important to examine the positive aspects of the patient's personality, as well as his or her resources, areas of mastery, and social supports. In contrast, many long-term therapists often emphasize deficits, deep-seated weaknesses, and pathology. A recent magazine cartoon showed a picture of an analytic patient lying on the couch, with the analyst behind him saying, "I would say your feelings of inadequacy represent progress. When you first came here, you thought you were pretty hot stuff."

5. The brief therapist takes the patient's presenting problems seriously and hopes to help make changes in some of the areas that the patient specifies or comes to clarify as important. Of course, many people come to therapists and cannot identify the source or focus of their distress. For others, the problem may be erroneously defined—for example, "My neck is always hurting," instead of "I feel terribly grieved by my father's recent death." In these cases, the therapist and patient must first define the problem collaboratively and consensually and then develop a treatment plan.

6. The brief therapist realizes that he or she may not be thanked for changes that have occurred after therapy, and may not, after relatively few visits, ever see the patient again. Furthermore, if the therapist is called again, it may be *after* major changes have already occurred. We have recently come to realize that although some patients have "amnesia" for their brief therapy experiences, there are a substantial number for whom even one visit becomes a live and ongoing interaction. One of us recently saw a short-term therapy patient again after a 2-year hiatus. As she sat down, she said to the therapist: "As you were saying the last time we met . . ." The pace picked up from there as if no break had ever occurred.

7. The brief therapist assumes that psychotherapy may be "for better or for worse" and that not everyone who requests treatment needs or can benefit from it. Frances and Clarkin (1981) have recently discussed when to prescribe the briefest of brief therapies—that is, no therapy at all—as the treatment of choice. The short-term therapist realizes that in certain circumstances therapy may do more harm than good (e.g., the chronically dependent, treatment-addicted patient who cannot or does not use therapeutic input in the service of making changes), and that in these cases withholding anything beyond the most minimal intervention may be advisable. Cummings (1977), in discussing realistic versus ideal psychotherapy, indicates that there is a population for whom significant increases in the amount of psychotherapy lead to marked deterioration in functioning.

8. Finally, and most importantly, being in the world is seen as far more important than being in therapy. Most brief therapists are present-oriented. They are interested in emphasizing current relationships (Klerman *et al.*, 1984), present-centered problems, and ongoing life situations. This type of orientation has major implications for determining the style of therapist intervention and the use of significant others in the treatment process.

Patients' Attitudes in Long-Term and Short-Term Therapies

By the time a person first seeks therapeutic help, his or her attitudes about length of therapy have already been affected by factors such as the following:

1. Familiarity with mass media portrayals of the therapeutic process. (We have yet to see a movie that portrays brief therapy. Perhaps this is because most actors, directors, and screenwriters are in long-term treatment. In any case, most media portrayals of psychotherapy seem to imply a long-term continuous treatment relationship.)

2. Previous personal experience in therapy.

3. Whether or not the patient is a mental health professional.

4. An implicit view of psychological health and pathology. Some sophisticated patients arrive as "friends and supporters" of long-term therapy. On the other hand, those less "sophisticated" or with no previous experience as mental health patients often arrive expecting to be helped in relatively few (usually fewer than 10) sessions (Garfield, 1971).

Obviously, clarifying and negotiating the duration of treatment are essential in short-term therapy. Moreover, clarifying patients' expectations of what can be achieved in such a brief treatment is very important.

Some patients who are "friends and supporters" of psychotherapy refuse to improve under any circumstances other than one or two sessions per week of time-unlimited therapy. In general, however, such people are in the minority. In fact, if a time frame is established for the treatment, if treatment is kept focused on a clear central theme, and the patient is allowed to return as needed, most patients' relationships with their psychotherapists will approximate their relationships with other professionals, such as lawyers, family physicians, and accountants (Bloom, 1981; Cummings & VandenBos, 1979; Rabkin, 1977).

Institutional Factors in Brief and Long-Term Therapy

Only when and if strong institutional supports exist do planned short-term therapies become the major modes of treatment in a given mental health setting. If such supports do not exist, therapy will probably be either unplanned and brief (because so many patients drop out or unilaterally terminate), or, for a smaller number of patients, continuous and open-ended.

Until recently, in all but a few settings, organizational incentives for brief therapy were virtually nonexistent. Indeed, continuous and time-unlimited services fit better with the organizational needs of many settings. In many areas of the country, for example, therapists in a private fee-for-service group practice or in solo practice have very little incentive to see individuals briefly. Rent, overhead costs, and salaries must be paid. Similarly, at a treatment center oriented toward training (with the exception of a minority of patients seen in the "brief therapy clinic"), it is often argued that trainees should attempt to include in their caseloads patients who are likely to remain in treatment for a year or longer. Only by having such experiences, the argument goes, can neophyte therapists come to understand the complexity of people and begin to develop a "rich" appreciation for the subtleties and intricacies of ("real") psychotherapy. It is also our impression that geographic and related "therapist density" factors are often important incentives or disincentives to longer or shorter therapy length. There are data to support the contention that on the East and West Coasts (where therapist density is greatest), patients with comparable problems are seen for a far greater length of time than in areas of the country where there are fewer therapists (G. L. Klerman, personal communication, 1984).

From the perspectives of the system, the therapist, and the patient, one of the major factors operating against planned brief therapy is that it is simply easier neither to plan nor to ration treatment. It is nearly impossible for a system to police how long therapy will be; it is difficult for a therapist to be planful and organized in determining durations of treatment and to terminate treatment with many patients so frequently; and it requires much more personal responsibility for change on the patient's part if he or she is seen in briefer treatment.

TECHNICAL TREATMENT ISSUES IN BRIEF THERAPY

Although, as we have said, attitudinal factors are central in the practice of brief therapy, technical treatment issues are, of course, also very important. At a meeting of the Society for Psychotherapy Research, Kernberg (1981) stated that there is really little technique required in brief (as opposed to long-term) therapy; he went on to conclude that short-term treatment merely provides the patient with a friendship. However, when the same criticism was made of psychoanalysis, Hanns Sachs, a noted Boston analyst, is reported to have responded, "Ah, but where would you find such a friend?" (Budman & Gurman, 1983).

We now describe some of what we believe to be the most salient technical elements in brief treatment. Although some of these factors have been noted as more important in short-term therapy approaches than in time-unlimited treatment (Butcher & Koss, 1978), they may be equally powerful in all types of effective psychotherapy.

Maintenance of a Clear and Specific Focus

Setting and maintaining realistic goals are very important in the brief therapy process (Budman & Gurman, 1983; Butcher & Koss, 1978; Small, 1979). We place much emphasis in this book upon the development and maintenance of therapeutic focus. At the same time, the attitude of "not having to do it all right now" allows the therapist to centralize a particular problem or set of problems without becoming mired in the task of total personality reconstruction. Recent research data offered by Sachs (1983) further support this notion. She related therapy process to outcome for 18 neurotic male college students treated for a maximum of 25 therapy sessions by highly experienced psychotherapists. Her research demonstrated a strong and consistent relationship between what she called "errors in technique" and outcome. A major component of such errors in technique was the failure of the therapist to *structure* or *focus* the treatment sessions.

High Level of Therapist Activity

Because time and the maximal use of time are so important to the brief therapist (Budman & Bennett, 1983), extended periods of therapist inactivity are unwise. There is a greater need than in time-unlimited therapies for the therapist to structure parts of the session, offer suggestions, collaboratively assign homework, ask "leading" questions, and so forth.

Maintenance of an Awareness of Time

Even though patients can and do come back for additional courses of brief therapy, each and every session should be seen as important, just as the matter of the total number of sessions contracted for in a given course of treatment is important. In brief therapy, the therapist and the patient view time differently than they might if therapy unconsciously holds out the possibility of continuing "forever" (Mann, 1973). The awareness of limited time in therapy also makes the clinician and patient acutely aware of existential issues (Budman, 1981b). For example, for whom does thinking about an important ending not stir up feelings about other losses, deaths, and indeed one's own mortality and existence? To illustrate, the reader might try a brief exercise suggested by James Bugental and described by Yalom (1980): "On a blank sheet of paper draw a straight line. One end of that line represents your birth, the other end your death. Draw a cross to represent where you are now. Meditate upon this for five minutes" (p. 174). Whatever else is focused upon during treatment, the brief therapist must maintain a constant ancillary focus on the time issue.

Therapist Encouragement of the Patient's "Being"
Outside Therapy

A number of important technical factors follow from the emphasis on the patient's "being in the world":

Liberal Use of Homework Assignments

The patient should be given various tasks to carry out between sessions, if possible, so that the approach expands treatment beyond the consultation room and promotes a generalization of change. One example of this type of homework is not only to tell a patient that he or she is harsh on himself or herself and ought to give himself or herself more credit for various successes, but to suggest that for 1 week the patient should make a list of ways to treat himself or herself better and the next week should try to implement one or two of those items. Of course, patients are not "assigned" between-session tasks like schoolchildren; the patient must collaborate in the design and timing of such out-of-therapy experiences.

Involvement of Relatives and Significant Others in Treatment

With few exceptions, an adult seen in brief therapy should be seen with his or her spouse, parents, siblings, and so forth, at least as part of the evaluation process. This is appropriate for several reasons. Frequently the patient's focal problem, relates either overtly or covertly to a problem with others. Input about a patient from relatives or significant others may be quite useful. Furthermore, the patient's interaction with these significant people in their lives may represent the unspoken focal problem or may be a visible and changeable microcosm of the patient's interaction with others. When specific interpersonal relationships, such as marriage and the family, are emphasized by the patient as central problems, assessing "the problem" by seeing it in action and in context almost always leads to a useful shift away from defining the problem as within an individual toward defining it as between or among individuals. Moreover, research suggests that under these circumstances, direct intervention with the family system is more effective than individual psychotherapy (Gurman & Kniskern, 1978b). Finally, when one is dealing with highly dependent patients, who are often seen as extremely difficult to treat in brief therapy (Wolberg, 1965), the involvement of significant others may dilute what would under other circumstances become a highly dependent and needy transference.

Use of "Naturally Occurring" Therapies in the Environment

Therapeutic experiences can and do occur outside a psychotherapist's office (Bergin, 1971). The tense and anxious business executive, for example, may benefit substantially from regular physical exercise (Folkins & Sime, 1981). Joining a club or social organization can be a valuable group experience for the shy and retiring young adult. Also, self-help organizations for people with various types of problems and concerns abound (Lieberman & Borman, 1979). In addition to better-known groups such as Alcoholics Anonymous (AA) and Overeaters Anonymous, there are groups for those with phobias (e.g., The Boston Phobic Group), those who want more experience in public speaking (e.g., Toastmasters International), bereaved parents (e.g., Compassionate Friends), and so on. Such self-help groups often remain available to the patient as long as he or she wishes, are far less costly than professional psychotherapy, and can become and remain part of the patient's real world much more easily and appropriately than can a therapist, thereby helping maintain the durability of change.

The Inextricability of Evaluation and Treatment

To make the arbitrary decision that a specific number of sessions will constitute a pretreatment evaluation period is not cost-effective. Such a view is also naive in a system-analytic context, in that it assumes a linearly causal model of therapeutic influence (i.e., the therapist "acts upon" or influences the patient, but is not influenced by the patient).

Brief therapy sometimes has the same number of treatment hours as an extended evaluation. The brief therapist must "hit the ground running." That is, each comment made by the therapist should have some potential therapeutic benefit, and should also be an attempt to gather information about the patient. From the first session, the therapist should test hypotheses and therapeutic formulations. If wrong, these formulations should be modified. These formulations, in turn, must also include the therapist as a real and salient aspect of the unique system that evolves in each patient–therapist relationship. A common error in such formulations is the therapist's failure to see how he or she could attempt to influence the system of the therapeutic encounter while remaining "outside" that system.

Flexible Use of Interventions and Time

If therapy is to be maximally effective in a brief time period, therapeutic flexibility is essential. Gurman (1981), in describing what he calls "integrative marital therapy," calls for an amalgam of techniques from various schools of family treatment. The problem-centered orientation of the brief therapist requires that he or she tailor interventions to the needs of a specific patient at a given time. Cummings and VandenBos (1979) describe the discontinuous brief treatments of a man over a 7-year period; during this time he was seen individually, in a short-term group, and in couples therapy. It is probably most useful for a brief therapist to operate out of a systematic and coherent conceptual scheme, and yet to use a variety of interventions derived from "other" models of therapy (Beutler, 1983; Garfield, 1980). Gurman (1981), for example, has shown how common behavior therapy techniques, such as communication training with couples, can be meaningfully integrated within an object-relations schema of intimate relationships.

Time is the major commodity that we sell as therapists. It comes, however, in very few sizes: The 50-minute hour for individuals and the 90-minute session for groups appear to be sacrosanct. There are, however, an infinite number of ways to slice time. Every patient does not need a full hour of therapy in a given week. For some people, a weekly 30-minute session or a biweekly session may be optimal. For others, a 2-hour meeting three times per year may be better than the rigid approach to time into which we often lock ourselves.

Planned Follow-Up of Brief Therapy

Many research studies of brief therapy indicate that within a year of terminating a course of treatment, a substantial percentage of patients (both "successful" and "unsuccessful") return for additional therapy (e.g., Budman, Demby, & Randall, 1982). It is also probably true that many people experience numerous courses of "long-term" continuous therapy. Henry,

Sims, and Spray (1971), in studying the lives of therapists, found many who had had even five or more courses of multiyear treatment themselves! Grunebaum (1983) found that among experienced therapists, only age correlated with total number of times in psychotherapy. That is, the older the clinician, the more courses of (often long-term) therapy the clinician had had. Unfortunately, it has often been assumed that a returning patient has failed or relapsed. In part, this is a function of Freud's early (1916/1961; 1917/1963) belief that psychoanalysis has prophylactic qualities and that a successfully analyzed patient should be immunized against future stresses. Indeed, a more appropriate model for this dimension of the doctor–patient relationship in psychotherapy is to be found in the practice of internal medicine, in which, for example, the successful treatment of a given infection does not lead to the conclusion that the patient should never again experience any other infection.

In assuming a more realistic role *vis-à-vis* the returning patient, Wolberg (1980) advises a planned reunion with the patient after about a year. We have found this approach extremely useful at the Harvard Community Health Plan (Budman, Bennett, & Wisneski, 1981). It serves several important functions: The patient feels that the therapist maintains a continued interest even after the "end of therapy"; the patient realizes that the relationship with the therapist is not lost forever; and since a return is planned, the patient does not feel overwhelmed or as if he or she has failed if he or she comes back.

PATIENT SELECTION FOR BRIEF THERAPY

Although Bennett and Wisneski (1979) and Cummings and VandenBos (1979) have been optimistic that the vast majority of outpatients seen in their HMO settings can be treated using brief therapy approaches, other therapists do not share as optimistic an outlook. Sifneos (1978a) has set rather stringent selection criteria for his brand of brief treatment, "short-term anxiety-provoking therapy"; these include above-average intelligence and psychological-mindedness, a clear chief complaint (which can be formulated as having an Oedipal focus), a history of at least one meaningful relationship, motivation for change, and an ability to relate flexibly to the interviewer and to collaborate actively in the therapy process. About 20% of outpatients are appropriate for this approach (Sifneos, 1978b).

Mann has not set out the same sort of criteria for his 12-session, time-limited approach, but by requiring that patients have a capacity for rapid emotional involvement and for rapid separation as well as good "overall ego strengths," he also seems to be setting requirements that exclude many of the troubled individuals who visit psychotherapists (Mann, 1973; Mann & Goldman, 1982).

The Tavistock group, whose major spokesmen have been Balint (Balint, Ornstein, & Balint, 1972) and Malan (1976), exclude patients from their mode of dynamic brief therapy on the basis of the patients' responses to what Malan calls "trial interpretations" and the therapist's quick interpretation of patient resistances. Malan sometimes considers his approach to be contraindicated if a patient cannot use such interpretations effectively, but rather becomes more hostile, withdrawn, intellectualizing, or in other ways more defensive. Silver (1982), examining Malan's published work, has estimated that 20% of outpatients are suitable for this approach.

Marmor (1979) has reviewed the literature on patient selection for short-term dynamic psychotherapy and cited seven major criteria: evidence of ego strength; at least one meaningful interpersonal relationship; the ability to interact with the therapist in the first session; the ability to be psychologically minded (and insightful); the ability to experience feelings; the existence of a focal conflict; and motivation to change. He concluded that "the critical issue [in selection for short-term dynamic psychotherapy] is not diagnosis so much as the possession of certain personality attributes plus the existence of focal conflict and a high degree of motivation" (p. 152).

It is our impression that many of the attributes recommended in the past for patient selection have excluded those individuals who are most difficult and problematic in *any* form of psychotherapy. The vast array of selection criteria for brief psychotherapy have developed over the years despite a lack of empirical data to support the contention that some types of patients are better suited to brief treatment than are others.

Lambert (1979), reviewing the empirical data on patient characteristics and their relation to outcome, has written:

> Unfortunately, the tendency is for clinicians to specify, on the basis of intuition and theoretical bias, the clients that are most suitable for particular brief therapy interventions, without evaluation of these assumptions in a formal research design. Thus, there has been a failure to test the suitability of these treatments with some patients who are presumed unsuitable, but who may very well profit from such an approach. It does not appear that acute onset, good previous adjustment, good ability to relate, a focal problem, high initial motivation, lower socioeconomic class, current crises, or a host of other determining variables related to the patient have been shown to be any more highly related to outcome in brief therapy than in longer term therapies. (p. 27)

In other words, such criteria do not discriminate between those who would benefit differentially from short-term and long-term therapies, but rather may exclude those deemed least desirable by clinicians practicing in any modality.

Recently, however, the demarcation between those suitable for brief therapy and those suitable for longer-term therapies has become even more blurred. On the dynamic psychotherapy front, Davanloo (1978a, 1980) has developed an approach to short-term therapy aimed at patients with severely entrenched obsessional character problems. With such patients, Davanloo is a self-described "relentless healer," using activity and confrontation to ultimately break through the patient's "character armor."

Strupp and Binder (1984) have developed a carefully defined brief dynamic therapy approach for the "more 'difficult' patients, that is, individuals whose problems are intertwined with characterological trends and who may not become so readily involved in a collaborative relationship with the therapist."

In a recent article of great interest, L. W. Lazarus (1982) has discussed his approach to the brief psychotherapy of narcissistic personality disorders based upon the work of Kohut (1972, 1977). Leibovich (1981, 1983), working in Boston, has come to view a time-limited approach (short-term integrative psychotherapy) as the treatment of choice for many types of borderline patients. He believes that short-term therapy (in this case, 9–12 months) for these patients allows them a greater sense of control, autonomy, and accomplishment. Furthermore, their fantasies of timelessness and distorted sense of reality can be effectively challenged by the structural clarity of this approach.

In the area of nonpsychodynamic therapies, where a problem-centered approach has always been prevalent, selection criteria have in general been less stringent. For example, in the treatment of depression, McLean's behavioral social skills program (McLean, 1982), Beck's cognitive therapy (Beck *et al.*, 1979), and Klerman's interpersonal therapy (Klerman *et al.*, 1984)—all brief treatments—the only exclusions are of those most severely disturbed. That is, by implication or by direct statement of the authors, these approaches exclude only those depressed individuals suffering predominantly from organic brain syndromes, alcoholism, or bipolar affective disorders. In some clinical trials (e.g., Weissman, Klerman, Prusoff, Sholomskas, & Padian, 1981), patients are excluded because they are *not* severely depressed enough to participate.

The question that we ask in initially seeing a given patient is this: Might this person make substantial gains in brief, discontinuous courses of therapy, or *must* he or she have a continuous long-term relationship with a therapist in order to change in ways that are significant for his or her life? In determining the answer to this question, we partially agree with Wolberg's (1965) advice:

> The best strategy, in my opinion, is to assume that every patient, irrespective of diagnosis, will respond to short-term treatment unless he proves himself refractory to it. If the therapist approaches each patient with the idea of doing as much as he can for him, within the space of, say, up to twenty treatment sessions, he will give the patient an opportunity to take advantage of short-term treatment to the limit of his potential. If this fails, he can always resort to prolonged therapy. (p. 140)

Instead of referring to "failed" brief therapy followed by the need to "resort" to longer treatment, however, we would frame our approach differently. First, 20 (we assume) continuous sessions with a patient can be viewed as quite an extended period of treatment. Various sources indicate that reasonably good predictions of responsivity to a particular brief therapy situation can be made on the basis of one to three therapy or pretherapy "trial" sessions (Budman, 1981a; Budman & Clifford, 1979; Budman, Clifford, Bader, & Bader, 1981; Sachs, 1983).

Second, to assume that a particular patient has failed at brief therapy because of a poor response to a trial of such treatment and now has no alternative other than long-term therapy does not take into account a variety of other possibilities. It has been, for example, a long-held belief, with some research support, that therapist–patient compatibility on a variety of personality characteristics is an important determinant of the quality of the therapy relationship (Parloff, Waskow, & Wolfe, 1978). If progress seems unlikely or there is deterioration after a trial of treatment with one therapist, it may be reasonable for the patient to have another trial of treatment with a second clinician whose approach is somewhat different, who is the opposite sex of the first clinician, or who is older or younger. It is also possible to vary the modality of treatment, the duration of sessions, the therapeutic orientation, the focus, the interval between visits, and so on.

Assuming that a variety of briefer options has been explored with a given patient and has not appeared to be useful, does one then "resort" to long-term treatment? This is an intriguing question. Presented in this manner, "resort" has negative implications for the patients (i.e., that he or she could not succeed with less treatment) and very positive implications for the therapy (i.e., that long-term therapy may be the most powerful treatment—"It's our last resort"). We have yet to see persuasive research evidence indicating that particular types of patients clearly do better in long-term continuous therapy than in short-term courses of therapy over extended periods of time. Rather, the research seems to indicate that there is a type of patient who does better than another type of patient, regardless of treatment duration. In fact, virtually the same characteristics viewed as desirable for a good brief therapy candidate (high motivation, ability to verbalize feelings, minimal acting out, etc.) are seen as most suitable in a psychoanalytic candidate (S. Levin, 1962; Zetzel, 1968).

Rather than "resorting" to long-term therapy, the therapist may consider examining a patient's responses to more open-ended and continuing treatment. A trial of longer, open-ended therapy is done not because the clinician believes that if nothing else succeeds long-term treatment will, but because the interpersonal styles, family histories, or interactional experiences of some patients seem to make it difficult for them to change in a limited time or with discontinuous courses of treatment, and it is reasonable to explore other alternatives.

Although at this point we would like to list contraindications for brief therapy, it is not possible to do so. On the surface, many patients who seem to be poor brief therapy prospects may, with an appropriate patient-therapist match or with the correct brief modality, do extremely well in short-term treatment. Our recommendations in patient selection are to monitor the patient's response to treatment on a trial basis; to be prepared to make creative modifications as necessary (two such modifications may involve the patient's seeing another therapist or including the patient's family); and to be prepared to use various alternatives, including longer and more open-ended treatment.

2

Initiating Brief Therapy

Give me a place to stand and I will move the earth.
    —Archimedes

For most people, even those with clear psychiatric diagnoses, seeking the assistance of a psychotherapist is not a usual state of affairs (Dohrenwend *et al.*, 1980; Goodman, Sewell, & Jampol, 1984). Such a move often indicates a failure in one's environmental supports and/or an arrest of individual, couple, or familial developmental processes. This is true even for the most severe forms of psychiatric disorders. Indeed, Zola (1973), describing Clausen and Yarrow's (1955) study of first psychiatric hospital admissions for schizophrenics, writes:

> Most striking about their material was the lack of any increase in the objective seriousness of patient's disorder as a factor in the hospitalization. If anything, there was a kind of normalisation in his family, an accommodation to the patient's symptoms. *The hospitalization occurred not when the patient became sicker, but when the accommodation of the family, of the surrounding social context broke down. . . .* it seemed very likely that people have their symptoms for a long period of time before ever seeking medical aid. (p. 3; italics added)

Though Clausen and Yarrow's research was done over 30 years ago, it seems to have anticipated the very recent findings of C. M. Anderson, Reiss, and Hogarty (1986) and Falloon, Boyd, and McGill (1984) on the important role of family interaction in the course of major psychiatric disorders such as schizophrenia, as well as the developmental life cycle view of family theorists such as Haley (1976).

There are, of course, some instances of "recreational psychotherapeutics," in which mental health treatment is sought not because of a particular problem or constellation of problems exists per se, but for a variety of other reasons. For example, in some areas of the country and among particular populations, having one's own "shrink" seems to be a prerequisite for social acceptance. Never having had a therapist is akin to never having been divorced or never having smoked marijuana. For now, however, it can be safely assumed that *most* people seek out therapy because they are in pain and are hoping to see change in their everyday experiences and interactions with other people.

THE ISSUE OF FOCUS IN BRIEF PSYCHOTHERAPY

All major brief psychotherapy theories share the belief that such an approach must be "focal" (Butcher & Koss, 1978). In general, this means that the therapy should have a central issue, topic, or theme that is dealt with over the course of treatment. For some brief therapists (Malan, 1976; Sifneos, 1979), the focus is psychodynamic in nature and may entail, for example, examining historical issues such as the Oedipal triangle, especially in terms of its current interpersonal manifestations with the therapist. Others (e.g., Klerman *et al.*, 1984) emphasize interpersonal themes outside the therapeutic encounter, and still other clinician/theoreticians (Beck *et al.*, 1979) focus on the patient's examination of the nature of his or her "erroneous cognitions." The more interactional brief therapies, which may or may not include nonsymptomatic family members, emphasize what is often the problem-maintaining nature of the attempted "solutions" to problems (Watzlawick, Fisch, & Segal, 1982) and the discovery of concrete alternatives to problem-maintaining feedback cycles (De Shazer, 1982, 1985).

The variety and breadth of possible foci for brief therapy are obviously quite great. Before we discuss the clinical development of a therapeutic focus further, however, it is important to consider why the establishment of such a focus is essential in brief therapy. Without such a central theme, the therapy is likely to lose its sense of purpose and may lack a coherent and targeted sense of direction. Furthermore, a lack of focus does not permit either the therapist nor the patient to be able to gauge progress clearly or to keep their "eyes on the ball" as treatment proceeds.

An approach to the discovery and establishment of a therapeutic focus is suggested here that is neither overly restrictive nor so vague as to lack clinical utility. In addition, it is our impression that for many brief therapies, the general domain of initial foci that we present—that is, the interpersonal–developmental–existential (I-D-E) domain—is either explicitly or implicitly of great relevance. The I-D-E approach in brief treatment is an attempt to capture and understand the core interpersonal life issues that are leading the patient to seek psychotherapy at a given moment in time, and to relate these issues to the patient's stage of life development and to his or her existential concerns. (Existential concerns include factors such as the meaning and values of one's life, and ultimately the issue of confronting one's own mortality.) Th I-D-E approach is neither exclusively symptom-oriented nor exclusively intrapsychic or interpersonal. Rather, it is an amalgam based upon currently evolving principles of individual, couple, and family development (Carter & McGoldrick, 1980); existential theory (Yalom, 1980);

theories of interpersonal relationships, particularly those regarding attachment, loneliness, and social supports (Parkes & Stevenson-Hinde, 1982); and models of human potential (e.g., Lankton & Lankton, 1983).

The (I-D-E) focus is a frame of reference to help the therapist conceptualize the answer to the central question in brief therapy (see below). In graphic form, the I-D-E focus may be pictured as a straight line. If this line is imagined to be the course of our lives, with one end representing birth and the other representing death, each of us is somewhere along this line (the developmental component). We are all interactional beings, and our difficulties, symptoms, joys, and sorrows can usually, at least in part, be understood in terms of these interactions (the interpersonal component). The fact that we are mortal and our lives are finite gives each of us a "hovering awareness" of our own mortality and that of those around us. This awareness of finiteness and limitation carries with it the final component to our tripartite model of focus (the existential component). Whenever we consider any of the possible foci for brief therapy (described later in this book), we attempt to keep in mind these three issues.

The Central Question: "Why Now?"

The major question (not necessarily voiced) for the brief therapist upon seeing or hearing from a prospective patient for the first time should be, "Why now?" Of all possible moments that this person could understandably have sought treatment, why did he or she choose to do so at this point in time? With the answer to this question, the therapist will often have found at least a partial focus for treatment. This "Why now?" position will lead, as we shall explain, to a developmental, problem-oriented, and systemic perspective. In contrast, simply assuming that entrance into psychotherapy occurs "once the pain is great enough" ignores the fact that many people choose to see a therapist only if and when they are beginning to feel *less* desperate or upset, or healthy enough to recognize the value of treatment. Zola (1973), describing why people seek medical care for physical illness, makes the same point and cites the following example:

> A rather elderly woman arrived at the Medical Clinic of the Massachusetts General Hospital three days late for an appointment. A somewhat exasperated nurse turned to her and said, "Mrs. Smith, your appointment was three days ago. Why weren't you here then?" To this Mrs. Smith responded. "How could I? Then, I was sick." (p. 1)

It is important to realize that entrance into therapy is *not* a random event. Rather, it usually occurs in the context of interpersonal, existential, and developmental changes within and around an individual. In this regard, research indicates that the majority of people entering therapy have experienced one or more major life events (usually undesirable ones) in the 3 weeks to 6 months preceding treatment (Barrett, 1979; B. B. Brown, 1978; G. W. Brown & Birley, 1968; G. W. Brown & Harris, 1978; Paykel, 1974; Thoits, 1985).

If a therapist does not maintain an investigative stance regarding "Why now?", it is easiest to assume the "flawed-personality" perspective. From this point of view, weak or vulnerable individuals simply succumb periodically (e.g., in periods of unusual stress). The inherent-defect or flawed-personality point of view leads readily to "total overhaul" therapy. By omitting questions regarding current changes both within the patient and between the patient and his or her environment that have led to the desire for mental health treatment, the therapist often neglects the strengths, inputs, and social network supports and/or impediments that have allowed or caused the patient *not* to be in therapy for some period of time, or the previous barriers to such care. Furthermore, the therapist may fail to use the leverage that comes with the answer to "Why now?"

Richard, for example, was a 19-year-old who called for an appointment in desperation. He had been feeling depressed and upset and was for the first time in his life thinking about suicide. "I don't believe that I would ever really do it, but sometimes the thoughts are too real." When the therapist saw him for the first time, he appeared to be either a precocious 14-year-old or a youthful 30-year-old. He was small, slight, and childish-looking, while at the same time he had a new but already heavy growth of beard. Richard told the therapist that he had been forced to repeat his final year of high school because of truancy and poor grades. He also explained that he hated going to school during this, his fifth year there. His grades, however, had improved and were better than they had ever been.

When first seen by the therapist, Richard was 3 months away from graduation, but felt that he was so lonely, depressed, and unhappy that he would have to drop out. He explained that he had no one to spend time with at school and was too old to be there. In exploring his family history, Richard described himself as the youngest of five sons. His father had abandoned the family when Richard was 6 years old, and his mother, a rather depressed and anxious woman, had managed to raise the boys alone on her meager salary as a clerk at a department store. When Richard was 8 his father had been murdered in a distant city, leaving no life insurance.

Although Richard had been seeing a counselor at school, whom he liked and who he felt cared about him, his depression had worsened. The counselor's interpretation of Richard's problem was that he "feared success" and that this prevented him from letting himself graduate. The therapist told Richard that it was not clear whether or not he feared success. The therapist did know that Richard was a good son and could not now bear to leave his mother alone, feeling anxious and depressed, after all she had done for him.

He proposed that Richard come in with his mother for one session to see whether "we could be helpful to her" in what must be a very tough time in her life. "It's not easy to lose your youngest son," the therapist explained. After one joint session with his mother, focusing mostly on her concerns but also on her strengths, Richard's symptoms were reduced; he finished the term and successfully entered college in another city the next fall. This example illustrates, in part, the contrast between a "flawed-character" viewpoint (i.e., "You fear failure") and an I-D-E focus examining why the patient is seeking care at this time.

Dimensions of "Why Now?"

How and why do people decide that the time is appropriate to seek mental health care? For the most part, people do so when they reach a state of existential–developmental crisis (Prochaska & DiClemente, 1982). This state is frequently described by the patient as having *always* been present (thus immediately, though unfortunately, "confirming" the flawed-personality perspective). Indeed, from the patient's point of view, he or she may feel as though the distress experienced *has* been present forever. We believe that for most patients this is a cognitive distortion along the lines of those that Beck *et al.* (1979) describe for people who are depressed. For many people, and particularly those who experience psychic pain intensely and dysfunctionally, a dysphoric state will quickly be perceived as a pervasive trait (Peplau, 1982). The therapist should remain skeptical about the patient's claims of having *always* been a particular way. Even if it is true that a specific behavioral and/or cognitive style is most characteristic of a given patient, it is almost certain that such behaviors and/or cognitions are not totally static and immobile.

For example, Clara, a 31-year-old unmarried woman, consulted one of us because of her increasingly interfering sense of "guilt" over the "irreparable damage" she had caused Dan, her ex-husband, whom she had divorced almost 1 year earlier. On closer inquiry, it became evident that since their divorce Dan had not only been getting along quite well in life, but indeed had made major advances in the range and depth of his relationships with others; had gotten a promotion at his job; and, as far as Clara knew, was psychiatrically symptom-free. In the initial interview, she broadened the basis for her guilt to events that were either largely unavoidable or trivial (e.g. several years earlier she had rolled over in her sleep onto her kitten, suffocating it; more recently she had spent a couple of hours talking to an auto salesman about purchasing a new car, only to make the actual purchase from a different dealer in town). In large measure, as it emerged, her increasing sense of guilt about divorcing Dan (and about these other recent and distant actions) was found to be arising in the context of becoming much more emotionally committed to Mark, the man with whom she had been living for several months. Moreover, it became clear that her guilt about *"always* hurting other people" was not consistent with her easily perceptible empathy, caring, and sensitivity toward most people in her life; her love of animals; and so on. In a therapy without clearly established time limits, the therapist might have been tempted to leave Clara's exaggerated sense of guilt unchallenged initially, rather than, as he did, to focus on the meanings and function of her guilty feelings *now*, in the context of her anxiety about making a long-term commitment to her new lover. Without such a developmental focus, the therapist might have been misled into focusing on Clara's view of herself as insensitive and uncaring.

In seeking the I-D-E focus, the brief therapist can assume a particular set of attitudinal guidelines that may be of assistance.

1. Many adults (of similar age, sex, and socioeconomic cohort) expect to follow a relatively clear set of developmental pathways across their life span (Cohler & Boxer, 1984). Obviously, such developmental expectations have different nuances and connotations among individuals and between the sexes, as well as across socioeconomic classes and cultures. Furthermore, there are probably people whose anticipated modes of development fall largely outside of the beaten path (Vaillant, 1977). However, as a first rough attempt at answering the question "Why now?", the clinician might examine the hypothesis that birthdays, deaths, marriages, job changes, and so on, or the anticipation of these events, may confront the patient with either a sense of developmental retardation or one of inappropriate developmental acceleration (being "off time"). It is also true that the death of a friend or relative, or the forced anticipation of one's own death due to severe illness or crime victimization, acts as a catalyst for taking stock of one's life and the finiteness of existence (Yalom, 1980).

2. The patient wishes to overcome the obstacles to growth that impede developmental progress. The homesick and lonely college freshman would like to separate from his or her parents and get closer to peers; the 26-year-old man who has never dated would enjoy having an ongoing intimate relationship; the depressed 35-year-old married woman who cannot conceive would like to catch up with her age-mates who are raising children. There are certainly people who feel ambivalence and fear about developmental changes, or people for whom developmental milestones may require somewhat different kinds of progress (e.g., those who choose to remain childless or those whose sexual orientation is homosexual). The general impetus in almost all people is toward growth and development. As Milton Erickson (quoted in Lankton & Lankton, 1983) has stated, "Sick people do want to try—usually they don't know how" (p. 13).

3. Human beings are inherently social animals (Scott, 1981). A major

drive on the part of the overwhelming majority of people is to be close to and engaged with others. Indeed, Harry Stack Sullivan (1953) wrote, "There is no way that I know of by which one can, all by oneself, satisfy the need for intimacy" (p. 271). Many personality theorists such as Murray (1938) have postulated intimacy and the need to be with others as a universal drive or motive. The types of interpersonal "supplies" that one needs and desires from relationships may vary greatly, however, across the life cycle (Vaillant, 1977; Weiss, 1982) and according to sex (Gilligan, 1982). For example, young men in our society (and, according to anthropological data, in other societies as well) tend to be more centered upon power, control, and dominance issues in interpersonal relationships. It is only in the second half of their lives that many men find themselves increasingly concerned with issues of loving, friendship, and tenderness (Gutmann, 1977; Jung 1930–1931/1960; Levinson, Darrow, Klein, Levinson, & McKee, 1978; Vaillant, 1977). This may be illustrated by the male patient who, after more than 30 years as a hard-driving and successful businessman, tearfully confided to one of us: "In the last couple of years it's occurred to me that I worked so hard that I never had a relationship with my wife and kids. No time together; no closeness; no nothing. Now that I'm starting to need that stuff, everyone is gone." In contrast, for most women there appears to be a lifelong concern and involvement with issues of nurturance, support, and caring for others, sometimes at the expense of their own interpersonal needs (Gilligan, 1982). It may be that for women, as they get older, as children grow up, or as they move along an occupational track, there is an increasing concern with their own needs rather than with the needs of others (Lowenthal, Thurnher, & Chiriboga, 1975).

4. The I-D-E focus is frequently obscured by the symptomatic nature of the patient's presentation or by characterological concerns addressed by either the patient ("I've *always* been depressed") or by the therapist ("This is obviously a lifelong pattern for you"). It is also often the case that the patient views himself or herself as being in a crisis state but fails to comprehend the developmental nature of that crisis. Again, it is all too easy for the therapist to miss the developmental aspects of the crisis situation.

5. There may be some circumstances in which the characterological and/or symptomatic aspects of the problem are markedly prominent, or in which the patient's history and/or behavioral patterns preclude any focus other than on symptoms or aspects of character. These foci do not necessarily rule out an I-D-E orientation, but may require some modifications in intervention and technique. These are dealt with in Chapters 8 and 9.

The Value of an I-D-E Focus

Personal change is plentiful, yet rare. Each of us is constantly in the process of growing older and moving along the life course. At the same time, impediments to growth that may halt or delay maturation frequently come across our paths.

For some people who come to see therapists, blocks that prevent growth are relatively minimal and easily circumvented or removed, while for others these blocks are substantial and have prevented change for extended periods of time. In any case, discovering and using the I-D-E issues that explain the patient's current decision to seek treatment will provide substantial leverage. According to Archimedes's principle, with enough leverage any degree of change is possible. In understanding the I-D-E focus, the therapist is more able to understand where and how to maximize leverage. For example, in discussing how smokers decide to quit, Prochaska and DiClemente (1982) write:

> [M]any smokers begin to contemplate stopping smoking seriously as they approach age 40 and feel pressured to face the finiteness of their lives. Another group of individuals appear ready to change not because of internal developmental changes but because their environment has changed. Perhaps a spouse or child h?s reached a new developmental stage and asks or demands that they stop dri   smoking. (p. 286)

Milton Erickson, who based his treatment on developmental life stage principles (Haley, 1973), was a master at using these principles in the service of therapeutic leverage. For example, Van Dyck (1982) discusses the following case of marital therapy by Erickson:

> . . . Erickson tells about a couple from Pennsylvania who consulted him. The husband was a psychiatrist who, after 13 years, had not organized a successful practice. Both he and his wife were in individual therapy with the same analyst for several years. They traveled to Phoenix seeking marital therapy from Erickson. Erickson mentioned that he took no systematic history and, following a brief conversation, he sent them to complete separate tasks without explaining whether or how the task related to therapy. The husband was to climb Squaw Peak, investing three hours in the project. Similarly, the wife was to spend three hours at the desert botanical gardens.
>
> The next day they reported their experiences to Erickson. For the husband it had been "the most wonderful thing he had done all his life"; climbing Squaw Peak changed his perspective. The wife, on the other hand, reported that she spent the most "boring three hours" of her life at the gardens; all she saw was "more and more of the same old thing."
>
> Without further comment, Erickson sent the couple to complete new tasks. Now the wife was to climb Squaw Peak and the husband to visit the botanical gardens. Their report the next day showed the same discrepant pattern. The husband found it wonderful and awe-inspiring to see all the different desert plants. His wife, who climbed that "goddamned" Squaw Peak, cursing Erickson and herself for doing so, still cursed when she reported about it. Only briefly did she feel some satisfaction upon reaching the top. Erickson then asked them each to choose a task next afternoon, admonishing them to do

it *separately*, and then he told them to come back the following day and report to him. When they came in the next morning, the husband said that he returned to the botanical gardens and again had enjoyed every minute of it, regretting having to leave. To her puzzlement, the wife decided to climb Squaw Peak again. She did so, cursing even more fluently than she had before, both on the way up and on the way down. Again, she felt only a momentary satisfaction upon reaching the top. After they had given these comments, Erickson said: "All right, glad to hear your reports. Now I can tell you your marital therapy is complete. Go down to the airport and return to Pennsylvania." This they did.

A few days later, Erickson received a telephone call from the couple, detailing the following: Upon returning home, they had each separately gone for a ride "to get the cobwebs out of their minds." Next, they had each separately fired their analyst. In addition, the wife reached the decision to file for a divorce which was eventually the outcome of this marital therapy. (pp. 39–40)

Clearly, Erickson quickly realized that this couple perceived themselves to be in an existential, interpersonal, and developmental crisis. They had come to Arizona from Pennsylvania for marital therapy; they had been married for an extended period of time, and presumably had been holding their marriage together by an attachment to their shared analyst. It is our assumption that the partners in this couple were in their 40s or 50s and were dealing with midlife issues. Through indirect hypnotic suggestion, symbolic tasks, and working briefly, Erickson helped the couple achieve what Yalom (1980) has called a "boundary situation"—that is, an "event, an urgent experience, that propels one into a confrontation with one's existential situation in the world" (p. 159). Going all the way across the country to see Erickson for treatment after having had years of analysis, having their differences emphasized to them, and coming to feel that they were at a point in their lives where it was either a matter of taking action now or finding themselves 65 and still unhappily married apparently allowed them to become unstuck.

Discovering and Establishing the I-D-E Focus

In Chapter 3, we describe the major foci that we believe are most frequently treated by brief therapists using an I-D-E perspective. These foci include the following:

1. Losses
2. Developmental dysynchronies
3. Interpersonal conflicts
4. Symptomatic presentations
5. Personality disorders

Each of these areas can and should be understood within a developmental life span context, and as related to a patient's current interpersonal milieu. It is only when the therapist fully considers the developmental, the interpersonal, and the existential aspects of the problem that he or she is able to maximize therapeutic leverage and to reach a clearer understanding of the patient's current motivation for treatment. The following examples may help to clarify the perspective we are describing.

Ron, a 39-year-old philosophy professor, presented with severe depression and a general sense of malaise. The patient felt unhappy much of the time, could not focus on his work, and got pleasure out of little that he did. He had "always" been a fairly depressed person, but had begun to feel more unhappy about 5 months before. At that time, he had accidentally met at a professional conference a young woman with whom he had previously worked and had had a 2-year sexual relationship. This woman, Lisa, was only one of "a dozen" women with whom Ron had had affairs over the course of his 14-year marriage. However, Ron felt that Lisa was the only woman he had every really cared about (including his wife). He had seriously contemplated divorcing his wife, Margie, and marrying Lisa during their affair, but was "too guilty and scared to do it." When he again met Lisa at the conference, she was married and 5 months pregnant. He had become increasingly depressed since that contact.

Ron and his wife, Margie, had been in a great deal of marital and individual therapy as well as psychoanalysis, all to no avail. Treatment would drag on while Ron attempted to "understand" why he was "so angry at my mother." In the first visit he explained to the therapist that he wished to "learn why" he stayed put in "a terrible marriage" that wasn't going anywhere and that made him feel so unhappy. The therapist replied, "You seem like a bright man who has been in enough therapy to understand the whys and wherefores of your anger toward your wife. You and I could probably sit here for months or years and talk about this. Because you are so bright and intellectual, I don't imagine you would do anything particular with this knowledge. I think that you have come in *now* because having seen Lisa makes you realize where you are in your life. You are nearly 40. You've been playing at relationships with women for years. The relationship with Lisa felt different, more real and genuine. Maybe you could stay with your wife for another 10, 15, or 25 years, but you wonder what you will feel like if this is where your relationship and life are when you are 50 or 60." The therapist set a five-session, once-a-month contract with Ron to focus upon what he would do in regard to his marriage.

Christine's 34th birthday was approaching. She and her husband, Adam, had arrived in Boston about a year before because of a major job promotion for him. In Colorado, Christine had been a special education teacher, but had had difficulties finding suitable work following their move.

After several months, however, she had obtained a reasonably good part-time position. It was her hope that after their arrival she would quickly become pregnant and have a child. This had not occurred, and the couple was being medically examined for infertility problems. The first time the therapist met with Christine she was tearful and depressed. Over the previous 4 months, she had lost considerable weight and was sleeping poorly. When asked what she thought was most depressing her, she responded that it was "just everything. The move, the lack of friends, frustration about the pregnancy issue, conflict with my husband, and the fact that I am just a very depressive type of person."

The therapist told her that he thought that all those things were at issue, but that most central appeared to be the infertility problem and her husband's lack of support in regard to this issue. "Women are often affected in a very profound way by infertility problems. Sometimes men are as well, but for women there is a most intense sense that the biological clock is running out. I am sure that this issue is taking its toll on you." In reply, Christine told the therapist that her husband's reaction was to tell her that she was being foolish and irrational to worry about her ability to have children. As it turned out, he had, in fact, considered remaining childless by choice. In the first interview, the therapist spoke with Chris at length about her great pain and fear that she would be unable ever to become pregnant. The therapist set an appointment with her and her husband to discuss this issue in particular and referred Chris to RESOLVE, a national support organization for women and men having problems regarding infertility. After two additional conjoint sessions, therapy was interrupted for 3 months. At that time Chris was feeling much better, and the depression had lifted. She said, "Your talking with me and Adam about what a big issue infertility can be helped a lot. I felt like I was crazy. It meant so much to me, and seemed to mean so little to him. You really helped me validate my feelings. Meeting together also got us talking about the issues. We had been avoiding them before."

AN I-D-E CHECKLIST

The I-D-E frame of reference maintains that frequently the reason a patient seeks therapy at a given time consists of a particular conjunction of interpersonal, developmental, and/or existential events. The events leading the patient to seek therapy (or, in other words, to desire change) may be frequently obscured by the intensely symptomatic or chronic characterological nature of the patient's initial presentation. The I-D-E perspective allows for a rapid clarification of focus for the clinician, and, most importantly, is of great value in maximizing therapeutic leverage. If the central reason why a patient is seeking treatment *now* can be understood, therapeutic force can be greatly increased in the area in question.

It should be noted that although an I-D-E framework attends mainly to current here-and-now or there-and-now issues, historical concerns may be reactivated, and therefore may need to be addressed. This is particularly true when the anniversary of a past loss or a current set of losses has triggered past issues. When past issues are examined, this should be done because the therapist intends to relate these issues or events to the current I-D-E focus. The purpose of historical inquiry is not to excavate the past, but to clarify the present.

Even under circumstances in which the therapist chooses to address a more "purely" symptomatic focus (Chapter 8) or to focus upon characterological issues (Chapter 9), the I-D-E factors remain tremendously important. They provide a context within which to understand the symptomatic or characterological impairments in question, and to help the therapist go about his or her work more efficiently and with greater empathy for the patient's circumstances.

The brief therapist seeking to locate an I-D-E focus should consider the following questions in particular:

1. *What is the patient's (or family's or couple's) reason for seeking therapy at this time?* This is a different question from only identifying the presenting symptoms or problems (which certainly are themselves important). Although the patient may have difficulty in clarifying any changes that have led to his or her seeking therapy, the therapist should assume that either readily observable or more subtle psychosocial changes have contributed to the patient's entrance into care. C. M. Anderson *et al.* (1986) has suggested that people enter therapy not to change, but in response to change. At times, a patient will very clearly identify such changes, thus greatly simplifying the process of clarifying a focus. Frequently this rapid clarification of focus occurs under circumstances in which some type of obvious crisis has occurred. For example, a recent death, discovery of an extramarital affair, relationship loss, illness, job change, accident, crime victimization, and so on can lead to acute symptomatology and the decision to enter into therapy. (Even under "clear" circumstances, however, the developmental, interpersonal, and existential issues should still be kept in mind. That is, the existential impact of a given crisis such as the death of a parent or a personal illness has different meanings at different stages of life and is affected by the nature of the patient's interpersonal supports.) As an example of such a "stage-related" response to crisis, Lowenthal *et al.*, (1975) found that serious illness in adolescence often appeared to be conducive to growth, while in middle age or later it was more likely to be accompanied by psychological regression. Milton Erickson himself displayed such "growth" in the face of physical disease when, both as a child and as an adolescent, he was twice stricken by polio and used his period of infirmity to sharpen his perceptual abilities and sensitivity to the world around him.

The patient who enters therapy with a self-identified clear (often crisis-related) focus has frequently been viewed as the ideal candidate for brief treatment (Small, 1979). In cases in which the focus is less readily identifiable—when the therapist must answer the question of "Why now?"—this allows for the treatment of a much wider diversity of patients than has often been considered appropriate for brief treatment.

2. *What is the patient's age? Date of birth? Approximate developmental stage?* We believe that more adults enter therapy in the months surrounding their birthdays than during other parts of the year, although we have seen no research data regarding this specific hypothesis. It is certainly the case, as Zusne (1986) indicates, that approaching birthdays affect mortality rates in what is called the "birthday–death day" phenomenon. That is, statistically there appears to be a decrease in the probability of death as a birthday approaches and an increase in mortality afterward. Even people who consciously choose to ignore the fact know that their birthdays are coming and going (with what feels like ever-increasing speed). Often, a patient will arrive shortly before or after a "significant" birthday. A childless woman may feel that each birthday in her 30s and 40s is a signpost indicating her diminishing opportunity to become a mother. For the single and unattached young adult with unfulfilled yearnings to enter into a long-term relationship, birthdays can also be markers highlighting loneliness and frustration in being unable to find a special person with whom to be intimate.

Even if a given patient's birthday is not of major importance, his or her developmental stage is always central. Any specific symptomatology must always be considered in light of developmental level. Anxiety, depression, and even characterological complaints have different implications in the context of the developmental phase of the patient in which they occur. In clarifying the patient's normative expectations accompanying a given stage of adult development, the therapist often understands more clearly either why a specific symptom has appeared for the first time, or why a long-standing or intermittently present complaint has returned. Developmental issues also frequently explain why a problem that has been present for a long period of time has finally caused the patient to seek therapy.

Moreover (except for hermits, who are not often likely to seek psychotherapy), the developmental and existential context of help seeking for most people is more fully understood not only as an event within the boundaries of a person's physical and psychological self, but as one level of more inclusive systemic phenomena involving the life cycle of interpersonal relationships—usually, though not exclusively, involving marriage and the family. (Indeed, from a systemic perspective, it has been said that even a hermit needs a crowd to stay away from!) For example, a man's reaching age 40, while certainly an "individual" event, also may mark simultaneously the impending graduation (both literally and figuratively) of the man's eldest child, his wife's return to the work force, and so on. Developmental events involving the coming and going of people in a person's (or a relationship's) life (e.g., births, deaths, graduations, promotions) are particularly important to attend to in the beginning of brief therapy.

3. *Are there any significant recent or upcoming anniversaries for this patient?* Unconscious processes can help many people to forget, and can protect them from events that feel too painful to acknowledge. Often, however, these events will continue to have implications for and a significant impact upon their lives. Frequently, a patient may come to therapy because of feelings of malaise, depression, anxiety, and so on centering around the date of a painful anniversary for which the person may overtly be amnesic. Or, if the patient does realize the date of the anniversary, he or she may not connect the symptoms and that event (e.g., "It happened too long ago to mean anything to me now").

A significant but forgotten or minimized anniversary may provide a very clear and useful focus for brief therapy, as is illustrated in the cases below; again, such a focus should always be considered in light of developmental and interpersonal issues.

Tom and Valerie R., both in their mid-30s, sought couples treatment after their verbal fighting began spilling over into physical violence between them. They had been married about 8 years and had dated for 3 years before their marriage. They described themselves as "hot-blooded Italians" who "always" argued. In the past 2 months, their fighting had become increasingly explosive and intense.

Both partners felt concerned that they would ultimately damage Rhonda, their 2-year-old daughter. In the first interview with them, it became clear that the escalation of their fighting had occurred in the month prior to the fourth anniversary of their first child's death. Lilly, who had been frequently ill from birth because of a very rare immuno-deficiency disease, was 3 years of age when she was suddenly stricken by a rapidly spreading pulmonary infection. Neither the doctors nor her parents realized the gravity of the situation. Within hours of the first flu-like symptoms' appearing, Lilly was dead. In the months following Lilly's death, Tom and Valerie alternately blamed themselves, the doctors, and each other for the tragedy. After about a year, they became more civil to each other, felt less depressed, and began to suppress the death and the events that surrounded it. As they reported a chronology of events, it became clear to the therapist and then to them that February had been a time of great tension each year since Lilly had died, with this year being the worst. The focus chosen with this couple was to examine at length their relationships with Lilly and with each other in the period just prior to and following the death.

Jenni, age 34, entered therapy because of a feeling of extreme crisis. For many years she had felt chronically sad, anxious, and lacking in self-esteem; however, over the past several weeks she had been feeling even worse and "like I can't survive." Jenni had had serious thoughts of suicide and "finally ending all the pain." She attributed her desperation to an "off-again, on-again" relationship with a married man at her office, which had continued (with great difficulty) for 10 years and now appeared to be very shaky once more. In talking with Jenni, it became apparent that much of her symptomatology (which included frequent and sharp intestinal pain with no physical basis) had begun shortly after the birth of an illegitimate daughter 17 years previously, when Jenni herself was 17. This child, who had been born deformed and brain-damaged, had been immediately given up for adoption and had never been seen by Jenni again. In dealing with Jenni, it rapidly became clear that she felt terrible guilt and responsibility regarding this baby. The immediately focus for treatment, which was chosen in the first session, was the issue of this child and how her birth had affected Jenni's attitudes about herself and the people around her. (Jenni's mother and father, for example, could never bring themselves to utter a word about the baby or its birth.) It is also most interesting to note that Jenni had called regarding therapy just days before her child's 17th birthday.

Anna, a divorced computer programmer, called one of us for an appointment several days after "breaking down" while at a singles bar with one of her female friends. She had begun to cry uncontrollably and felt an overwhelming sense of despair and anxiety. Anna was an extremely attractive 35-year-old who spoke about her disgust with the "bar and dating scene." Over the years since her separation, she had gone out with dozens of men (having no problem whatever getting dates). All of these "flings" were inappropriate or unfulfilling. This patient did not remember (until it was pointed out to her by the therapist) that the third anniversary of her divorce was 3 days after her "breakdown." Anna's divorce and separation had been traumatic. Her husband walked out (without informing her that he planned to leave or even indicating that he was dissatisfied) 2 days after she found out that she was pregnant for the first time. He had almost immediately moved in with another woman, told Anna that he was out of love with her, and told her to have an abortion (which she did). The patient had reacted to all of this pain by simply "blocking it out" and launching into a frantic but unsatisfying social and sexual life. The focus of the treatment became Anna's unresolved grief over the end of her marriage and undesired abortion. Noting the anniversary reaction proved to be an important event in the treatment, helping to establish a strongly empathic alliance regarding the patient's deeply felt but unexpressed pain.

4. *Has this patient experienced any major social support changes (improvements or deteriorations) recently?* Although most patients will recognize recent changes and variations in their interpersonal environments, at

times such changes will not be clearly linked to symptoms or to the decision to seek therapy. This is especially true if the interpersonal changes lack the suddenness, intensity, or enormity of a crisis. As previously noted, cognitive distortions often lead the depressed or anxious patient to assume that "I have always been this way," rather than to seek a precipitating event or set of events. It is also true that the patient who suffers from self-esteem problems will feel that he or she is "getting off too easily" if precipitating events are "blamed" instead of himself or herself. The brief therapist should clarify not only interpersonal changes indicating recent losses, but also those indicating recent gains. For some individuals, the decision to seek care comes only after they are feeling better and more able to "deal with" therapeutic input. For others who have clung to their deficiencies and inadequacies over many years of hard work, being involved in a romantic relationship, for example, may lead to a loss of homeostasis and uncertainty about how to proceed. It has been said, "You should not wish for something too much, because you just might get it." Obviously, for some, getting what they wish for may be as disruptive as not getting anything at all.

5. *Is the patient drinking and/or using drugs at this time?* This question must be answered in the first or second visit. It is our strongly held belief that any patients who are alcoholic and drinking during a given course of mental health therapy, or any patients who are psychologically or physically dependent upon drugs and using these addictively, will make few or no therapeutic gains unless or until their addiction is treated. This alcohol or drug dependency must be the primary focus for such individuals; what appears to be a superb course of brief treatment may have little or no impact if the patient is simply anesthetizing himself or herself throughout the therapy. In our experience, alcoholics who are drinking over a course of treatment add the therapy as another form of unproductive, addictive behavior. The easiest approach to attempt in dealing with drug or alcohol problems is to explain to such patients the importance of halting or greatly reducing their use of alcohol and drugs, because it will interfere with a beneficial outcome. If the patients cannot or will not modify their drinking pattern or drug usage alone, referring them to AA (if they are willing to become involved) should be the next step. Most patients whom we have referred to AA have benefited greatly, in regard both to altering their drinking behavior and to developing a useful social support system. A patient who will neither attempt to modify addictive drug or alcohol behavior on his or her own, nor will try to do so with the help of a program like AA, has a poor prognosis for improvement in brief therapy (or in long-term or intermediate-term therapy, for that matter). The focus on the addiction should take precedence over any other possible foci. Other problems are unlikely to improve as long as the patient is drinking or using drugs excessively.

Bretta, a 28-year-old librarian, initiated individual therapy after coming to a family therapy session with her adult brother, who was being treated by one of us. She had been drinking heavily for 10 years, at times missing work and being unable to function after particularly drunken weekends. The therapist saw her three times, each time setting a plan with her for attending AA and halting her drinking. It was even arranged for Bretta to call another patient of her therapist (also a librarian) who had been active in AA for 6 years. All these attempts to have her curb her alcohol intake proved futile. Bretta came to sessions with alcohol on her breath and even mildly drunk. After the third session, treatment was halted, and it was recommended to the patient that when she felt she could work on her drinking problem *before* dealing with other issues, that she should return. After nearly 2 years, the patient came back ready to start treatment. She had stopped drinking on her own and had been sober for 6 months. She felt appreciative that the therapist had not let her simply skirt the drinking issue.

6. *Is the patient initiating treatment because of outside pressures?* Many people are "forced" into therapy by other people in their environments, and have little self-motivation to change or respond to treatment. For example, a pattern frequently seen by clinicians is one in which a person "misdiagnoses" marital conflict as an individual issue residing in the problems of the "other" partner. The individual coming for treatment under such circumstances often either appears reluctant to engage in therapy, or spends his or her time discussing the absent spouse. In a similar vein, some people are "pushed" by attorneys, judges, or others in the legal system to seek therapy because it may "help their case" to have been to a therapist. We have seen individuals with alcohol problems, criminal records, pending charges, and so on come to treatment for no good therapeutic reason whatever. Obviously, such situations are extreme examples, but it is essential to recognize that a focus may be unavailable under some of these conditions. There are approaches for dealing with low motivation or motivation from an external source. For example, regardless of who is labeled in a troubled marriage as the "sick one," the therapist should, early in therapy, see both partners together to get a sense of what the "healthy" spouse wants to gain or lose from the other's therapy, and what type of motivation for change exists in the marital system.

It must also be considered as a possibility that the patient simply does not have sufficient motivation *at this time* for therapeutic change. *Everyone coming to see a therapist need not be engaged in treatment.* In some circumstances, excluding a patient with minimal motivation from treatment has the effect of a paradoxical intervention (L. F. Seltzer, 1986). This is particularly true under circumstances in which other therapists or change agents have spent time trying to *convince* the patient to attempt to change. As Watzlawick *et al.* (1982) have emphasized, it is probably never appropriate to argue with a patient, and we think this principle should be extended to never trying to argue a person into becoming a therapy patient.

7. *Is the patient addicted to psychotherapy and/or using treatment as a reason not to change?* For some people, psychotherapy becomes a way of life, no longer associated with the process of change or the amelioration of distress. The evaluating therapist may often recognize such patients by the fact that they are virtually never out of therapy. Often they wander from one psychotherapist to the next without stopping to live life outside of treatment. Some may even arrange to see a number of therapists simultaneously—one for psychoanalysis, one for marital therapy, one for family therapy, and one for group treatment. Often the most helpful intervention a therapist can offer under such circumstances is either to help the patient to determine which of these multiple therapies is likely to be most helpful *at this time*, and/or to convene all the clinicians involved in a meeting with the patient toward the same end.

These patients will make statements such as this: "Although Gloria and I have lived together for 15 years, I can't really get married until I work out my childhood neurosis about not trusting my mother." Milton Erickson (quoted in Zeig, 1980) received a letter from a therapy-addicted patient as follows:

> Concerning my problem I began to stutter somewhere between the ages of four to four-and-a-half. The onset of the stutter was pretty nearly coincident with the birth of my sister (my first sibling), and a tonsillectomy sometime early in my fifth year. As to how these events related to my stutter, I have never quite pieced them together. I have made many attempts to unravel childhood traumas, including conventional psychotherapy, unsuccessful attempts at hypnosis (Dr. L. thinks I can be hypnotized), "scream" therapy with C. D., the Fisher–Hoffman Process. I have tried various "body" therapies, i.e., Rolfing, Lomi body work, polarity therapy, acupuncture, bioenergetics, and breathing techniques. I have tried mechanical devices. I have done EST, as well as many meditative, spiritual and yogic practices. My stutter still remains. Some of the things I have tried have helped me in varying amounts, but I have the feeling that there still remains some highly charged material from the past which I am mortally afraid to face.
>
> Several Bay Area psychic friends of mine have told me that my relationship with my mother is still unresolved. I am also aware that I have difficulty dealing with anger. Although I am 30 years old, people tell me that I am childlike (many people find it hard to believe that I am over 20), and many still regard me as a child. I want to grow up and get on with my life. I am tired of living my life in this emotional soup.
>
> The pattern of my life has heretofore been as follows: In all of my undertakings, initially there is the promise of dazzling success. Things go well until the going gets a little rough. This is when I usually give up and fail.
>
> I am particularly hopeful to give up the pattern of stuttering, because it really has prevented me from flowing freely with other people and sometimes

even being with them. I have also allowed it to prevent my expansive movement in the world. Since it is a childhood trait, to an extent it keeps me feeling like a child.

My life right now is entering upon a period of change, but at present I am still unable to manifest my skills in the world and earn my living. My current situation is wracked with existential guilt. The only jobs presently available to me are semiskilled or unskilled labor jobs. This is painfully unsatisfactory to me in light of my past. I sailed through graduate school (in operations research and theoretical statistics) dropping out before I got a Ph.D. in order to pursue music. Then I stopped playing for awhile, and when I resumed I felt that there was less consciousness and more rigidity in my left side. From that point on my music has been deteriorating, and I no longer consider myself a serious professional musician. With my diminished ability to play music, my self-hate has increased, as did my consumption of drugs. It has only been in the last two years that I have been tapering off drugs (was taking them pretty regularly for seven years).

I feel like I am in a stronger place now and have an ardent desire to make my life work. I am hopeful about the prospect of working with you, although I am consciously aware of a strong resistance to being healthy, which still continues to haunt me. This resistance is part of my ego-pattern too. Perhaps out of fear or mistrust, I subtly resist cooperating with people.

I hope to hear from you soon. I look forward to working with you if you will take me on. I will be available at your convenience after the first of April (except Tuesday evenings through April). Respectfully yours, George Leckie. (Zeig, 1980, pp. 202–203).*

Erickson commented, "Here is one of those professional patients who *never* is going to get well, and who will play me for a sucker to get all my time and energy and have it result in a failure" (Zeig, 1980, p. 204). He continued:

> I got a letter from a woman once who said, "I've been in active psychoanalysis for 30 years. I am now completing four years of Gestalt therapy. After that, may I be your patient?" There is no hope for those people—they are professional patients. That is their sole goal in life. (Zeig, 1980, p. 209)

8. *Does the patient desire symptomatic change only?* Some patients enter therapy with a very clear desire to change this or that specific problem, but "not to talk about anything else." For example, some patients seek to change a particular habit disorder or discrete symptom, but state that they really do not desire any other changes, and are quite clear about their specified focus. Under such circumstances, one should assume the position that "the customer is right." Although the "Why now?" question may be easily answered, the therapist should use this answer to help himself or

*This quotation is taken from *Teaching Seminar with Milton H. Erickson, M.D.* by J. F. Zeig, 1980, New York: Brunner/Mazel. Copyright 1983 by the Milton H. Erickson Foundation. Reprinted by permission.

herself clarify the case, rather than for interpretive purposes. To try to convince a patient that he or she really wants to understand things better, if the patient is telling the therapist that the only thing desired is very specific symptom relief, sets off an unfortunate transactional spiral. The patient feels misunderstood and coerced, while the therapist feels like a high-pressure salesperson. In our experience, once the discrete symptom is addressed and dealt with seriously, the patient may find that he or she feels a sense of empathy and alliance with the therapist and may wish to discuss those interpersonal and developmental factors that give this symptom greater current urgency.

Ken, a 30-year-old real estate manager, sought therapy after he experienced a severe sleep disturbance over a 2-month period. Although his problems clearly related to a recent major business failure, Ken wished only to discuss his insomnia. He was treated successfully in three biweekly sessions using hypnosis. Several times over these meetings he began to address other issues, only to close up and become frightened as he found himself expressing intense pain about his sense of failure. The hypnosis was highly effective for him, and a year later he reported continued success using it to fall asleep.

Thirty-year-old Edith, a stockbroker, entered therapy regarding a compulsion to scrape away the skin on the inside of her navel. This area was chronically raw, red, and inflamed. At times, it would become infected and require medical treatment. Edith was quite adamant about not wishing to open up all of the "cans of worms in my family." She had been treated a number of times as an adolescent for this compulsion, by psychodynamically oriented therapists as well as some behaviorists, all without noticeable success. Although the reason for her current attempt at therapy appeared to relate to her recently turning 30, and her inability to form even relatively short intimate relationships with men, this was not addressed in early sessions. Rather, a variety of behavioral methods (counting the number of times she scraped, diaries, rewards for not scraping, etc.) and hypnotherapy were used to address the problem on Edith's terms. It was only after some initial and rapid great success as her navel began to heal, and equally rapid failure as she "fell off the wagon" and began to scrape at it again, that the therapist started to explore with her some of her feelings about relationships. The "Why now?" question then began to come into focus.

As we have mentioned previously, to argue with a patient is futile. One must use the "currency" with which patients are entering treatment, rather than forcing a particular point of view upon them. The strength of the I-D-E focus is that most patients can rapidly perceive their concerns within that context. If the therapist can become clear about "Why now?", there is a rapid and powerful empathic bridge with the patient. The patient feels understood and correctly perceived. As has been stated, however, such a focus is too threatening and overwhelming for some subgroups of patients, or is perceived as irrelevant. These patients must be treated in accordance with the (usually) specific symptomatic orientation they present.

There are two major reasons why therapists who refuse to treat patients' face-valid symptoms demur. The first, and most obvious, is that some such therapists genuinely (though mistakenly, in our view) believe that symptom-focused psychotherapy is "inferior" to personality reconstructive aims; that is, it does not address the "real" or most important issues confronting the patient. The second reason why some therapists "pass" on their prospective patients' requests for symptom-focused treatment reflects the unpleasant and therefore rarely acknowledged fact that many therapists simply do not know how to treat such symptoms with a direct, problem-solving approach. A lack of such specific technical skill on the part of the therapist does not, of course, justify persuading a patient that what he or she "really" wants (or, usually, needs) is something different from what is being sought.

MAXIMIZING THERAPEUTIC LEVERAGE DURING INITIAL CONTACTS

The initial contacts in brief therapy are critical. One simply does not have the time or opportunity to sit and wait endlessly for treatment to evolve. In addition, research and clinical findings seem to indicate that the early sessions of therapy have the greatest impact, while later sessions appear to show somewhat diminished returns (Howard *et al.*, 1986). Figure 2-1, from Howard *et al.* (1986), indicates that it is over the first six to eight sessions that much individual psychotherapy has its greatest impact.

This phenomenon of early treatment sessions' having maximal impact can probably best be explained by the concept of "therapeutic leverage." Therapeutic leverage is the increased thrust toward change that comes from the therapist's creative and judicious use of his or her influence, situational factors (such as novelty or surprise in a given setting), and the patient's readiness or desire for change. When people enter a new therapeutic situation (or one in which they have not been involved for a period of time), they are maximally available for change. They often wish to change and are expectant. They may be in a state of existential and developmental flux. They have greater environmental distraction because the setting is novel or different for them (leading to a somewhat lowered resistance level or greater openness to influence). In addition, simply being in "the therapist's office" may initially carry with it a certain degree of power and persuasiveness. Finally, fantasies and consciously held beliefs about the particular therapist

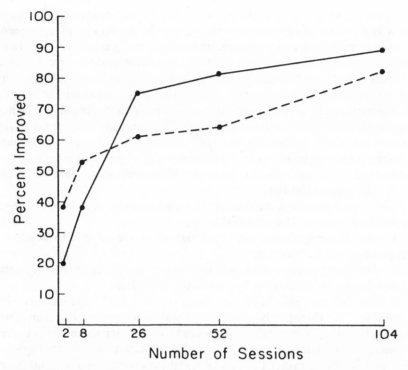

Number of Sessions

Note. Objective ratings at termination are shown by the solid line; subjective ratings during therapy are shown by the broken line.

Figure 2-1.   Relation of number of sessions of psychotherapy and percentage of patients improved. (From "The Dose–Effect Relationship in Psychotherapy" by K. I. Howard, S. M. Kopta, M. S. Krause, and D. E. Orlinsky, 1986, *American Psychologist*, *41*, 159–164. Copyright 1986 by the American Psychological Association. Reprinted by permission.)

to be seen may further enhance the likelihood that change can be successfully initiated.

There is probably, however, a "window of opportunity" after which the patient's resistances begin to increase; interpersonal, existential, and developmental concerns move from foreground to background; and the relative influences of the therapist and therapeutic setting are lessened. It would be difficult to state conclusively how large this "window of opportunity" is. Moving out of this "window," however, may be experienced by the patient as feeling that therapy is dull, stuck, and stilted. "It's just part of my routine to go to therapy every Tuesday morning at eleven." For the therapist, therapy with the particular patient may come to feel slow, unfocused, routine, and lacking in direction.

In order to maximize leverage, the brief therapist should attempt to use each and every early contact with the patient in the service of movement toward therapeutic change. Since optimal use of time is centrally important, there is no firm distinction made between evaluation and therapy. In some settings, long periods of valuable therapy time are spent on three- and four-session "evaluations" before or after which patients sit on extended waiting lists. Such practices, in our experience, lead to patients' "going sour"; if they arrive at all for the first "official" session of "real therapy," they arrive angry and with decreased motivation and high resistance. Evidence from a study by Budman and Springer (in press) indicates a strong relationship between treatment delay in individual treatment and patient dissatisfaction at the end of time-limited therapy.

There are a variety of ways in which a therapist can maximize leverage, and we list a number of such possibilities:

1. The therapist should use the initial telephone contact to begin the therapy and focusing process.

2. The therapist should listen closely and carefully for the I-D-E theme that is bringing the patient in for therapy *at this time*.

3. The therapist should not be afraid to share trial formulations with the patient. If the therapist is "wrong," the patient will make this clear; if the therapist is "right," the patient may begin to reconsider some of his or her preconceptions. In any case, the patient should come to see the therapist as active and involved, rather than passive and expectant. Sharing trial interpretations even if some are wrong, according to traditional views, necessarily decreases the patient's confidence in the therapist; on the contrary, it may actually convey to the patient the important messages that therapy is a collaborative effort, and that the patient's active contribution (including helping to correct the therapist's misunderstanding) is essential. Such messages are essential to the practice of effective brief therapy.

4. The therapist should quickly involve significant others where possible. Spouses, siblings, parents, lovers, friends, and roommates can all make meaningful contributions to the therapy. Also, actively influencing the patient's social system may have a more lasting influence than attempting to influence the patient alone. Moreover, it is probably true that a therapist almost never influences only the patient who is physically in his or her office; resistance to change in an individual can be attributable to the "significant others" in the patient's life as often as it can be attributable to the patient himself or herself.

5. Initially, it may be wise to use extended or more frequent visits. For some patients, we have experimented with the use of one, two, or three 2-hour sessions on a weekly basis before moving to less frequent 1-hour, 30-minute, or 15-minute sessions. Meeting on a less-than-weekly basis (weekly meetings are routine in therapeutic practice, and thus expectable to many patients) may simultaneously convey the therapist's optimism about

the patient (i.e., indicate that the patient does not need to be seen as often as the patient may expect), send an important message about the need for change to occur outside the therapist's office, and implicitly counter powerful conscious and unconscious fantasies about the therapist's role as a healer.

6. The patient should usually have some type of mutually agreeable task or homework assignment to accomplish between early sessions. This can take any of a variety of forms—thinking about something, reading or writing about a given issue, talking with someone, or traveling somewhere. One function of such tasks is to keep therapy and change from becoming events that only occur in the therapist's office.

7. The brief therapist's stance, from the very first communication with a given patient, should be that unless it is clearly demonstrated to be impossible, this individual can and should be treated in psychotherapy that is both cost- and time-effective. In order to enable clients to work in a time-intensive manner, the therapist must have first examined his or her underlying therapeutic value system (see Chapter 1), and in fact must believe that change can be initiated by a relatively brief series of contacts.

Some of these suggestions are discussed in more detail below, and the chapter ends with a transcript from an initial interview that exemplifies many of them.

The First Telephone Call

Upon the very first phone contact with a potential client, one can and should begin the process of clarification and focusing. In general, the patient's first contact with the therapist is by telephone. The patient, having decided to seek therapy, or with the support and encouragement of another individual (such as a spouse, friend, nurse, or physician), calls to make an appointment for evaluation and/or treatment. Clearly, although there are variations in how the therapist and patient first make contact, the most common mode of entry into mental health systems remains patient-initiated contact.

Patient: Hello, Dr. Smith, this is Ann Jones. I'm a friend of Jim Taft, whom you treated, and I'd like to make an appointment to come and see you.
Therapist: That's fine, but could we talk for a few moments now on the phone about the problem you are experiencing?
P: Sure.
T: Tell me just a little about what has made you decide to come in now.
P: I've been having terrible headaches and dizziness. My doctor says there is no real physical basis.
T: Have you ever had this problem before?

P: Yes, when I was a teenager. After I started college they got better.

T: Do you live with anyone now? Are you in a relationship?

P: I'm married and just had my second child 8 months ago.

T: What does your husband make of the headaches?

P: Lenny says I'm doing it to myself. He's pretty angry that they're not getting better.

T: I wonder how you and Lenny would feel about coming in together for at least a first interview?

P: I can ask him. I've seen therapists myself a few times in the past. He has never been. He might be uncomfortable.

T: I find it most useful to see people together, at least initially. It gives me a much better sense of what is going on. If Lenny has any questions or problems about that, please ask him to call me. Otherwise, let's plan to meet jointly for that first visit.

In just a few moments on the telephone, the therapist in this example has been able to gather some potentially useful data. The presenting patient has had previous therapy, has presumably experienced substantial tension in regard to college and separation, has recently given birth to a child, and is dealing with some marital conflict. The therapist also initiates two strategies that may be most valuable at a later point: Dr. Smith (1) begins the patient thinking about the question of "Why now?", and (2) places the problem in a social/interpersonal context by immediately trying to engage the patient's spouse in the evaluation process.

The Collaborative Context

A brief therapist may be technically proficient, but may do treatment that is of minimal utility. All therapy takes place within a collaborative interpersonal context, without which treatment will fail. It has been maintained by some theorists (Bordin, 1979) that this context is actually the basic curative element in all modes of psychotherapy. In our view, however, a collaborative relationship between therapist and patient is a necessary but not usually a sufficient condition for change. Although many theorists address this issue to one degree or another, those who view it as being secondary (as opposed to those who view the alliance as primary) have said little about how one builds or enhances therapist–patient collaboration.

The neglected aspects of the collaborative relationship may be the elements which differentiate exceptional therapists from adequate or poor therapists. In this regard, a story told by Yalom (1980) may be illustrative:

Once, several years ago some friends and I enrolled in a cooking class taught by an Armenian matriarch and her aged servant. Since they spoke no English and we, no Armenian, communication was not easy. She taught by demonstrations; we watched (and diligently tried to quantify her recipes) as she prepared an array of marvelous eggplant and lamb dishes. But our recipes were imperfect; and, try as hard as we could, we could not duplicate her dishes. "What was it," I wondered, "that gave her cooking that special touch?" The answer eluded me until one day, when I was keeping a particularly keen watch on the kitchen proceedings, I saw our teacher, with great dignity and deliberations, prepare a dish. She handed it to her servant who wordlessly carried it into the kitchen to the oven and, without breaking stride, threw in handful after handful of assorted spices and condiments. I am convinced that those surreptitious "throw-ins" made all the difference. (p. 3)

The alliance-building "throw-ins" offered by the outstanding therapists of our times are probably not even recognized by them as central aspects of their techniques. Rather than dealing with specific methods of enhancing patient–therapist collaboration, many brief therapy authors simply indicate that such relationship factors are important and desirable in brief treatment (Flegenheimer, 1982). A clear exception has been the work of hypnotherapists and Ericksonian psychotherapists (Erickson, Rossi, & Rossi, 1976). We believe that various aspects of hypnotic induction provide us with useful and clear models for the establishment and development of the alliance in brief psychotherapy. Further, induction procedures can be examined at a microscopic level, and this understanding can then be applied to psychotherapy approaches. Readers who are familiar with hypnotic techniques will recognize various aspects of these in our descriptions of approaches that may be useful in enhancing the collaborative context.

Using One's Eyes and Ears

Because all of us are bombarded by so many stimuli all of the time, the mind usually becomes trained to focus on certain aspects of our environments while ignoring or limiting that which is consciously attended to. For example, a person reading these words is probably not attending to the sensations of his or her feet where they are touching socks, stockings, or shoes, and probably does not consciously realize that every few seconds his or her eyelids are gently touching in a natural blinking response. In a similar fashion, it is easy to meet new patients and never really *see* or *hear* 90% of what they are communicating. This is, we believe, particularly true if one is attempting to validate a theory in each interaction with a patient. The family therapists Fred and Bunny Duhl (Duhl & Duhl, 1981) have said that "you don't kiss a system." Similarly, one cannot treat a theory. Thus, the therapist looking *only* for signs of Oedipal conflict, or *only* for cognitive distortions, can easily ignore major aspects of the patient's experience that are being communicated. As a concrete example, the reader should quickly glance at the sentence below and then state aloud what it says:

I love Paris in the
the spring.

It is very easy to miss "the the" because one reads the sentence with an intuitive sense of what it sounds like and because of previous acquaintance with the phrase. Part of Milton Erickson's remarkable skills as a clinician certainly related to his uncanny ability to notice and perceive even minute aspects of his environment. Lankton and Lankton (1983) described just such an experience with him:

> One group of his students, discussing and arguing about the range of Erickson's perceptual skills, set up a test by turning a very small figurine of an owl on its side where it sat on a very crowded shelf in the back of the office. They waited expectantly, wondering if Erickson would notice the small alteration and, if he did, how he would respond. He said nothing about it all day and apparently hadn't noticed it. As the students were filing past his wheelchair to leave the office, Erickson casually remarked, "Oh by the way, that other thing you want me to mention, I don't give a 'hoot' about it." (p. 16)

It is very important that the successful brief therapist listen to the patient and observe as much about him or her as possible throughout the treatment. However, in the early stages, as one attempts initially to "tune in to" the patient to clarify a focus ("Why now?") and build rapport, careful observation is a *sine qua non*. This intensive observation begins with the very first communication, be this by letter, by phone, or in person.

Some time ago, one of us received a telephone call from a woman who was a friend of another person whom he was then treating. "I've been to 11 therapists in this area and I've wasted my money with each of them. None of them gave me what *I* wanted or helped in the way *I* wanted. I have heard a lot about you from Liz. I'd like to come in and *see* you. However, I'll only come in if you don't charge me for the first session." The therapist had no interest in providing her with a money-back guarantee or free trial offer, so they could not come to an agreement. She called the therapist again several weeks later and said she was now reluctantly willing to pay for the first consultation. A time was arranged and the patient came in. She walked into his office, looked at him for 15 seconds, and then said, "I won't come to see anyone who takes notes." (The therapist had sat down with his pad and pen on his lap to get some specific information.) Thereupon, she suddenly stood up and walked out of his office, never to be heard from again. She had gotten what she said she wanted to get in their very first 3-minute conversation: *She saw him once for free.* If one listens and looks carefully enough, people will often communicate something of what they want with even the most minimal contact.

Work with hypnosis teaches one to observe small differences and changes in behavior. For example, when one is inducing a trance state one watches for slowed breathing, relaxation and flatness of facial muscles, eyelid flutter, and so forth. The same type of observational stance should be applied to nonhypnotic therapies. Does the patient move toward or away from the therapist in conversation? What is the reaction to the therapist's input (both verbal and nonverbal)? Does the patient blush or become flushed at any point in the interview? Is the patient rigid or relaxed? Are there any tremors or repetitive movements?

Tracking the Patient

As an initial approximation, it may be valuable to begin sessions by internally pacing and tracking the patient. This means trying to keep one's body posture, breathing, speech rhythm, and so on approximately linked to those of the patient. The therapist should watch the patient's facial expressions, skin color, repetitive movements, and so forth for clues to his or her affective state. Often, nonverbal behavior is most easily observed when it contrasts with or is at odds with verbal behavior. The woman who talks about loving her husband and children while slowly shaking her head conveys a contradictory message. Similarly, the man who says that his divorce no longer bothers him, while his eyes well up with tears, communicates in an important way.

For Helmuth Kaiser, the famous existential therapist, it was precisely this lack of congruence between the verbal and nonverbal that typified psychiatric patients. He wrote:

> [They] did not talk straight. They were never completely, never wholeheartedly behind their words. Listening to them required a very special effort. . . . Listening to them caused some inner struggles, almost as if one has to listen to two speakers simultaneously. There was a strange duplicity about their communications. There were words and sentences and whole stories which were quite understandable and made sense in themselves; but the accompaniment of the tone of voice, facial expressions and gestures interfered subtly and sometimes grossly with the total communication effect. (quoted in Fierman, 1965, pp. 30–31)

The therapist can also make links to the patient by expressing interest in (and, one hopes, feeling an interest in) those nonproblematic areas that are of importance to the patient. Patients are more than a series of presenting complaints. By eliciting information regarding those things that the patient values and enjoys, the therapist learns about strengths that can later be utilized in treatment, and also builds rapport. A patient who is athletically oriented should be questioned about his or her skills and interests in this area. The writer or artist may be engaged about issues related to his or her craft. The same concept holds true for those interested in business, the outdoors, children, science, and so on. Most people like, enjoy, or have some proficiency at something. Obviously, this issue should not, under most circumstances, be the only thing discussed in a session; however, many therapists consider such factors unimportant side issues that have little impact on or value for the overall treatment. In fact, with some patients, engaging them regarding their strengths and the healthier sides of their personalities may be *the* most useful strategy for rapidly establishing a collaborative context.

Several years ago, one of us observed a master hypnotist, who was a dentist by profession, demonstrating his various trance inductions with a number of patients. He had very little formal knowledge about psychology or psychiatry, but was tremendously skilled and successful at treating patients with chronic and severe pain problems. Before beginning to induce a trance in any patient, he would have "a little chat." In this brief conversation, he would rapidly learn a great deal about the patient's hobbies, interests, and leisure-time activities. Later, in his induction and trance utilizations, he would skillfully weave the information together and use it to enhance the hypnosis and his rapport with the patient. Like Yalom's Armenian cooking teacher, described earlier, this man believed that his "little chat" was a "throw-in" and that he was successful at his work because of other, more formal factors in the hypnosis. We have our doubts. The therapist should always bear in mind that most patients have interests and involvements outside of the treatment that they will enjoy talking about; these may provide a useful entree into a collaborative relationship, as well as information regarding how this person sees the world and what is meaningful and valuable to him or her.

Initial Interview with Helen

The transcript that follows of an initial visit illustrates some of the elements we have described as important in initiating brief therapy. The patient, Helen, was an attractive 25-year-old woman who, as she put it in the course of the interview, felt as though she were "12 going on 65."

Therapist: How can I help you?
Patient: I've seen many therapists without any real help for myself. One man told me I was very anxious, and that I needed to become less so. He felt like biofeedback was what I needed. I felt like it wasn't really so much that. I saw someone else a few years ago (*laughs*); he gave me a bunch of tests—I tell you, loads of them, and he told me I have low self-esteem. I knew that before. I saw him about five or six times, but nothing was really going anywhere. I heard about you from my friend Judy. It's real hard, you know, to find a reputable therapist these days.

I thought you might give me some names when we're through, you know, somebody closer to [her home town].

[The patient presented herself with great hopelessness and demoralization. She indicated that she had not been understood by therapists in the past and that her contacts with them had not been helpful. If she had not offered information about her previous experience with mental health treatment, it would have been most valuable to ask her about this, insofar as her underlying attitudes about treatment might be very important in determining how she would use therapy. It is also interesting to note that even before beginning to discuss her issues she was talking about seeing "somebody closer to home," thereby defending herself against rejection.]

T: What's the problem you're having right now?

[The therapist tried to refocus on the *current* issue that was bringing the patient to therapy.]

P: I feel sometimes (*becomes slightly tearful*) like I suffer from a terrible depression. I feel like maybe I won't be able to get out of bed in the morning, you know. It's like I don't want to go to work, face the day, or do anything. I don't know how I do it from one day to the next. I'm working at two jobs and going to school part-time. I've got a degree in biology. I never feel like my work is at all enjoyable. My whole life . . . it's so lousy. Sometimes it seems to me it would be best to just end it all. But I know how much my family would be hurt, so I probably never would really do it. I hold onto the thought [of suicide] though, because it's comforting to think about when the pain is too terrible.

[Here, and for the next several statements, the patient described her symptomatic state. Although this was important information, and is important in general, we do not believe that this alone represents an adequate therapeutic focus in most cases. The aim of the initial interview is to begin to understand why the patient is seeking therapy *now*.]

T: It sounds like you're in terrible pain most of the time.
P: (*Nods*) I'm always indecisive; I can't decide what to do. And my mother says, "You should be happy."
T: What do you mean?
P: "In this day and age, having *any* job should be OK," she says, but I just feel disappointed most of the time—in my life, in myself, in everything. I finished college, but that got me nowhere either.
T: When did you graduate from college?
P: In 1977 [3 years earlier]. But it's just all so frustrating. I was working in a drug abuse program, but . . . [She spoke here about conflict with other

staff, teachers in the program, her boredom, and so on, and described
other jobs she had had in very negative terms.] When I graduated from
high school, I thought of many careers, but somehow I soured on all of
them. I was fourth in my high school class. Teachers said that I was
brilliant, and should be capable of anything, but I just never knew what
I wanted.

T: What happened after high school?

P: I went to ——— College, then to ——— College. [Both colleges were very
near her home.] But I just couldn't find the right direction, I just never
felt satisfied.

T: What about your interpersonal and love life? Do you have girlfriends,
boyfriends, lovers?

P: (*Laughs*) I have plenty of girlfriends, but I've just never felt like I really
needed a boyfriend. I just don't need it.

T: Tell me about your living situation. Where do you live, and with whom?

P: With my mother and two brothers, in the country.

T: What about your father?

P: He's deceased.

T: Can you tell me some more about that? When did he die?

P: [She gave the year of her father's death.]

T: How old were you? How did he die?

**[Anniversary grief reactions are frequent. It is important to be quite specific
and precise about all issues related to significant losses.]**

P: (*Begins to well up with tears.*) He died when I was 6 years old, no, 5 years
old. He had a brain hemorrhage in his sleep. It just happened like that,
suddenly. I don't really remember.

T: It's very painful for you to think about it all.

P: (*Begins to sob*) It was just hard without a father. I'm sorry I'm crying. I'm
really embarrassed. It's just that I'm so emotional about this.

T: Tell me more about that time, whatever you remember.

P: I really can't remember. It's really weird. Maybe I'm crazy. I can't
remember really much at all. My youngest brother was only 2 months
old. He [the father] had taken us all out to the beach, then he went up
to bed and never got up in the morning. I don't remember anything,
really.

T: What kind of work did your father do?

P: He was a mechanic.

T: What else do you remember?

P: My mother closed the door on her life when he died.

T: Maybe you did as well?

P: I don't know. No one supported my mother at the time. No one was there
for her at all.

[The death was clearly an issue of tremendous importance for her. It could represent a partial focus for therapy. However, the question still remained as to why she chose this time to deal with the loss.]

P: [At this point, the patient described how her uncles and aunts on both sides of the family did not help her mother. She also stated that most members of her father's family had been opposed to the marriage of her parents.] I tried to help Mother, but she had no confidence in me at all. She was always afraid I would get hurt. She protected me from everything. She was always so full of shoulds and shouldnots. "If you'd just been a nurse, everything would be fine." Or she'll say, "If you'd done this, or if you'd done that, everything would be fine."

T: When did your father die? What was the exact date? What was his date of birth? How old was he at his death?

[Was this an anniversary grief reaction?]

P: (*Smiles*) My father died on the first of June, I remember that date well. We'd just had a day away from home. He was born on ———— [gives date]. It'll be 20 years ago very soon [about 3 months after this interview].

T: How old were your brothers?

P: The youngest was 2 months old. The others were 9 and 3. I just recall that (*starts to cry, softly*) Mom used to get real negative. She would say, "If you don't all just straighten up, I'll just leave you all at an orphanage." Sometimes I think she was really serious. She had it hard, but she was really always a martyr.

T: How did your brothers deal with her while growing up?

P: My older brother never did the, you know, work that a man should have done around the house. There was always grass cutting, garbage dumping, cleaning up and Fred [the older brother] would not do it, so Mom just went and did it herself. She really was a martyr. She'd suffer, but let you know how badly she suffered. I'd do what I could. My brother ended up fighting with Mom for years. He got into drugs and trouble with the law, you know. Now he's okay—he got married, and he's working with computers.

T: What are your other brothers doing?

P: [The patient explained that one brother was in college, and the other brother was an accountant.]

T: It seems to me that your father's death had an enormous impact on your whole family. Maybe nobody's really recovered yet. One can never be certain about such things, but it seems to me that this early loss had a terribly profound effect. Did you discuss the death of your father in your other therapies?

P: No, the therapists didn't seem to be interested. One guy was into biofeedback and told me not to be anxious, and the other guy gave me dozens of tests and told me that my self-esteem was low (*laughs*). I knew that already. I just stopped going to them, because nothing was really happening.

[The death was a very powerful issue that had to be addressed, because it had been so central and important in her growth, and also because the therapist's recognition of its importance was beginning to establish an alliance.]

T: Have you ever left home for any period of time?

P: No (*starts crying*). I'm not crying because of my father. I'm crying because I get emotional when I release all these feelings. I don't usually talk about this stuff with anyone. No, I've not really left home, because me and my brother know that if we left, Mom would have to sell the house. She doesn't think so, but I know it. It's hard for me to even go away overnight. I always wonder how she will do without me.

[The separation issue began to emerge clearly as an important focus.]

T: You've carried a large part of the responsibility in the family.

P: (*Now sobbing*) But I've lost a large part of my life. I'm 25, and there seems to be so much I've missed . . . (*Trails off*)

T: What you've lost is the most painful to you. [Her father.]

P: Yes, my depression is sometimes so awful, and it's been there so long. My mother always says things that make me even more depressed. She doesn't believe in me; she says, "If you only went to this or that school, you'd be okay now." Also, she doesn't believe in therapy. She tells me, "Therapists can't help you. You're only wasting your money and your time. It's just foolishness. If you'd just enjoy your job, you'd stop being depressed."

[The fact that the mother was against therapy needed to be remembered and to remain important to the therapist. The therapist at this point meant a lot less to the patient than her mother did.]

T: Do you believe that your mother is right—that you can't really be helped?

P: Sometimes.

T: I think you also feel, at times, like things can't change. You don't know what you're capable of.

P: I just so often feel guilty, and like I feel so tired and unhappy. I wish someone could just tell me about why I feel so badly. I just can't tell why. If somebody only knew.

T: Do you want to know what's happening, and why? (*Laughs*)

P: (*Laughs as well*) Yes, please give me "the answer."

T: Obviously it's not the whole "answer," but it's part of it. You're a bright, attractive woman of 25 who always has felt without direction or purpose. You've not had a good idea of career, and you've been without a love relationship. You feel terribly stuck and trapped in your life. Are you attracted to men?

P: Yes, but I just don't want the trouble.

T: I think that you have been profoundly affected by your father's death. You were just a little girl when this occurred. You must have felt terrified, helpless, abandoned—just alone in the world.

P: (*Very tearfully*) I tried to step into my father's role. I tried to help Mother all the time. I tried to be like a husband to her. I feel guilty and sorry for her. I always worried about her.

T: And you don't want to be an orphan, either.

P: That would be awful.

T: What are you planning for next year?

[The separation and loss issue was so prominent and repetitive that it was increasingly apparent that the patient was trying to prepare to leave home.]

P: I want to go to graduate school on a full-time basis. The schools that I'm considering are all far away. I need to go, but I don't know if I can do it.

[*This*, then, appeared to be the issue leading up to therapy.]

T: Let me suggest to you that we focus on your father's death and how this affects you now. Let's especially think about this issue of your going off to school in August in relation to your father's death—how you can be helped to take that step of going if that's what you want to do. I'm certain that you can get a good deal out of treatment in a relatively brief period of treatment, say 4 months or so, perhaps on an every-other-week basis.

[The focus was offered here. In addition, the therapist expressed hope that therapy could and would succeed in a relatively circumscribed period.]

P: I'd like to try it, but what do you think my father's death has to do with my problems now?

T: There are many different ways of dealing with death. Some people talk about it and confront it directly, while other people just avoid it completely. I'm sure people in your family didn't really talk much about their feelings, and don't do so now.

P: That's so right.

T: Your mother must have been in terrible pain, with much fear. Obviously, that stuff about the orphanage came from her own terror about being alone in the world.

P: It sure does. She was also orphaned at 5 years old, when her father died suddenly.

T: Everyone in the family was terrified, so that all of the feelings got pushed away. When people go through such a trauma, they at times throw out the baby with the bath water. All feelings get pushed away. I think this is what you did. You've sort of frozen yourself in time. You don't allow much feeling. The only thing that comes through is depression, and no real connections or attachments. I think if you can do some mourning that you need to do, maybe you can move on and become a young adult, and really feel 25 years old.

P: What you're saying really fits. I feel different than when I came in, better, a lot less burdened. I wish I could feel 25. Right now it's like I'm 12 going on 65; there's a whole piece of my life missing.

T: I'm going to propose several things to you. These aren't orders, but suggestions. I'd like to suggest to you that if it's possible, we look at photographs of your family the next time, which go back as far as you can. Maybe even to your parents' childhoods. About 30 or 40 photos would be good. I'm especially interested in seeing pictures of your father and the family together. If we have the opportunity, let's try and make a visit to your father's grave. We can do that together, or you can do it alone, if you have the chance. And third, what I'd like to do is have at least one session with you, your mother, and your brothers, together. All of these don't need to be done at once, but a piece at a time. Let's start with the photos first. We can do that next time. Let's meet for five sessions, and then re-evaluate.

[A series of focal and active interventions was quickly offered. The patient was beginning to feel as though something *would* happen. There was a sense that things could and would change. It is often useful to offer several tasks at the same time; the patient can then reject several and still undertake one or more. Furthermore, it is frequently best to start with a very short, renewable contract of two to five sessions, so that all parties can decide whether and how therapy should continue.]

P: I'd like to think about some of that. I can certainly bring in the photos next time, though.

T: [The therapist asked the patient whether she had any questions or comments about the session, and they discussed some incidental issues.]

P: (*Handing the therapist a dollar bill*) Do you have any change for the turnpike? I don't think I can get change at the toll booths.

T: (*Smiles*) It always pays to be cautious when you're away from home, huh?

This patient was treated initially in a total of nine sessions over a period of approximately 20 weeks, at the end of which she entered a distant graduate school. The first three sessions (two of which were 2 hours long) were spent discussing her father's death and the patient's relationship with her mother. Although Helen never would agree to come in with her brothers or mother, in the fifth session she spontaneously decided that she would be willing to ask her closest female friend to come to the following session. This proved to be very productive and useful. The patient described herself as very much helped by treatment. She was far less depressed, no longer contemplated suicide, and felt more self-confident. Her friend reported in their joint session that Helen was happier, more communicative, and more outgoing. She also stated that the patient had ceased isolating herself and instead would reach out and discuss issues when she began feeling down. When the patient was questioned closely about the most useful events in the treatment, she said that talking about her father and mother helped her feel less guilty and less responsible for "my mother's state of affairs."

It is our experience that although some patients seem quite clear in regard to what has been helpful to them, for others (like Helen), a great deal of change has occurred at an unconscious level and is not directly available to the patient. Two years after therapy ended, the patient wrote to the therapist stating that she was continuing to do well and planned to take the next year off in order to travel. The therapist felt that this woman had improved because (1) mourning her father allowed her to express the deep and hidden pain about this loss; (2) the therapist recognized her fears and guilt about leaving her mother and her prospect of making the break; (3) he allowed her to examine some of her erroneous cognitions and patterns (e.g., "I can only be a good daughter if I take care of my mother," or "No one will want to talk with me if I am depressed; therefore, I will withdraw"); (4) a clear and explicit focus was maintained throughout therapy (on the father's death and the relationship of this death to the current interpersonal–developmental problem of separation).

In some ways, the last of these reasons may be the most important. This is because, as is often true with patients, numerous issues may be present simultaneously. If the brief therapist fails to find and maintain a coherent focus, or attempts to address all things at once, short-term treatment cannot succeed.

A Chasidic tale is told about the famous rebbe of Tsenz. When asked by one of his followers, "Rabbi, what do you do before you pray?", he replied, "I pray that I might pray well." The brief therapist must, like the rebbe, be single-minded in his or her maintenance of a focus. In Chapter 11, we return to Helen and discuss another course of therapy she had with the same therapist 4 years later.

3

Common Foci in Brief Therapy and Some Basic Assumptions

Round up the usual suspects.
    —Captain Louis Renault, in the film *Casablanca*

All forms of brief therapy emphasize the importance of having a clear area of focus for the treatment. The theoretical inclinations of the developer of the treatment determines the major focus or foci.

What is meant by "treatment focus"? How does one stick with the focus? And what are common foci in brief therapy from an I-D-E perspective? These are some of the questions we attempt to address in the following chapters.

Human behavior is so complex, and can be organized according to such a wide variety of principles, that the therapist has literally an infinite number of choices regarding the potential core focal issue or issues. Kinston and Bentovim (1981), in describing the value of a therapeutic focus for brief treatment, have written:

> A focal hypothesis refers to an "ad hoc clinical theory" developed to clarify or bring into focus a large number of disparate and apparently unrelated phenomena. It integrates and provides continuity to the manifestations of the person or family. It also serves as a beacon to guide the therapist as he or she becomes involved in the detailed specifics of work with the individual or family. For this reason, it must be brief and highly pertinent. . . . (p. 367)

As described in Chapter 2, we believe that a focus relating to interpersonal, developmental, and existential factors has the greatest potential for being quickly relevant to the patient, closely related to his or her reason for seeking therapy, and useful to the therapist as a theme around which to organize his or her interventions. The foci we describe in this chapter are frequently seen in the general outpatient practice of psychotherapy with adults. Except for our final category, severe personality disorders, they generally relate to events or states of being that may be relatively independent of diagnostic category. As such, they represent what we view as the most prominent and immediate feature in the patient's life, which is directly

62

related to the patient's decision to seek therapy at this particular point in time.

In considering any of the possible central foci proposed below, the therapist should always taken into consideration the patient's life stage as a factor affecting the significance of the given focus for that person. For example, the death of a spouse has very different meanings for a 30-year-old widow and for a 75-year-old widow. There is intense pain and mourning in both circumstances. However, the 75-year-old woman may have friends who have also lost their husbands; there may have been more of an expectation that her husband might die before her; the couple's children are probably grown adults; and so on. For the 30-year-old woman, there would have been no expectation nor anticipation that she would be widowed at this point in her life; there are likely to be young children to raise alone; the support systems for young widows or widowers are likely to be minimal; and so forth.

In addition, the therapist should remain attuned to the interpersonal context of the patient. What supports exist? What are his or her familial and friendship networks like? What and who are the most powerful interpersonal influences in the patient's life?

THE FIVE MOST COMMON FOCI

We describe here the five most commonly occurring foci, which are discussed more extensively in later chapters.

Losses

Past, present, or impending losses often constitute a major reason for seeking psychotherapy. Examples include the loss of an attachment figure through moves, separation, divorce, or death; the loss of one's own health and well-being through illness, accident, or victimization; the loss of a home or a job; and so on. Not infrequently multiple areas are affected at once, as when an illness or disability leads to the loss of a job. It should be borne in mind that losses are not always dealt with directly by the patient at the time of their occurrence. That is, for a variety of reasons at the time of a particular loss, the patient may be unable to acknowledge the full meaning or power of that loss. It may take months or years before the impact manifests itself overtly. By that time, the patient has detached the original experience from its now manifest symptomatology. The symptoms are therefore viewed as mysterious, as unrelated to events in the present, and often as indicative of characterological deficits. In a similar manner, the patient who realizes that a loss will soon occur may deny its importance, thereby excluding from consciousness the cause of his or her discomfort.

Developmental Dysynchronies

Development throughout life is a dynamic process, with a variety of changing hopes, expectations, and role demands at various points. When our expectations at transition points are not fulfilled, and in particular when our age-mates are moving to achieve things that we ourselves have been unable to achieve, a disequilibrium occurs that may lead to help seeking.

For example, the single, unattached 28-year-old man or woman who finds that more and more of his or her friends are becoming involved in long-term, committed relationships, are living with lovers, or are getting married may feel an increasing sense of loneliness and heightened desire for such a relationship himself or herself. Similarly, the 64-year-old man who is quickly moving toward retirement without any real savings, sense of security, or plan for how he will spend the remainder of his life may be filled with fear, anxiety, and depression. This may be especially true if he has friends who have saved money and/or who are better organized to deal with retirement. When the therapist fails to take a dynamic (not psychodynamic) view of adult development, it may be easy to forget that the same symptomatology in those of different ages may have very different meanings and causes. We believe that for the patient to realize that the therapist can truly understand and empathize with his or her plight is of enormous value. Therefore, for many patients it is not as effective simply to comprehend that the patients are depressed as it is to convey an understanding of their developmental and existential pain.

Interpersonal Conflicts

A third major area of difficulty that frequently brings people to psychotherapists is the exacerbation of interpersonal conflicts. Frequently such interpersonal conflicts occur within the context of an intimate relationship. At times, conflict relates to different developmental sequencing between partners in that relationship, as when, for example, a woman feels ready to have children while her spouse does not. However, severe interpersonal conflicts certainly may occur with friends, employees, coworkers, and so on. Although conflicts may relate to potential losses or to developmental factors, they also may occur independently of either.

Symptomatic Presentation

Another major reason for presentation to a therapist is in regard to a particular clear and discrete symptom or set of symptoms. Not infrequently the patient has suffered with the symptom for an extended period of time, but chooses to seek therapy after a major loss or when he or she has just passed or is about to pass a particular developmental milestone. Unlike those circumstances in which understanding a particular loss, grieving for it, and so on is helpful, it is our impression that if the patient presents exclusively or almost exclusively with a symptomatic concern (e.g., "I have been an insomniac for 10 years and it has nothing to do with the circumstances of my life"), the patient *must* be treated first and foremost around that symptom. Even if other issues are clearly (to the therapist) the pivotal factor(s) driving the patient to seek help at this point—and they almost invariably are—the patient must be accepted on his or her own terms. This means an immediate focus upon the presenting discrete symptomatology. The range of symptomatic presentations is enormous, but usually includes habit disorders, sexual dysfunctions, fears, and phobias.

Severe Personality Disorders

There are some patients who simply never make progress when therapy deals with the major foci described previously. In addition, their presentation to a therapist often ceases to be clearly tied in to the losses, transitions, and conflicts described above. Rather, such patients present repeatedly for mental health therapy, with little indication that any change has occurred after any brief intervention. They present with constant reports of loneliness, isolation, depression, anger, and so on. Their pain is rarely alleviated by a problem-focused intervention. Moreover, such patients' characterological impediments often interfere with their abilities to relate productively with a therapist. The portrait that usually emerges is one of a patient with severe (at times borderline) character problems. It should not be assumed, however, that such a patient cannot be treated in brief therapy. We have seen such patients briefly using one or more of the major foci described for numerous courses of brief therapy, and this has appeared to be the treatment of choice. There are, however, other patients for whom the usual format does not appear to have sufficient useful effect and for whom other approaches (to be described in Chapter 9) seem to be more beneficial. For such patients, it may be necessary to focus on characterological issues per se if any change is to occur. This does not preclude brief therapy, according to our definition, for these patients; rather, it may indicate a longer but still cost-effective and time-effective intervention.

A Note on Substance Abuse

In choosing any of these five frequent foci, the therapist must always be aware of the problems of drug addiction and alcoholism. If, as the therapist is beginning treatment, it becomes clear that a major issue for the patient is that of a severe (alcohol or drug) addiction problem, this problem must take precedence over all others. A patient who is drinking heavily or using illicit drugs is unlikely to be able to profit from treatment, regardless of the therapist's best efforts. It is essential that the issue of addiction be addressed just as soon as the therapist is sure that this is a significant disruption in the patient's life. Enormous amounts of time in therapy can be wasted if the therapist neglects, ignores, or misses a substance abuse problem.

THE PROCESS OF FINDING A FOCUS

Figure 3-1 illustrates the process of finding a focus for the therapy. It is conceivable that more than one of the areas mentioned above may constitute the therapeutic focus. Once, however, the major focal area is clarified and agreed upon, it is most important that it be made the central theme of the therapy that follows. Whereas other issues may, of course, come up and be discussed, it is the responsibility of the therapist to keep the major theme of the treatment always at the forefront of the interaction. This has a number of important implications:

Figure 3-1. Major foci in brief therapy.

Key question: Why now?

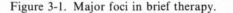

Is this visit related to any of the following?

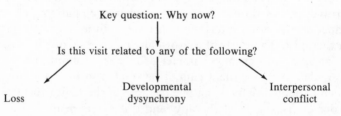

Loss   Developmental   Interpersonal
                          dysynchrony   conflict

If the patient does not view the above focal areas as relevant, *or* if the patient defines the symptom itself as the major issue,

Symptomatic focus

If the patient has had repeated presentations around any or all of the foci above, without clear benefit, *or* if character issues preclude these foci because of constant interference with the therapeutic process,

Character focus

Warning: Under circumstances of active alcohol or drug abuse, this problem *must* be addressed before or simultaneously with the development of any other focal area.

1. As early in the interviews as possible, the therapist presents the focus as he or she sees it and seeks clarification from the patient regarding whether or not the proposed focus appears consonant with his or her experience of the problem and goals for change. For example, one might say to a 48-year-old widower, "I believe that your wife's death from cancer 2 years ago left you feeling in enormous pain. I know that you originally said that you were depressed about your current relationships and did not know why these were going so poorly. But I think that the issue of your wife is central here. Perhaps we can, at least initially, focus on that and see if it is helpful to do so. What do you think?"

2. Once a relevant focus is established and accepted, the therapist deals with digressions by always maintaining clarity for himself or herself about what the central theme for this patient is. Some patients may have to be urged or guided to stick with the theme even after accepting it, whereas for others this comes easily. Certainly there are occasions when a particular crisis or real-life event may preclude dealing with the focal theme. For example, a young woman whose therapy was focused around a particular habit disorder (picking and scratching the inside of one of her nostrils) developed a very critical situation at work. The therapist under such circumstances should not behave as an automaton and must maintain empathy with the patient. However, even during a crisis or a temporary change of focus, the central theme can be brought up briefly and its importance remembered.

3. Sessions should end with some summary statement from the therapist regarding what has gone on during that session and how he or she views the situation in regard to the central theme. For example, "You've spoken a good deal today about the death of your brother. I know it's hard for you to do, but it looks to me as though you are really becoming more able to recognize just how much he meant to you and how much his loss hurt you."

Thus, the individual session and a given course of sessions are both like a fine fabric, woven together by the thread of the central theme. The theme opens the session, maintains a unity within the session, and closes the session. It is also part of what keeps a coherence between different sessions. Although people's lives tend to be multifaceted and complex, and we believe that it is quite important to give credence to this complexity, we also feel that without a focus brief therapy cannot exist. Were we to treat whatever came up for patients without tenaciously maintaining a focus, there would be no target, no direction, and no clarity about the utility of the treatment.

BRIEF INTERVENTION: SOME ASSUMPTIONS

In describing an I-D-E model of brief therapy, it is most helpful to begin with some theoretical assumptions about how psychopathology and other psychological difficulties develop and are maintained, since such views should directly influence what the brief therapist does in the face of such problems.

1. *It is our first assumption that the patient-to-be has been subjected to faulty learning at some point during his or her early growth and development.* This faulty learning may take a variety of forms and/or relate to various aspects of the child's life. It may be direct and cognitive (as when a parent states; "Sex is dirty and you should stay away from it"), and/or subliminal, symbolic, and emotional (the parent grimaces whenever sexual issues are portrayed on TV or in movies, etc.). Furthermore, it may be and remain conscious, or may be unconscious and not readily available to the individual. In any event, a cognitive–emotional map of the world is internalized and to a greater or lesser degree becomes a template for future behaviors and relationships. It is supposed that the greater the intensity of the faulty messages, the greater the psychopathology subsequently displayed. It is also assumed by psychoanalytically oriented clinicians that the earlier the occurrence of the faulty learning, the greater the psychological disturbance that results.

Many major systems of personality and psychotherapy make similar assumptions regarding the issues of faulty learning. Writing from a social learning perspective about internalized belief systems, Bandura (1982) states:

> People seek and hold firmly to beliefs because they serve valuable functions. Indeed, life would be most taxing and chaotic if people had no conceptions of themselves and the world around them. Their experiences would lack coherence; they would cede the substantial benefits of foresight, which requires a system for predicting conditional happenings in daily affairs; they would lack guides for action with situational influences pulling in all directions; and finally, they would be without basic goals for organizing their efforts over long time spans. Belief systems thus help to provide structure, direction, and purpose to life. Because personal identity and security become heavily invested in belief systems, they are not readily discardable once acquired. (p. 753)

Strupp and Binder (1984), from the perspective of object relations theory, likewise conclude: "Every current relationship is more or less influenced by past relationships which have become organizing themes in the personality structure and, as such, are reenacted in the present" (p. 34). From the Ericksonian viewpoint, Lankton and Lankton (1983) also present a very similar set of concepts:

> [Milton] Erickson believed that "maps" or rules for recombining experience, are so automatized that they become unconscious and the experiences and perceptions attached to them become automatized. Since the map is rarely in a person's conscious awareness, it is not scrutinized and updated with the passage of time. It is, instead, reinforced by the outcomes of the person's selective behavior and perceptions. Symptoms are generally the result of the client's

making the best choice among options determined unconsciously by those associations available in his or her map. (pp. 34–35)

2. *The person and his or her environment are in constant interaction and are reciprocally influential.* Many theories of personality, until more recent years, were based upon what Bandura (1977) has called "unidirectional determinism." This model maintains that either the environment acts upon the person to structure and shape behavior and experience, or, as the alternative, that the individual's mind creates reality. This point of view fails to consider the fact that the person, behavior, and the environment are in constant interaction and determine one another in a process of "reciprocal determinism" (Bandura, 1977). This can also be described as a nonlinear systems perspective. The individual operates within a particular, or at least relatively consistent, belief system; however, he or she is also changing and being modified over time as are his or her environment and behavior. Each aspect of the human ecology interlocks with all others, making it nearly impossible to effectively separate the elemental parts from one another.

A simple illustrative example might be the training of a young gymnast. Due to a variety of factors, such as the child's physical attributes, parental interest and support, recollections of champion gymnasts on TV, and so on, a child might begin gymnastics training. Skill level achieved might lead to further training and improved environmental supports and to the child's modification of her belief system regarding what she is capable of. However, it may also be that modified environment (e.g., going to a better gym) precedes improved skill level and modified belief system ("I am a very good gymnast"), or that beliefs, environment, and skills change simultaneously and are synergistic to one another.

Because even the most basic reciprocal systems are in fact highly complex, most psychotherapy theoreticians have chosen to deal with only one aspect of interpersonal systems (i.e., either behavior, environment, *or* beliefs). It is our contention that the effective brief therapist will have in his or her repertoire interventions that may modify the system at any of these three levels, and will choose from among intervention possibilities by trying to consider where the greatest leverage can be exerted with the least expenditure of time or effort.

3. *The patient's existing, current interpersonal environment (and his or her view of that environment) either may provide a buffering effect in the management of major or minor stress and distress, or may be a factor leading to the exacerbation of these factors. The interpersonal environment is never neutral.* Everyone, other than hermits or those who are living alone on isolated deserted islands (who, for obvious reasons, are rarely seen by psychotherapists or anyone else), exists as part of some social interpersonal systems. These systems are often central factors in mitigating the effects of adverse life experiences, or may be exacerbating factors, or may themselves

be the adverse life experiences that contribute to symptomatology. In our view, the patient's real interpersonal system is obviously of great importance in a number of ways. However, of at least equal importance is the patient's *perceived* interpersonal system. Until recently, it was simply assumed that those with the fewest social contacts and the most impoverished social systems would be the most highly susceptible to psychiatric symptoms. Contemporary epidemiological research has indicated that *perceptions* of the environment are as important in the development of neurosis as, if not more so than, actual number of contacts or relationships. Henderson, Byrne, and Duncan-Jones (1982), reporting the results of a major study of the relationship between neuroses and the social environment, conclude:

> [T]he actual availability of social relationships probably has little to do with the causes of neurosis. The perceived adequacy with which others meet the individual's requirements, especially under adversity, seems much more important. . . . Under adversity, it is those who construe their social relationships as inadequate who are more likely to develop symptoms. (p. 197)

This means that patients can be helped in a variety of ways (which we describe later) to re-evaluate their social environments. Furthermore, a social system that the individual patient has initially described as impoverished often includes many more supports than are readily apparent to the patient.

4. *Although personality, character, social supports, and so on play an important part in contributing to an individual's life pattern, chance encounters are also prominent factors in shaping the life course.* Both psychoanalytic and humanistic theorists assume that the individual is the major determiner of his or her life course, either because of early development or through free choice. The role of chance encounters is either minimized or ignored. Bandura (1982), in presenting a psychology of chance encounters, defines such events as "an unintended meeting of persons unfamiliar to each other" (p. 748). As an example, he presents the story of Paul Watkins, who was

> . . . a talented teenager headed on a promising course of personal development—He enjoyed a close family life, was well liked by his peers, excelled in academic activities, and served as student-body president of his high school, hardly the omens of a disordered destiny (Watkins & Soledad, 1979). One day he decided to visit a friend who lived in a cabin in Topanga Canyon in Los Angeles. Unbeknown to Watkins, the friend had since moved elsewhere and the Manson "family" now lived there. This fortuitous visit led to a deep entanglement in the Manson gang in the period before they embarked on their "helter skelter" killings. To an impressionable youth the free flow of communal love, group sex, drugs, spellbinding revelations of divine matters, and isolation from the outside world provided a heady counterforce that launched him on a divergent life path requiring years to turn his life around. (p. 748)

Bandura continues:

> In the preceding case the initial meeting was entirely due to happenstance. Human encounters involve degrees of fortuitiveness. People often intentionally seek certain types of experiences, but the persons who thereby enter their lives are determined by a large element of chance. (p. 748)

In a similar vein, a recently popular foreign film, *The Return of Martin Guerre*, is based upon the true story of two 16th-century French peasants who meet, fortuitously, as comrades in arms. The two look very similar and are often mistaken for each other. One of the peasants, Martin Guerre, has run off and abandoned his wife, child, and village many years before as a youth, and tells his comrade that he will never return to them. Thus, the other, upon leaving the army, surreptitiously goes to Guerre's village, masquerading as the true Martin. He is accepted as genuine, moves into his old comrade's house, lives with his wife and has children by her, works his fields, and totally assumes Guerre's identity, until another series of chance encounters lead to the imposter's unfortunate discovery and ultimate execution.

The assumption of chance encounters is not meant to imply that one has no control over one's own life. Rather, we believe the following:

a. All of our lives are determined, at least in part, by good and bad fortune, which cannot be fully under the individual's influence and are not predetermined by experiences up to the age of 4.

b. Chance encounters may be significant events (for better or for worse) in shaping the individual's life.

c. There are probably ways in which individuals can be helped both to put themselves in circumstances where positive and useful chance encounters are more likely to occur, and to maximize the benefits of such environmental events.

A final example in this regard comes from Bergin and Lambert (1978), who call positive chance encounters "naturalistic therapy":

> One example of a naturalistic therapy process comes from our experiences in conducting extensive personality assessments of normal persons for a governmental agency. During these evaluations we have occasionally noted an exceptionally effective person who has come from a chaotic and ordinarily pathology-inducing family life. A young college graduate illustrated this well. He came from an extremely disturbed home setting in which every member of his family except himself had been hospitalized for severe mental illness; and yet he had graduated from a renowned university with honors, had starred on the football team, and was unusually popular. During his government training he was held in the highest esteem by staff members and was rated as best liked and most likely to succeed by his peers.

In examining this young man's history we discovered that during his elementary school years he had essentially adopted a neighborhood family as his own and spent endless hours with them. Certain characteristics of this family appear most significant. They were a helping family in the sense that love emanated from them and was freely available to all. Of special significance for the fellow under consideration was his relationship with a boy in the family, a year older than he, who formed for him a positive role model with whom he closely identified and whom he followed to his considerable satisfaction.

An even more crucial factor was his relationship with the mother in this family, who became his guide, counselor, and chief source of emotional nurturance. His reports indicate that while this relationship was intense, it was not symbiotic, and seemed to foster his independence and self-development. This particular woman was apparently the prototypical mother and influenced more than one stray youth toward security, resilience, and accomplishment. It is difficult to deny the potent therapeutic impact of this woman, at least as it was portrayed by her protege's report. Although there are probably few like her, she represents a dimension of socially indigenous therapy that may be more significant than is usually recognized. Her home became a neighborhood gathering place. It might be characterized as an informal therapy agency, a kitchen clinic! Certainly, it makes the possibility of "spontaneous" remission more believable. (pp. 149–150).*

5. *Experience is always understood by the individual (at least in part) on the basis of his or her stage of life development.* It is clear to us that one's stage of life development is an important lens through which experience in the world is viewed. A 24-year-old with obsessive concerns about death may be viewed as having a serious psychiatric problem, whereas a 75-year-old with major concerns in this area may be normative. Symptoms such as depression, loneliness, problems with intimacy, and so on all have different meanings, depending upon the patient's stage of life development. Although each of us follows an individual and unique life course, there are similarities regarding what most people in a given age cohort value in regard to issues such as intimacy, financial stability, and so on.

6. *Our final assumption is that little or no therapy will actually occur unless or until the patient is ready for change.* Ability to profit from treatment is far more closely related to this concept of readiness than it is to diagnosis or psychopathology. We emphasize the notion of "Why now?" because it is the question most central in clarifying patients' readiness to work on change. Patients with very severe diagnoses, levels of pathology, and long-sustained problems may be confronted by developmental mile-

*This quotation is taken from "The Evaluation of Therapeutic Outcomes," by A. E. Bergin and M. J. Lambert, 1978, in S. L. Garfield and A. E. Bergin (Eds.), *Handbook of Psychotherapy and Behavior Change* (2nd ed., pp. 139–190), New York: Wiley. Copyright 1978 by John Wiley and Sons. Reprinted by permission.

stones or find themselves dealing with other events that make them "ready" and available for treatment.

CONCLUSION

In finding a focus for treatment the clinician helps to clarify where the push for change is from, so that this healthy thrust can be capitalized upon and enhanced. As we have indicated, alcohol and drug abuse *must* be addressed early in therapy, and it may be necessary to delay or refuse therapy to a patient who is actively drinking or abusing drugs.

The common foci and the six assumptions that we have described provide the clinician with a conceptual frame of reference in the practice of brief therapy. Clearly, patients come to us with their own unique personalities, areas of conflict, and ways of being in the world; however, we believe that the overall perspective we are providing offers the brief therapist a method for determining the area or areas that may be most readily and beneficially addressed in treatment. The assumptions provide a general orientation to our theoretical position, which in turn lead to our intervention strategies.

4

Losses

That loss is common would not make
   My own less bitter, rather more:
Too common! Never morning wore
   To evening, but some heart did break.
         —Alfred, Lord Tennyson, *In Memoriam A. H. H.* (1850/1979)

In this chapter, we assume a rather broad view of the types of significant losses that cause people to seek the help of psychotherapists. Such losses include not only the loss of a loved one or loved ones through death or separation, but also the loss of long-held beliefs about one's invulnerability or immortality as a result of trauma, impaired physical functioning, or illness. Thus, the two major classes of losses that we most commonly see in those coming for psychotherapeutic help are (1) losses regarding significant people in one's life (interpersonal losses), and (2) losses regarding ideas or beliefs about oneself or one's world (existential losses). Clearly, these two types of losses are not mutually exclusive and may often occur together. For example, the man whose wife dies suddenly of cancer loses that relationship, along with its closeness and interaction; he also loses (sometimes temporarily, sometimes indefinitely) the ability to deny his own mortality and that of those around him.

INTERPERSONAL LOSSES

Attachment: The Research Background

Understanding the impact of the loss of significant people in one's life requires us to examine the concept of attachment. There is now a vast body of data both from animal research (Rosenblum, 1984) and from the observation of human infants under a variety of circumstances (Bowlby, 1973) supporting the notion that attachment is an instinctual mechanism.

   In most primate infants, there appear to be distinct and successive phases of reaction to a sudden separation from the mother (Rosenblum,

1984). In the first of these phases, the baby reacts with anxiety and protest, which include high levels of motor activity and loud, repetitive cries. This so-called "protest phase" is followed by a period of "despair and depression." During this phase the infant often loses interest in the surrounding world, and becomes very passive and withdrawn. In what has been described as the "detachment phase," if the infant is reunited with the lost caregiver, both human and nonhuman infant primates behave "strangely." The baby generally appears distant, remote, and even somewhat fearful when approached by the mother. Rather than enthusiastically welcoming the return of the mother, the baby is hesitant and avoidant. Both Main (1977) and Bowlby (1973) suggest that this is how the infant copes with the conflictual feelings of attachment to and anger toward the lost parent.

It has been postulated that attachment is an extremely important survival mechanism. Weiss (1982) has hypothesized that those who display such behaviors are more likely to survive and have progeny in successive generations who also demonstrate such behaviors. He writes:

> Attachment in children contributes to children's keeping close to protective adults, particularly in apparently risky circumstances. Attachments in adults contributes to the adults' keeping close to potentially helpful fellow adults, again particularly in apparently risky circumstances. Insofar as attachment is reciprocated, it provides a basis for pairing. (p. 181)

Types of Attachments and Losses

Researchers and theoreticians have examined the development of attachments and the response to their loss over the life course. Interestingly, a large number of surveys have repeatedly indicated that there is a consistent *inverse* relationship between loneliness and age, (Lowenthal *et al.*, 1975; Rubenstein & Shaver, 1982), with adolescents showing the greatest degree of loneliness and the elderly displaying the least. It appears that most adolescents have an almost overwhelming hunger to be with others much of the time (usually with a significant group of friends). Without social contact, they feel lonely and isolated. In contrast, for an aged population, extensive periods of solitude may be viewed with some sense of relief and as a respite.

Weiss (1974) speculates that for adults there are six basic "provisions" provided by social relationships and close contacts with others. Relationships tend to be specialized in the type of provision they supply. Thus, for example, a close intimate relationship with another adult provides "attachment." One's family offers "a sense of reliable alliance"; "social integration" comes from being part of a community of friends; coworkers and colleagues can provide "reassurance of worth." From mentors and teachers one can get "guidance," and offspring offer an "opportunity for nurturance." In a number of interview studies, Weiss (1974, 1975) found that those experiencing particular types of losses were not relieved of the pain of that loss by social provisions in another sector of their lives. For example, those dealing with a marital separation were distressed and uncomfortable, whether or not they had close friends. Similarly, in a study of married women who had just moved to a new area, Weiss (1974) found that a supportive marriage did not really alleviate their sense of alienation and loss of friends and community.

Just as Weiss's "social provision theory" indicates that we get different types of supplies from different types of relationships in our lives, it should be noted that different types of losses may have different impacts upon us. Furthermore, a particular loss (e.g., the death of a parent) may have a different impact, depending upon when in the individual's life course it occurs.

Losses of significant attachment figures occur with great frequency in our society. Divorce occurs in about 40% of all married couples (Kitson & Rashke, 1981). In 1976, census data indicated that there were over 7 million currently divorced men and women in this country (U.S. Bureau of the Census, 1977). Since there are many more separations in marital relationships or serious nonmarital relationships than there are actual legal divorces, we have strong indications that the loss of a significant other through the disruption of a relationship is a problem of great magnitude.

The loss of a loved one through death is, according to Osterweis, Solomon, and Green (1984), a "fact of life." They go on to write:

> Only those who themselves die young escape the pain of losing someone they love through death. Every year an estimated eight million Americans experience the death of an immediate family member. Every year there are 800,000 new widows or widowers. There are at least 27,000 suicides in the country annually, and probably more, since suicide is underreported.

In addition, in a mobile society such as ours, frequent moves are not uncommon. For a large segment of the population, friendships and romantic ties will often be made and broken, leaving many people without ongoing or sustained social support systems for periods of time. Furthermore, because relatively few people live near their families of origin, the loss of this type of support is also pervasive.

.

The Consequences of Interpersonal Loss

There are strong indications that the emotional and health status impact of separation and bereavement is highly adverse (Solsberry & Krupnick, 1984; Weiss, 1975; Windholz, Marmar, & Horowitz, 1985). Although studies correlating marital separation and its health and mental health consequences are thought to be possibly confounded by issues of adverse selection—that is, perhaps those who are less mentally or physically healthy are more likely to get divorced (Bloom, Asher, & White, 1978)—epidemiological studies of the impact of bereavement are not as subject to the same confounding factors.

Klerman and Clayton (1984), in summarizing the data regarding the impact of bereavement upon health, conclude:

> Following bereavement there is a statistically significant increase in mortality for men under the age of 75. Although especially pronounced in the first year, the mortality rate continues to be elevated for perhaps as long as six years for men who do not remarry. There is no higher mortality in women in the first year; whether there is in the second year is unclear.
>
> All studies document increases in alcohol consumption and smoking or greater use of tranquilizers or hypnotic medication (or both) among the bereaved. . . .
>
> Depressive symptoms are very common in the first months of bereavement. Between 10 and 20 percent of men and women who lose a spouse are still depressed a year later. . . .
>
> Perceived adequacy of social support and remarriage protect the bereaved from adverse outcomes. (pp. 39–40)

One's immediate reaction to a major loss may be to realize its importance, to "deal with" and confront its pain, and to attempt to "work it through." It is also possible that, because of the magnitude of the loss and its shock (particularly in situations where the event has not really been expected), the loss will be "set aside" for some time before an attempt is made to confront it. In some cases, in fact, this approach may be highly functional. That is, a "delayed" grief reaction following a major loss may allow the person who is experiencing the loss to shore up his or her defenses before dealing with the difficult situation in question.

It may also occur, however, that in "setting aside" a loss the person is never really able to return to it. What may occur instead is what has been described as the "tar baby" phenomenon, after an Uncle Remus story by Joel Chandler Harris: The more one tries to get away from something, the more one may "stick to" it. Ideas, feelings, or behaviors that become associated with the major but unexamined loss also are avoided. This was most certainly true in the case described at the end of Chapter 2. The patient's long-avoided feelings about the loss of her father many years previously did not allow her to separate either physically or emotionally from her mother. She only became more aware of her ungrieved loss as a function of her treatment.

It is also possible for an anticipated future loss to trigger entry into psychotherapy. The patient's fears about survival without the attachment object may lead to anticipatory grief, depression, and/or anxiety—again, for a variety of reasons the patient may believe that he or she should *not* feel worried about (e.g., moving out of town, or being left by an abusive husband). Therefore, the symptomatology may remain separate from the issue causing the difficulty. Thus, the patient may arrive symptomatic, but without a clear sense of why he or she is experiencing such discomfort.

EXISTENTIAL LOSSES

Assumptions Threatened by Existential Losses

For most of us, unless or until we experience an event or series of events that causes us to come face to face with our own mortality and vulnerability, there is at an unconscious level the belief that although others may become seriously ill, grow old and infirm, be hurt in accidents, be victimized by criminals, or die, we will somehow be the exception. In this regard, Yalom (1980) states:

> Each of us, first as child and then as adult, clings to an irrational belief in our specialness. Limits, aging, death may apply to *them* but not to oneself, not to *me*. At a deep level one's convinced of one's personal invulnerability and imperishability. (p. 96)

Janoff-Bulman (1985) theorizes that in order to make sense out of our world, each of us functions from day to day on the basis of various assumptions and personal theories. These allow us to set goals, plan activities, and order our behaviors. The three major assumptions that may become deeply threatened or impaired in situations of existential loss are as follows:

1. The assumption of invulnerability
2. The assumption of the world as meaningful
3. The assumption of positive self-perceptions

In assuming invulnerability, people tend to believe, as Yalom (1980) has described, that "It may happen, but not to me." Weinstein (1980) has found that most people overestimate the possibility of their achieving positive outcomes in life and underestimate their achieving negative outcomes. This overoptimism appears to be shattered for those experiencing various traumas. Those who are robbed tend to be overly frightened of future robberies (Stinchcombe *et al.*, 1980). Rape victims develop great fears that this event will happen again (Burgess & Holmstrom, 1974). Those who have recovered from severe medical illnesses such as cancer (Burdick, 1975) are more likely than others to overinterpret discomfort and normal symptomatology as indicating a recurrence of their disease process (Kellner, 1985). It has also been found that bereaved individuals sometimes develop a profile of physical symptoms resembling that of their deceased relative (Parkes, 1964; Parkes & Brown, 1972) and fear that they have a similar illness.

A second basic assumption which is shattered by an existential loss is that of the world as meaningful. Janoff-Bulman (1985) writes in this regard:

> Our world "makes sense," for we have constructed social theories that enable us to account for specific occurrences. One way for us to make sense of our world is to regard what happens to us as controllable (Seligman, 1975). For example, we believe we can prevent misfortune by engaging in sufficiently cautious behaviors (Scheppele & Bart, 1983). At a fundamental level, we also believe we are protected against misfortune by being good and worthy people. According to Lerner's (1970, 1980) just-world theory, we believe people deserve what they get and get what they deserve. People appear to operate on the basis of such just-world assumptions even when they verbally deny a belief in such a "social law" (Lerner & Ellard, 1983). . . . The world does not appear meaningful to victims who feel they have been cautious and good people (Scheppele & Bart, 1983; Silver & Wortman, 1980). The victimization simply doesn't make sense. . . . In the case of serious crimes, accidents, and diseases, the problem of loss of meaning often seems to focus not on the question, "Why did this event happen?" but on the more specific question, "Why did this event happen *to me*?" . . . Victims often feel a total lack of comprehension regarding the whys and wherefores of their misfortune. Particularly if they regard themselves as decent people who take good care of themselves and are appropriately cautious, victims are apt to find themselves at a loss to explain why they were victimized. (pp. 20–21)

In regard to the assumption of positive self-perceptions, Janoff-Bulman (1985) cites research indicating that although most people operate with the belief that they are good, decent, worthy individuals, this is also modified for those who have suffered existential losses. Victims generally see themselves as weak, needy, helpless, and not in control (Horowitz, Wilner, Marmar, & Krupnick, 1980). There is also a strong sense of deviance, which again serves to strengthen negative self-perceptions (Coates & Winston, 1983). Thus, a person suffering the death of a loved one, crime victimization, serious illness, or other similar traumas that call into question basic life assumptions may find himself or herself feeling highly symptomatic, tense, and apprehensive. The victim's sense of the world as a comfortable, predictable, and stable environment is shattered. Sometimes this "dis-ease" is brief and self-limited; at other times, the victim's well-being is altered for an indefinite period.

Although the alteration of a victim's assumptions about the world is very central, at a basic level the most primitive fear for each of us is that of dying. The fear of death has pervaded the human psyche throughout history: "The fear of death plays a major role in our internal experience; it haunts as does nothing else; it rumbles continuously under the surface; it is a dark, unsettling presence at the rim of consciousness" (Yalom, 1980, p. 27). Although most people are able to keep fears of death and vulnerability at bay much of the time by using a variety of defense mechanisms, such defenses will typically break down, at least to some degree, following a traumatic experience such as crime victimization, serious illness, or the death of someone significant. The closer and more important this relationship, the greater the likelihood that it will be experienced as an existential loss. Again, although the person experiencing the existential loss and the ensuing symptomatology may readily connect the two, this may not always be the case. The personal experience of one of us (Simon Budman) may be illustrative in this regard.*

While in the process of writing this book, I had a sudden, unexpected, and quite nearly fatal aortic aneurysm. One pleasant fall morning as I was preparing to go running, I suddenly experienced a severe tearing pain in my back. A complicated series of medical transactions ensued, the ultimate outcomes of which were two emergency open-heart surgeries and aortic repairs. Each of these surgeries was risky, with my survival uncertain for weeks afterwards. I was fortunate, did well, and recovered almost completely from the physical impact of the illness. However, for months I remained anxious and preoccupied with my health status and the health of those close to me. A cold was a disease entity to be studied and followed carefully. I found myself gravitating to the health care section of the book stores, which I frequented in order to learn as much as possible about various obscure disease processes. Vast periods of time were spent ruminating about such issues and trying to make a variety of differential diagnoses of my various normal aches and pains.

Although this behavior could initially be readily tied to the previous life-threatening event, I came to feel with the passage of time, and heard from those around me repeatedly, that "The worst is over" or "You must feel great now that you're through the awful part and are doing so well." In many ways, the pressures within myself and around me were in the direction of disconnecting the trauma and its residual affect.

Another clinical illustration may be useful here as well.

Fred, a 32-year-old married man, sought therapy during an acute and debilitating month-long episode of insomnia. He had never had such extensive sleep problems previously, and was beginning to feel that his work functioning was becoming impaired. Although he could not initially identify any clear precipitants of his difficulties, it did seem that the sleep he did get was often disrupted by a frightening and repetitive dream. In this

---

*For the sake of clarity, this description is written in the first person singular.

dream Fred was always chasing an unknown male figure. He would try repeatedly to catch this person, but was unsuccessful in his attempt. As Fred and his therapist spoke about the dream, Fred began to describe a situation that had occurred several months prior to his insomnia. A drunken teenager in his neighborhood had broken a window in Fred's house while he and his family were away. He had felt furious and violated. When the police minimized the matter, Fred had done his own investigation, discovered the culprit, and threatened him with violence if this recurred. Fred's history revealed that 10 years previously, while working as a lifeguard at a city pool, he had been set upon by two drunken teenagers. These assailants, using a broken bottle, had damaged one of Fred's eyes so extensively that it had had to be replaced by a glass prosthesis. He retained the sight in his other eye and was able, after recovering from the attack, to continue all of his usual activities such as driving and reading. Although the youths who had attacked him were subsequently caught and incarcerated, and although people saw him as "handling the situation very well" (i.e., without very much affect), Fred's repression of this initial event ceased to be as effective after he experienced the attack on his home.

"Normal" Recovery from Existential Losses

Taylor (1983), in studying the adjustment of women who were found to have breast cancer (and that of many of their families as well), has developed a model to describe adaptational tasks in the adjustment to threatening life events. It is her position that the victims of such events (1) search for meaning in the experience, (2) try to regain mastery over the event, and (3) attempt to enhance personal self-esteem. These three corrective factors tie in very closely with the three elements of Janoff-Bulman's (1985) model of the life assumptions challenged by existential losses, described previously.

In searching for meaning, the victim tries to make sense out of why this event has happened to him or her. The cancer patients studied by Taylor often attributed their tumors to stress, bad diet, poor relationships, and so on. Whatever they attributed their illnesses to, it seemed clear that all needed a way to understand why this had happened to them and what had gone on.

A second important phase of adjusting to such a major personal catastrophe appears to be an attempt to regain a sense of mastery over the loss. For the women in Taylor's study, this usually took the form of a change in life style and/or behaviors in order to prevent a recurrence of the cancer. Some women began to meditate, use biofeedback, or work fewer hours in trying to alter the factors that they felt had contributed to their disease.

A third aspect of the adjustment process was typified by the tendency of many of the women interviewed by Taylor to view themselves as handling the cancer and subsequent mastectomy, lumpectomy, and/or chemotherapy in a very effective way. That is, most made efforts to enhance their sense of self and to restore self-esteem. These cancer victims generally compared themselves to other women whom they knew or knew of, who had not handled cancer as well. The conclusions of these comparisons was generally that the women making them were better off than others in the same or similar straits.

It was most interesting to note that more than 50% of Taylor's respondents felt that their psychological adjustments were better *after* their cancer than at any time prior to their illness. Obviously, for some people, a traumatic existential loss is perceived of as leading to *greater* meaning, understanding, and satisfaction in life. Taylor concludes:

> My biological acquaintances frequently note that the more they know about the human body, the more, not less, miraculous it seems. The recuperative powers of the mind merit similar awe. The process of cognitive adaptation to threat, though often time-consuming and not always successful, nonetheless restores many people to their prior level of functioning and inspires others to find new meaning in their lives. (p. 1171)

Such findings support an optimistic perspective on the part of the therapist who is helping patients to deal with existential losses. Many people can and do overcome even highly adverse events. At times they may even feel that such circumstances have left them with a fuller and more comprehensive understanding of their lives. For some people there may be truth in Nietzsche's statement, "That which does not kill me makes me stronger" (cited in Frankel, 1961, p. 21).

THE BRIEF THERAPY OF INTERPERSONAL
AND EXISTENTIAL LOSSES

Interpersonal and existential losses often (but certainly not always) occur simultaneously. It is therefore important to bear in mind that the patient who is experiencing an interpersonal loss may also be dealing with existential issues related to the interpersonal loss. Generally, the brief therapist should consider the following as part of the process of dealing with losses:

1. Specifying and naming the relevant loss, exploring its meaning, and identifying for what other people besides the patient it is a loss.
2. Providing information about the frequent course of or response to this type of loss.
3. Encouraging a "regrieving" for the loss, both with the patient and with others who have suffered the loss in question.
4. Gaining some closure on the loss.

5. Addressing the loss in a social context. That is, when there are significant people in the patient's environment who are experiencing that same loss or are affected by the loss (e.g., brothers and sisters when a parent has died; other family members, lovers, etc., when a patient has experienced a major illness), they should be seen with the identified patient.

The overall goal of the therapist in situations of loss is to help the patient go through the transformation from being a victim to being a survivor:

> Victims and survivors are similar in that they both experienced a traumatic event. But while the victim has been immobilized and discouraged by the event, the survivor has overcome the traumatic memories and become mobile. The survivor draws on the experiences of coping with the catastrophe as a source of strength, while the victim remains immobilized.
>
> What separates victims from survivors is a conception about life, an attitude about the safety, joy and mastery of being a human being. Being a survivor, then, is making peace with the memories of the catastrophe and its wake. (Figley, 1985, p. 399)

It is important to note that although many or all of the interventions suggested below may be part of the treatment, they will not necessarily occur during the same episode of therapy. That is, part of the work described above may happen during an initial 1- to 2-month period of treatment (two to six sessions); other aspects may not occur unless or until the patient returns to treatment at another point. Furthermore, it may be important that in some situations of acute bereavement, for example, the therapist should treat the patient only minimally until the patient is out of his or her initial state of shock. In this regard, Polock, Egan, Vandenbergh, and Williams (1975) developed and studied an immediate crisis intervention program for families experiencing a sudden death. It was their conclusion that drawing people out too quickly and forcing them to confront their feelings about the deceased impaired or delayed "normal" grieving processes. It is our impression that on some occasions the clinician's best course of action may be to supportively explore the events around a given loss with the patient and then recommend that continued work in regard to the loss take place at some time (a few weeks or months) in the future.

Noreen, a physician in her late 20s, was seen by a therapist 5 days after her father's suicide. Her father had called Noreen, complaining of the increasing severity of his depression and the overwhelming pain of his bad back. By the time she reached his apartment, her father had died of a self-inflicted gunshot wound to the chest. Noreen attempted to revive him and called for emergency assistance. Although nothing could be done to save her father, she felt guilty and responsible that she did not get to him sooner. At the time that she was initially evaluated, Noreen was clearly in a state of shock. She could express little affect regarding her father's death, and seemed to describe the events centering around his suicide in neutral, almost uninterested tones. She was seen three times initially in a 3-week period. Following this, the therapist explained to her that she still appeared too close to the situation to be able to explore it thoroughly. An appointment was set up for her to return 2 months later. At that time, she was able to talk about her father's death with a great deal of intensity and much more profitably than might have been the case earlier.

Specifying and Naming the Relevant Loss

In the children's story "Rumpelstiltskin," the evil dwarf is vanquished when the princess is able to discover and to state his name. In a similar way, naming a particular problem and specifying what it relates to may have a significant detoxifying effect for the patient. For example, an acquaintance of one of us had major surgery for a disc problem. After the surgery, the patient began to experience severe arm and hand pain and numbness. His orthopedic surgeon and internist were baffled. It was not until an experienced neurologist was called in to consult on the case that any clarity was achieved. She said, "I have seen this situation before. I believe that you will be pain-free 6 to 8 weeks from now. This will not be a chronic problem." When she was able to clarify the situation, name it (as nonchronic), and specify its course, the patient felt tremendously reassured.

For the patient entering therapy who has had or is anticipating an interpersonal and/or existential loss, there is often a sense of depression, sadness, loneliness, anxiety, and perhaps fear. Sometimes the patient will be able to specify the difficulty as being related to the issue of loss, while at other times this will not be possible. Specifying the loss will be particularly difficult for the patient if he or she assumes a "characterological hypothesis" regarding his or her current discomfort: for example, "I have *always* felt this way; I'm just more aware of my depression now that my husband has left me."

In initially interviewing any new patient, it is one task of the therapist to explore with the patient the issue of recent relevant losses. If loss or anticipated loss appears to be an important precipitant, the therapist must explore the meaning of the loss to the patient. Once the therapist has a relatively clear sense that a particular loss or constellation of losses has resulted in the patient's seeking therapy at the present time, this information is shared with the patient and explored with him or her.

David, a man in his late 20s, had lost his wife nearly 2 years before he sought therapy. Kate, his wife, had died a painful, prolonged, and difficult death. For the last year of her life she was constantly in and out of hospitals with the sequelae of systemic lupus erythematosus. The enormity of Kate's suffering had been such that although she had been home nearly until the time she died, she had had to take huge doses of narcotics in order to be able to function in even a minimal way.

When his wife died, David was overwhelmingly sad and for a very brief period functioned poorly at work. After several weeks, however, he made what friends and relatives termed a "miraculous recovery," and by the end of 12 weeks was dating. Although he would see various women for periods of time, he would always feel dissatisfied and lonely in these relationships. He entered therapy while in the process of breaking up with a woman he had been seeing for about 6 months. In his first therapy session, David wondered aloud, "Why do these relationships constantly end up so lousy? Can't I be satisfied with anyone?" He recognized that Kate's death was an important factor for him, but he was not clear about its magnitude as an issue until the therapist said, "I believe that the central issue for you currently is the tremendous pain of Kate's death. Overall, you may feel like that is basically in the past, but it sounds to me like her death continues to affect you in a profound way in all of your romantic relationships with women. The ending of your current relationship is, I believe, tied into your continued feelings about Kate and her death."

Although the patient often believes that his or her loss may be having a profound effect, there is also a tendency in our society to value people who can "tough it out." Heroes are those who deal with pain and adversity without flinching. Therefore, the patient may tend to minimize the impact of the loss and begin to look elsewhere (often assuming a characterological focus) in order to explain his or her discomfort. Here is another example of this type of reaction:

Arthur, a 31-year-old accountant, was in treatment with his wife after a horrible set of medical crises. Six months prior to beginning therapy, he had been found to have cancer, which had spread into his stomach and bowels. For a period of 3 months, he underwent surgery, chemotherapy, and radiation therapy. Arthur was in and out of the hospital during this period. While undergoing an experimental form of chemotherapy he began to suffer major neurological deficits, was unable to walk or hear well, and lost manual dexterity. These neurological difficulties were caused by the anticancer drugs, and it was unclear to what degree normal functioning would return. The therapist, after reviewing the course of his illness with Arthur, said, "You've had an unbelievably difficult and painful 7 months. Something like this would take its toll on anyone." Arthur replied, "Was it really so hard? People go through a lot worse." To some degree he failed to recognize the magnitude and significance of his own suffering, and the courage with which he had coped with the situation.

Therapists who lack a sufficiently developmental–systemic view of behavior may often focus on the meaning of a patient's loss from a nearly exclusively phenomenological stance, usually emphasizing the meaning of the loss for the patient himself or herself. This approach, while appropriate and empathic, is unfortunately often incomplete, in that it may fail to consider the meanings of the changes in the patient's intimate relationships occasioned by the loss. Identifying who else is involved in what might be called the "loss network" is an essential part of the initial assessment. It is quite common to find that people continue to suffer from a loss at least as much because of the continuing rearrangement of their close relationships that has been set off by the loss, as because of the attachment to the lost object.

Providing Information about the Frequent Course of or Response to the Loss

Whereas naming the loss allows the patient to know what the trouble is, describing its course gives the patient some sense of how most people respond to this problem. For example, when treating a patient who is dealing with a recent marital breakup, we often give him or her information from Robert Weiss's *Marital Separation* (1975) and/or ask the patient to read the book. In *Marital Separation*, Weiss describes naturalistic research findings on the frequent course of separation and divorce. Generally, patients do not expect that losses will affect them for as long after the actual event as is usually the case. For example, Weiss (1975) believes that the major impact of marital separation may last for 4 or more years, with the first year of separation generally being the most difficult. He also stresses the "roller-coaster" quality of adjustment to separation, with the individual at times feeling free of an uncomfortable situation and excited about the future, while at other points (perhaps even in the same day) feeling a sense of despair, grief, and intense loneliness.

It is essential that those dealing with any type of loss be aware that the impact of losses is powerful and that their effect is often measured in months or years rather than days or weeks. At the same time, however, many people do recover from even those losses that would at first glance appear to be insurmountable. Such recovery is, we believe, best exemplified by Holocaust survivors. Many of these individuals lost family, friends, and homes, and were cruelly tortured and starved in Nazi concentration camps. Yet, remarkably, they went on in great numbers to begin new, productive, and fulfilling lives after the war. As we have mentioned previously, the patients with breast cancer whom Taylor (1983) studied often made extraordinary emotional recoveries from even dreadful circumstances, such as double mastectomies.

Without some clear information indicating that dealing with loss can be a lengthy process, patients often tend to expect that they should feel fine in a relatively brief period. After 6 months, when they still feel a profound sense of pain and sorrow, and when most friends have ceased to be overtly solicitous, people may assume that they "shouldn't still feel this way." Furthermore, when one is doing brief therapy with a patient who has experienced a recent loss, the patient should be aware that at the end of treatment the loss may not have been fully dealt with. That is, the treatment may help to encourage a process of healing and recovery, but such recovery may take extended periods of time after the patient and therapist are no longer meeting. Were therapy to be extended until the patient completely recovered from his or her loss, it could easily be interminable.

This attitude—that much therapeutic work occurs between sessions, or even after therapy has ended—is important in differentiating brief and long-term treatment. In the latter, for example, if a loss is being dealt with, the patient is treated until the loss is "worked through." On the other hand, the brief treatment of losses is seen by the therapist as the opportunity to help the patient to *begin* to confront the loss and its implications for his or her life. The brief therapist sows the seeds of change, but cannot follow these changes throughout their process of occurrence.

If the therapist lacks expertise or information on the course of and response to a particular loss (e.g., the long-term reactions of mastectomy patients), he or she can try to obtain information on the subject, and/or can refer the patient to resources in the community (e.g., as a mastectomy support organization). As a general rule of thumb, however, we have found that the impact of loss is unexpectedly long-lasting. David, the patient described earlier whose wife had died, felt some degree of surprise when during his first visit he began to weep as he described Kate's death: "I thought that I had this more behind me by this point."

Another function that is served by describing the usual course of response to loss is that the patient realizes that his or her sadness, pain, and discomfort will not last forever. A recently separated patient remarked after reading *Marital Separation*, "I certainly wasn't pleased to read that this [his pain] could go on for so long. But I was encouraged to learn that most people do get better."

Regrieving for the Loss

All major therapeutic approaches—behavioral (Keane, Fairbank, Caddell, Zimering, & Bender, 1985), cognitive (Melges & DeMaso, 1980), interpersonal (Klerman *et al.*, 1984), and analytic (Worden, 1982)—recommend some form of "regrieving" as a way of assisting the recovery process for those experiencing interpersonal or existential losses. Although the particular elements may differ (as do the theoretical underpinnings), the procedure for the most part involves the patient's recounting the traumatic event or events in extensive and at times minute detail, in a strongly affective way and under safe circumstances. There may be particular techniques added to encourage a powerfully emotional "reliving" of the loss, such as looking at photographs of the deceased or lost person, visiting significant locations such as gravesites or the site of a trauma, or using hypnosis to encourage time regression to the point of the trauma or before it.

As an initial therapeutic strategy, we believe that it is imperative to have the patient who has suffered the loss describe in as great detail as possible every aspect of the events leading to that loss. For example, Noreen, the physician whose father had committed suicide, was asked to detail everything that had happened in the days before the suicide and the days afterward. Such questions as "What went on during the phone conversation with your dad?", "Who said what?", "What did you do at that point?", and "What did you think and feel as you walked into your father's apartment?" were asked. To some degree, the detailed description of such events has almost a hypnogogic effect upon patients. As they begin to recall and search for significant details, many people take on the glazed, distant expression typical of those in an eyes-open trance state. Frequently, the regrieving may occur over a number of sessions, and at times these sessions may be spaced by many months or even many years. That is, it is not usually the case (but it may occur) that one cathartic session can negate the internal disruption caused by significant trauma or loss. The "working through" of the loss is begun by the therapist's interventions and may be periodically boosted by continued, detailed discussion of the loss; however, the therapist need not be present on a continuing basis in order for the regrieving to occur. The following case exemplifies this process.

Rita, whose father had committed suicide, could recall few details of this event when she was first seen by the therapist. She had been in her early 20s when she returned from graduate school for a brief planned visit. Upon arriving at her home, Rita became alarmed when she smelled the odor of gas emanating from the kitchen. When she entered that room, she found that her father, who had a long history of severe depression, had asphyxiated himself with gas from the oven. At the time that Rita was first seen by the therapist, 4 years following the death, she spoke about the suicide in a detached and distant manner, with little memory for the event itself or other related matters. She was seen initially for 10 sessions, with a major focus upon her father, his death, and her relationship with him.

When she returned for additional treatment approximately 18 months later, her father's suicide was again chosen as the focus. At that point her description was far more affective, intense, and detailed. She was able to discern how her father, his depression, and his suicide had affected her involvements with men in romantic relationships. Rita also vividly recalled finding her father on the day of his suicide. She remembered that she had experienced severe nausea and repugnance when she realized that as her father lay dying he had lost bowel and bladder control; his pants were soiled, and the kitchen floor around him was wet. It was clear that over the interim between the two courses of therapy, Rita had done a great deal of internal "working through." She was far more able to confront her pain, anger, and other reactions to her father's suicide during the second part of her treatment.

In terms of Janoff-Bulman's (1985) and Taylor's (1983) models of adjustment to existential losses, the regrieving may serve two major functions. It may give the patient the opportunity to try to give meaning to and to gain mastery over the loss. The intensive, affective analysis of "what happened" and "how it happened" allows the patient to build a theory about the reason why a particular loss occurred and to consider ways to prevent such losses in the future. For example, those who are experiencing a divorce or separation during the regrieving invariably develop a "story" (we do not wish to imply that the "story" is untrue) about why the breakup occurred. The story usually leads to actions that should or should not be taken in order to prevent similar outcomes in future relationships.

A number of techniques can be used to enhance the immediacy and intensity of the regrieving process. The techniques should be seen not as gimmicks of tricks, but as significant interventions occurring only within the context of a safe and empathic therapeutic interaction. Not infrequently, of course, the most potent enhancement of the regrieving process is achieved by sharing the grief with other family members. The intensity is greatest because a person's truly significant interpersonal losses are almost always experienced by someone else as well.

Photographs, Films, Diaries, and Tapes

The therapeutic task during the regrieving process is to have the patient review with affective intensity the traumatic events that have occurred. The chances that this will be done with emotional involvement may be increased by sitting with the patient, looking at and discussing photographs, home movies, diaries, audiotapes or videotapes, and so on, which relate to the trauma (Kaslow, 1981). The patient should be asked whether he or she has such items available and should be encouraged to bring them into the session, as was done in the following cases.

Edith had experienced a difficult and painful separation and divorce from her husband, Craig, 2 years prior to seeking therapy. Her initial complaint was one of severe depression and anxiety, as well as problems concentrating at work. Once the therapeutic focus on the divorce was established, Edith was encouraged to describe the events surrounding this occurrence in great detail. Craig had begun to see another woman shortly before the separation took place. At the same time, he had told Edith that he felt that their marriage was having problems and he was feeling interested in another woman, but that these difficulties could probably be worked out. Several days after this pronouncement, when Edith returned from work, she found a note from Craig saying that he was gone, would be moving in with his girlfriend, and would like to file for divorce as soon as possible. Early in the treatment, the therapist had Edith bring photos covering the course of her relationship with Craig. She also brought their wedding album into the session to look at and talk about.

Peter and Janet, a young couple whose child had died of sudden infant death syndrome several years previously, were encouraged to bring in the home movies they had taken of the child prior to her death.

David, the young man described previously whose wife had died of lupus, was asked to bring in the diary which his wife had kept during the last years of her life, and to read significant sections to the therapist. He also brought in and read aloud a eulogy he had given at his wife's funeral.

The general goal of the therapist in encouraging patients to bring in the types of materials described is to help them to experience emotions about their losses that have been hidden or covered over because of fears of being overwhelmed and consumed by the powerful feelings associated with such events. When family members of a patient participate, lasting change is likely to occur not only through a type of "cocatharsis," but through a realignment of relationships that often takes place in such powerful shared experiences.

Other Active Interventions Related to the Lost Object

It may be valuable to encourage an actual visit to a cemetery or gravesite in a situation where a patient is regrieving a death (Williamson, 1981). If this is not possible, or in other loss situations, using imagery and hypnosis may be helpful in similarly facilitating this process.

If a patient is encouraged to visit the grave of a significant person in his or her life who has died, it must be remembered that this can be a difficult and emotionally demanding task. It should be carefully planned with the patient; its purpose should be clarified; and any task or tasks to be accomplished should also be considered with the patient. In some circumstances, if it is feasible and appropriate, the therapist may wish to make the visit with the patient. In other circumstances, the patient may be asked to record his or her thoughts at the grave in a small portable cassette tape player.

A gravesite visit may be explained as follows:

> I think that your father's death has had a great impact on you. Ever since this happened, it has been very hard for you to trust men and to allow yourself to feel comfortable in an intimate relationship. I believe that you have some very strong feelings about that loss, which have been extremely difficult for you to express. Let's hope that you will gradually become able to express some of those feelings here in therapy. Perhaps you can do some things outside of here as well that can facilitate that occurring. Since your father is buried in a cemetery nearby, I'd like to suggest that if you feel up to it, between now and our next meeting you might visit his grave. Maybe you could think about some of the things you had wanted to say to him and talk to him about before or even after his death. If you could talk about some of those things when you are there, that would be good. When we get together again, we can go over just what the visit was like for you, so try to really remember everything that went on and just what you felt about it.

In a situation where either the gravesite is so far away that a visit is not really feasible, or the patient is emotionally unable to make the actual visit, a very beneficial alternative is the use of hypnotic imagery, as in this example.

Krista, a 25-year-old teacher, had suffered from severe depression for the 2 years since her mother's death from leukemia. Although she lived with her boyfriend, Rick, their relationship had deteriorated badly as she became increasingly withdrawn from him in the months following her bereavement. Following her mother's funeral, Krista found herself totally unable to drive into the cemetery where her mother was buried, even though her route between work and home brought her directly by its gates every day. At times when she was feeling particularly upset, she might drive far out of her way in order to avoid coming too close to the cemetery.

Because Krista felt herself totally unable to visit the gravesite, the therapist chose to implement a hypnotic approach. Over five sessions (spaced about 3 weeks apart), Krista was first taught self-hypnosis and imagery (see Chapter 8). She was then asked to visualize herself in progressive sessions coming nearer and nearer to her mother's gravesite. At first she saw herself doing so in her car, then by foot. She was also asked to try to replicate her imaginal progress in real life between sessions. This she was able to do. By the fifth session, she had actually walked to the gravesite and had experienced significant symptom relief from her depression, which was clearly evident to her boyfriend.

We have indicated earlier, when discussing Janoff-Bulman's (1985) perspective on the major personal assumptions that become impaired following existential losses, that victims often begin to view themselves in a negative light. It is therefore essential that the therapist in no way discredit the patient's previous efforts at grieving his or her loss, when a regrieving becomes the focus. That is, the patient should never be left with the impression that his or her previous attempts at coping with the traumatic situation are being in any way belittled. Victims of major losses are extremely vulnerable to such perceptions. Rather, previous efforts should be acknowledged as valid and often valiant attempts to cope with a difficult and painful set of circumstances.

Gaining Some Closure on the Loss

"Working through" a loss implies that the patient has a clearer sense of how the particular loss has affected or is affecting his or her life, as well as of the emotions that are associated with the trauma. In addition, although the loss is remembered, the pain ceases to be as consuming, intense, or debilitating. An important aspect of the working-through process may involve getting some sense of closure on the lost relationship or relationships. This may mean visiting a past lover in order to talk about "what really happened." One may write a letter to an estranged or even deceased family member or friend, or the patient may simply work on accepting the limitations that have come from a severe illness and determining how he or she can proceed with life from this point. A sense of closure involves an acceptance of the past trauma and loss and of the associated feelings. It also includes a view toward the future and an idea of how the person can proceed with his or her life in spite of all that has transpired.

Edith, the divorced woman described previously, whose husband Craig had left her suddenly and with little warning, was asked to write him a letter. It was initially recommended that the letter be written only for her "personal benefit," without any immediate decision about whether or not it would be sent. This decision was left to her. In this letter to Craig, Edith was asked to describe at great length her response to his method of breaking up with her, her emotional response to the separation, and any thoughts or feelings about these events that she had been "pushing away." In writing the letter Edith was able to express some of the anger and sense of betrayal she felt, as well as the great pain she had experienced and the love she still felt for Craig. Following the session in which the letter was discussed, Edith decided not to mail it to him. Shortly afterward, however, she began to have a greater sense of distance from Craig and felt less obsessed by her divorce. About 8 months after this session, she reported to the therapist that she had begun dating another man, with whom she quickly became very close. Approximately 6 months later they were married.

Addressing the Loss within a Social Context

We believe that whenever possible, those being treated in short-term therapy, regardless of the focus of therapy, should be seen with significant others for at least part of their treatment. The central differences regarding specific foci relate to the goals one hopes to achieve in bringing in the significant others. That is, in some focal situations, such as loss, the significant others are brought in to provide support or reinforcement, as well as to reflect upon their own reactions to the loss. Indeed, once one considers the possibility, it is quite common to find that the identified patient may be coping with a loss just as well as—and sometimes much better than—other people within his or her intimate social network, especially his or her spouse or family. At such times, the patient may usefully be viewed as a sort of "emissary" of the couple or family to the outside world, whose implicit task is to find help for others in the family. "Finding help" for others does not mean doing so literally. Rather, the patient, who may actually be adapting better than other family members to the loss, may have begun to reveal more distress of his or her own, and thereby may have lost some of his or her soothing, healing, or facilitating capacity for other family members. The "emissary" is then "dispatched" in order to be restored to his or her previous level of helpful functioning for others. Such an arrangement may be quite destructive to the "emissary" in the long run, if other family members do not cope well with their loss. Moreover, such an arrangement does nothing to empower the patient's family members and may bode very poorly for their handling of future stressors, including losses. Since these possibilities often cannot be assessed adequately by meeting with the patient alone, it is essential that his or her family members be present at least for the initial evaluative phase of the treatment, and often preferably throughout treatment.

In treatment situations where interpersonal conflict is the central focus, the significant others of the identified patient may be present in order to allow for a negotiation regarding the dispute in question. When there is a focus on character problems, the significant others may be able to provide the patient with important input about his or her problematic behaviors in a social/interpersonal context. Moreover, the "others" in the patient's life are often extraordinarily "significant" not in the mere sociological sense of the term, but because they may be a fundamental source of reinforcement for the most interpersonally maladaptive aspects of such character problems. Thus, although the therapist's behavior of asking the patient to come in with a sister, brother, father, mother, husband, wife, or lover may seem to be overtly the same in various circumstances, the goals that he or she is trying to achieve may differ considerably. Chapter 7 addresses such conjoint therapy in greater detail.

The goals of having significant others present when dealing with a focus on loss are, then, (1) to provide support and reinforcement for the patient regarding his or her loss; and (2) if the significant others have also experienced the focal loss, to have them talk about their reactions to the bereavement. In addition, (3) working face to face with these significant others may play an important preventive role in the family's capacity to cope with future stressors. There is a good deal of data indicating that experiencing social support under adverse circumstances has a protective effect (Henderson *et al.*, 1982; Klerman & Clayton, 1984), and that this is especially true in bereavement (Windholz *et al.*, 1985). In addition, having others present who have shared a loss may change the patient's perspective about this event. It may be viewed as an "act of God" that affects everyone in about the same way (J. P. Wilson, Smith, & Johnson, 1985), rather than something aimed solely at the particular patient.

It is also interesting to note that Kaltreider, Becker, and Horowitz (1984) found what they described as a "domino effect" for some adults experiencing the death of a parent. That is, they "noted the frequent rupture of a love relationship in the few months [following] the loss of a parent" (p. 243). This phenomenon they attributed to the activation of latent negative self-images, held in check while the parent was still alive. In any event, it is obvious that interpersonal and existential losses have implications not only for the individual most directly affected, but for significant others as well.

Finally, it appears that social supports are important mediating variables, in moderating the impact of many life crises and losses (Cohen & Wills, 1985; Kessler & McLeod, 1985; R. J. Turner, 1983). Interestingly, however, it is not the number of social supports per se which are most significant in reducing the impact of stressful events, but *one's satisfaction with those supports* (Henderson *et al.*, 1982). Thus, the goal of the therapist need not be to help the patient expand his or her social network following the loss, but rather to use existing social supports most effectively and to gain greater satisfaction from these, rather than becoming more angry, alienated, and withdrawn in one's grief.

In the case of Bea, a 31-year-old policewoman whose father had died suddenly under vague circumstances in a distant city, the therapist requested during the first telephone contact that she attend the initial session with as many of her six siblings as were willing to come. Mr. C, Bea's father, had left his wife of 40 years and his job 6 months prior to his death. He had taken off without warning, and had no contact with any of his children or his wife until 3 days before his death. At that time, he called to say that he was very ill and in a hospital with a life-threatening illness. It was also discovered that he had been living with a woman for most of the time he had been away. Before his children or wife could reach the hospital at which Mr. C was a patient, he died. After his body was returned, Bea discovered that her father had had several illegitimate children, by different women, over the course of his marriage, some of whom attended his funeral.

All of the painful revelations about her father proved unbearable to Bea. Two weeks after his death, she sought therapy in a severe and nearly incapacitating state of agitated depression. She came to the initial session with the three of her siblings (two sisters and a brother) who were in the area and willing to attend. During this first visit, the therapist got descriptions from all of the family members present of Mr. C, Mrs. C, and the nature of the family relationships. The focus was particularly upon the events immediately before and after Mr. C's demise. There had been severe upset and trauma for all of his children regarding Mr. C's abandonment of their mother, his death, and then the subsequent information concerning their illegitimate siblings. Bea was seen with her sisters and brother for four sessions. These sessions were an opportunity to discuss and mourn their father's life, death, and interactions with them. Bea and her siblings discovered how unsupported and uncared for they all had felt in growing up. They also shared a feeling of great anger at their deceased father for having seemingly been more involved with his illegitimate children than with them. Their shared intensive discussions in the therapy sessions were the most intimate conversations that they had ever had in the family, and proved to be enormously helpful to Bea and several of the others.

THERAPIST PITFALLS IN THE BRIEF TREATMENT OF LOSSES

Kushner (1981), in his book *When Bad Things Happen to Good People*, describes an intriguing Chinese folk tale: A woman's only son has died. In her grief she seeks out a holy man and asks him to magically bring her son back to life. The holy man replies by requesting that she bring him "a mustard seed from a home that has never known sorrow. We will use it to drive the sorrow out of your life." The woman sets out in quest of the seed. However, whether she goes to mansions or hovels, she is unable to find a home free of sorrow. She becomes so engrossed in helping to minister to the bereaved people whom she meets that she forgets about her own pain and her search for the magical seed.

Since none of us is immune to tragedy, and almost all of us will be faced with grief, crises, and losses over the course of our lives, the barrier between the therapist and patient in the treatment of such situations is a very fine line indeed. The major impediment to the effective brief therapy of losses is in the area of countertransference. What female therapist treating a young woman with newly diagnosed breast cancer does not feel an increased sense of vulnerability and fear? What male therapist treating a young man who has just had his first heart attack does not later become at least somewhat tense and concerned when he feels even a twinge of chest discomfort?

Just as many other authors have posited (Foreman & Marmar, 1985; Langs, 1975), we believe that countertransference may be a major impediment in brief therapy and psychotherapy in general. This can be particularly true when one is dealing with universal issues, such as loss. Countertransferential errors may develop in two quite different directions. On the one hand, the therapist can develop a negative and/or somewhat sadistic set of attitudes toward the victim. That is, most therapists, like most people in general, maintain a "just-world theory" (Lerner, 1970, 1980). Such a model posits that "you get what you deserve." A gay man comes down with acquired immune deficiency syndrome (AIDS) because of his promiscuous behavior. A colleague fails to get tenure because she didn't work hard enough. A neighbor dies of heart disease because he worked too hard. In order to make sense of the world, we attribute orderliness and causality to a world that may be at times incomprehensible and random. Such an exercise may also help distance us from the victim, and demonstrate to ourselves that we are different and will not be affected in the same way. Depending upon how powerful the therapist's need to differentiate himself or herself from the patient is, this process may be experienced as an angry coldness by the patient. On the other hand, a therapist may behave in a way that is overly solicitous or even condescending, in order to "save" the "poor" victim. This protective stance may prevent the clinician from being adequately direct and/or challenging, thereby shortchanging the patient of a good deal of potentially useful input.

Neither of these approaches will be particularly useful to the patient. In the former situation (i.e., the hostile response), the patient feels unsupported, hurt, and revictimized by the therapist. In the latter situation (i.e., rescuing the victim), the therapist feels so solicitous about the patient's plight that termination becomes inconceivable: "He's been hurt so badly in the past that I can't see hurting him again [by ending]." Under such circumstances, brief treatment can easily become interminable and can lose any sense of focality. Furthermore, the patient's view of himself or herself as weak and helpless may be reinforced, rather than the part of his or her personality that feels capable of overcoming the pain and misfortune of the loss.

5

Developmental Dysynchrony

PERSPECTIVES ON THE COURSE
OF EMOTIONAL DEVELOPMENT

The classical psychoanalytic perspective on emotional growth maintains that all subsequent development is based upon infant and childhood experience (A. Freud, 1965; Mahler, 1968). Little change in basic personality structure is believed to occur after these early points. Gergen (1980) calls this position the "stability account" of human development. Wachtel (1977), critically describing Freudian thought in this area, states:

> [It postulates] the persisting influence of certain childhood wishes and fears *despite later experiences that might be expected to alter them*. Repression, in the psychoanalytic view, does not merely prevent the individual from being aware of what is being repressed; it also prevents the repressed desire or fantasy from "growing up," from changing in the course of development as do unrepressed desires or fantasies. (p. 27, italics in original)

Research indicates, however, that a variety of characteristics such as IQ, temperament, and activity–passivity have little stability over time for infants and young children (Emde & Sorce, 1984). Kagan (1980) has noted that psychological profiles describing children at 2 years of age are minimally predictive of behavior 10 years later.

It is unlikely that most adults are rigidly enslaved by their childhood environments in the manner originally posited by analytic thinkers (Block & Haan, 1971; Elder, 1974; Maas & Kuypers, 1974). There are even indicators that under some circumstances children dealing with extremely difficult and adverse early life events may be strengthened by such experiences and may develop healthy and highly adaptive coping mechanisms as adults (Werner & Smith, 1982). Elder (1974), in a study of middle-aged adults who had been children during the Great Depression, found that those whose families had been financially deprived were better able to handle current life stresses than those whose families had had financial security.

In recent years, a theoretical position of increasing prominence has been that of the "adult developmentalists." According to this point of view, one's personality continues to develop after childhood and goes through a series of clear, orderly, invariant, and sequential steps that are related to the particular tasks associated with a given stage of life (Erikson, 1963; Gilligan, 1983; Gould, 1978; Kegan, 1983; Levinson *et al.*, 1978; Vaillant, 1977). Those who "get stuck" at an earlier step or follow deviant or unusual paths are viewed as troubled or abnormal. In line with Tolstoy's view in *Anna Karenina* (1878/1965), this perspective maintains that "Happy families are all alike; every unhappy family is unhappy in its own way" (p. 3).

This position, also called the "ordered-change account" (Gergen, 1980), although clinically and intuitively appealing, is highly evaluative in regard to how "normal" people *should* evolve. The authors presenting this viewpoint often fail to recognize that such evaluations are deeply rooted in a particular socioeconomic class, age, and gender cohort (e.g., American, middle-class, male, heterosexual adults born in the late 1930s). Furthermore, even the fact that within such a specified cohort the pathways to normal development may vary greatly is often not considered. In this regard, Offer and his colleagues (Offer, 1969, 1984; Offer & Offer, 1975; Offer, Ostrov, & Howard, 1981) propose a "multiple-pathways" model of development. In their longitudinal study of "normal" middle-class adolescent males, these researchers found what they believed to be three distinct developmental routes. In a more recent study by Petersen (1982), a similar set of routing patterns was found for adolescent females. Offer and Sabshin (1984) describe these three adolescent growth patterns as "continuous," "surgent," and "tumultuous."

The continuous-pattern boys in the study by Offer and colleagues were characterized by an absence of "even a mild behavioral or emotional crisis" (Offer & Sabshin, 1984, p. 417). They coped well with peers and with school work. They had good friends and were well liked by people in their communities. These boys "were favored by environmental circumstances" (p. 417). Their families were supportive and encouraging without being intrusive. In addition, and perhaps most importantly, these youngsters had not had to deal with deaths, losses, or serious illnesses in their families. All had nuclear families that remained stable and intact throughout their childhood and adolescence.

The development of those in the surgent pattern was marked by some periods of calm, smooth adjustment like that of the boys in the continuous-growth category, but at other times they would appear closed, stuck, and angry or depressed. These boys were more likely to have been affected by parental separation or death and/or by serious illness in their families.

The third pattern, that of tumultuous growth, was typified by considerably more emotional and/or behavioral strife than either of the other two patterns. These youngsters appeared more like those dealing with the "adolescent crisis" described in the psychoanalytic and social science literature.

They tended to come from troubled families, often with severe marital problems and major mental illness. Nonetheless, "as a group they were no less well adjusted in terms of overall functioning within their respective environmental settings than were the persons in the continuous- and sur-gent-growth groups" (Offer & Sabshin, 1984, p. 421). Thus, it appears that even within a fairly well-specified cohort, a variety of possibilities exist for normal development and alternative approaches to healthy growth.

Gergen (1980) adds another critique regarding those who propose a single pattern of smooth, clear development when, in what he describes as his "aleatoric account" of development, he emphasizes the flexibility of develop-mental patterns and the chance nature of influential events in people's lives:

> [E]xisting patterns appear potentially evanescent, the unstable result of the particular juxtaposition of contemporary historical events. For any individual the life course seems fundamentally open-ended. Even with full knowledge of the individual's past experience, one can render little more than a probabilistic account of the broad contours of future development. (pp. 34–35)

The aleatoric perspective assumes that chance or random events may have great impact upon our lives, and that it is not altogether possible to predict how someone will evolve either from their childhoods or from their more recent histories.

Bandura (1982), in an article on "chance encounters and life paths," states a very similar viewpoint. As two of many examples of the ways in which fortuitous circumstances may dramatically alter a person's life course, he cites the following:

> Nancy Davis met her future husband, Ronald Reagan, through such a turn of events (Reagan & Libby, 1980). While pursuing her acting career, she began to receive in the mail announcements of Communist meetings intended for another person bearing the same name, who appeared on a Hollywood list of Communist sympathizers. Fearing that her career might be jeopardized by mistaken identity, she voiced concern to her film director, who arranged a meeting with Ronald Reagan, then president of the Screen Actors Guild. Before long they wed. In this instance, a coincidental likeness of names and a postal mix-up altered the course of lives. . . .
> Sometimes the path-setting event involves a fortuitous symbolic encoun-ter mediated through another's actions. In his Nobel lecture, Herbert C. Brown (1980) recounts how he happened to decide to pursue doctoral research in the rare field of boron hybrids. As a baccalaureate gift, his girlfriend presented him with a copy of the book, *The Hybrids of Boron and Silicon*, which launched his interest in the subject. This was during the Depression when money was scarce. She happened to select this particular chemistry book undesignedly because it was the least expensive one ($2.06) available at the university bookstore. Had his girlfriend been a bit more affluent, Brown's research career would in all likelihood have taken a different route. (p. 749)

We view the phenomenological position on adult development taken by Cohler (1981a, 1981b; Cohler & Boxer, 1984) and Neugarten (1970) as integrating some of the strengths of the perspectives described above while suffering from fewer difficulties. We also perceive this position as highly applicable to clinical practice. According to the phenomenological point of view, people are "on time" or "off time" developmentally to the extent that they *feel* that they are subjectively doing what they and others expect for a given stage of their lives.

> Individuals create for themselves a set of anticipations; they carry with them a set of social clocks by which they measure themselves with regard to major life events (Neugarten, 1970) across the life course. Persons psychologically pre-pare, rehearse, and come to expect a series of life events, making subjective assessments of the extent to which they are "on-time" or "on-course" in terms of expected life events. For example, it is not generally expected in our society that men and women will marry by their mid to late twenties. If a first marriage should not occur until the forties, the marital partners themselves, as well as their significant others, would perceive the marriage as "off-course" in terms of the expected timing of life events. More important, the forty-year-old who expected to marry at twenty and still finds him or herself single is likely to feel "off course" with accompanying feelings of alienation and regret. If widowhood comes too early—that is, for a twenty-five- or thirty-year-old—such an unex-pected event is experienced as a particularly stressful life crisis (Lopata, 1979).
>   Feelings of self-esteem are tied to shared perceptions of being more or less "on-time" or "off-time" across the life course. Realization that an event is taking place at a time other than when it is expected leads to feelings of being "off-time" and often, lowered morale (M. Seltzer, 1976). Particularly impor-tant as a determinant of morale is the impact of the timing of life events in terms of the social support systems available (Atchley, 1975; Elder & Rockwell, 1978; Troll, 1975). A woman widowed in her sixties or seventies is "on-time" for this event. She is able both to look to friends of her own age, who are likely to be experiencing widowhood, as role colleagues sharing a common event and to learn from them the manner of negotiating this new role. A woman in her thirties does not have such a group of role colleagues available to help her; the fact that she is "off-time" for this event further increases her sense of distress; not only is she more isolated from possible sources of help, but, in addition, she senses that her loss is not expected in terms of anticipated life-cycle events. (Cohler & Boxer, 1984, pp. 150–151)

Although this position may be viewed as being based upon a relatively high degree of conformity to social standards and expectations, it is likely that among cohorts of a given age, sex, and socioeconomic status, there is a relatively high degree of uniformity in regard to personal life goals. When Groucho Marx was asked, "What if everyone thought the way that you do?", he replied, "Then I'd be a fool to think otherwise." What is central, however, is how the person views his or her life cycle. If his or her view of appropriate development is unique or idiosyncratic, then the problem of related discomfort and symptomatology may not arise, even if he or she is "off time," and this issue will be less likely to become the focus of therapy.

Another important point made by Cohler and Boxer (1984) is that we explain our lives in the form of a "personal narrative." This narrative, like other histories or literature, has a beginning, a middle, and an end. According to Cohler, the transformations or transition points in the narrative generally come (1) from early to middle childhood, (2) from childhood to adolescence and young adulthood, and (3) from adulthood to middle age. It is also Cohler's belief (1981a) that rather than reflecting the actual "truth" of the narrator's history, the story reflects a subjective meaning, telling us more about where the person is now or is expecting to go in the future. This perspective is supported by longitudinal research indicating a relatively high degree of inaccuracy on the part of respondents for historical "facts" about themselves (Vaillant & McArthur, 1972). Kegan (1983) relates a humorous story told to him by a rabbi, which captures this "changing perspective" on personal history:

A woman comes to see me, this is maybe thirty years ago. A woman who isn't a Jewish woman. She has fallen in love with a Jewish man. And, so that a lot of other people should be happy, she wants to make a conversion. If other people are happy she will be happy, this is what she says. She is very frank about this. Religion and politics and business—these things mean a lot to other people, she says. By her what matters is her husband and her friends, and one day, she hopes, her children. She is a good woman, a sincere person, but she has no real feeling about Judaism and I can't be much help to her.

Seven years later, comes to see me the same woman. But it's almost a different person. Yes, she converted. Yes, she got married. Yes, she has children. But something is not right. She loves her family but she doesn't love herself, this is what she says. "I'm thirty years old," she says. "I have three children and I don't even know who I am." She thinks maybe she can figure this out by learning what is this Jewish stuff. She wants to study by me. Not to make a conversion, she says. "I'm already converted." But to learn who she is.

For the next year she studies by me. What a workhorse! She learns Hebrew. She reads Talmud. She makes a Kosher house. Her husband, who I bar mitzvahed, is complaining to me, "Stop already, you're making my wife into a rabbi." But it wasn't me. She was taking every step on her own. She was finding out who she was. Then she starts to be concerned about her conversion. "It wasn't sincere, Rabbi." "It wasn't kosher, Rabbi." "I'm not really Jewish, Rabbi." What can I tell her? She didn't make an orthodox conversion, this is true, and, by her, this is now the only thing that counts. Do I have to tell you what happened? Almost ten years after she first comes to see me she is dipped in the ritual baths and I am signing her document, a legal convert, more orthodox than I am.

Ah, but that isn't the end of the story. Before the next High Holidays she decides how can she live with a Jew who would marry a Gentile and so she divorces her husband. (pp. 219–220)*

By means of the "personal narrative," we make sense of our lives. We can understand where we are, how we have done so far, and where we intended to go. As the rabbi's story so aptly indicates, our narrative perspective even on the same events may change dramatically, depending upon our current perspective. What is central to each of us is not so much that our personal narrative is "true" as that it makes personal sense. That is, we strive to achieve an understanding for how we got to a particular point in our lives, whether we are "on time" or "off time," and what we can expect for the future.

POINTS OF VULNERABILITY TO
DEVELOPMENTAL DYSYNCHRONY

People who enter psychotherapy because of developmental issues often appear to do so when they are experiencing life transitions, feeling that they are severely "off time," and losing a sense of coherence to their personal narratives. Cohler (1981a) believes that such a loss of coherence brings with it a feeling of fragmentation and disintegration. He writes:

> Actions and values are continually re-evaluated and reintegrated in the changing lifescript that contributes to the sense of individual identity which is vital for continued adaptation (Erikson, 1959; Loewald, 1978). This concept of internal consistency is an integral aspect of Freud's (1921) [*sic*] concept of the ego ideal and assumes major theoretical status in self-psychology, with its emphasis on maintenance of a cohesive self (Kohut, 1977). Indeed, the absence of this sense of self-consistency experienced as fragmentation or even disintegration is a major defining characteristic of serious psychopathology (Gedo and Goldberg, 1973). (p. 160)

A major goal of the therapy with people seeking help in these circumstances, as we describe later, is to help the patient to return a sense of meaning to his or her life, and perhaps to reassess the narrative as it now stands. Meaning is essential in our lives. As Nicholas Hobbs (1962) has written:

> Contemporary culture often produces a kind of neuroses different from that described by Freud. Contemporary neuroses are characterized not so much by repression and conversion . . . not by lack of insight but lack of sense of purpose, of meaning in life. (p. 742)

---

*This quotation is taken from *The Evolving Self*, by R. Kegan, 1983, Cambridge, MA: Harvard University Press. Copyright 1983 by Harvard University Press. Reprinted by permission.

We believe that there are several points at which those who are in developmental transitions, especially if they feel "off time" (according to their own experience and/or the experience of significant others in their lives), are particularly vulnerable to a major sense of crisis or "dis-ease." The following are some examples of such points.

1. When a late adolescent/young adult has been unsuccessful in attempting to separate from his or her parents (e.g., has been unsuccessful in going off to college).

2. When a young adult or middle-aged person has not been able to form a significant romantic relationship with another person.

3. When a woman moves toward the end of her childbearing years without having been able to have children.

4. When widowhood or significant illness occurs for a young adult or middle-aged person.

5. When a man or woman in midlife finds himself or herself increasingly aware of a long-standing lack of satisfaction in marriage or career.

6. When a person in late midlife or old age has an adult child or children who are still financially or very emotionally dependent.

A common element of all of these examples of developmental dysynchrony is often the patient's sense that a significant aspect of what he or she wished for at this point in life is not coming to pass, and that it may never come to pass. Some clinical examples will help to illustrate.

Adriana, a 34-year-old businesswoman who was a child of Holocaust survivors, sought therapy shortly after her mother was diagnosed as having untreatable lung cancer, and a man whom she had been dating for 6 months broke off the relationship. In early interviews it became clear that both for herself and for her parents, Adriana had dreamt that by her mid-30s she would be married and have children. Although her career was significant to her, she had always believed that marriage and a family would be a central aspect of her life. With her mother close to death and an important romantic relationship lost to her, she felt a great sense of emptiness and despair about her current and future life.

Victor, a photographer in his mid-30s, sought treatment a month after his birthday. He had, 1 year prior to this (also shortly after his birthday), been able to quit a three-pack-a-day smoking habit. He was deeply depressed about "my total immobility with women." Never had Victor been able to sustain an intimate relationship with a woman for more than 3–4 weeks. He would invariably become frightened and withdraw at that point. Occasionally, as his sexual frustration increased, he would seek out a prostitute and then find himself even "more deeply immersed in self-loathing."

Mildred and Ben, two married 68-year-old retirees, entered therapy several months before their only son, Stephen, was to be released from prison. Stephen had been incarcerated for 6 years on various drug charges. Although (or perhaps because) his parents were religious, law-abiding pillars of the community, Stephen had been in trouble with the police since his teenage years. Ben viewed with dread the prospect of his son, already 37 years old, moving back into the family home. "I've worked all of my life so that these could be relaxing years without responsibility—or maybe even he could help take care of us. I certainly never expected to still be taking care of him at this point."

For all of these people, their sense of developmental dysynchrony led to an experience of imbalance, confusion, and demoralization. Their personal narrative had a present (and therefore a future) that was undesirable and unacceptable to them. They sought therapy because their sense of being "off time" with their contemporaries was becoming more acute and severe. On the one hand, this acuteness signaled distress and fear that they would never be "on time." On the other hand, for their therapists, it should have indicated a new opportunity for change and modification.

THE BRIEF THERAPY OF
DEVELOPMENTAL DYSYNCHRONY

For the most part, those confronted by developmental problems related to a sense of being "off time" feel confused, uncertain, and demoralized. The major goal of the therapy for such individuals becomes helping them to learn whether they can modify themselves or their situations so that their developmental goals (such as an intimate relationship, parenthood, professional success, and so on) can be achieved—or, in some circumstances, helping them to learn how life can be significant and meaningful even without a major developmental goal (such as marriage) being met.

Many of the same principles that apply to the brief therapy of losses are also applicable to the short-term therapy of developmental dysynchronies. In addition, as we discuss elsewhere in this volume, all the interventions to be described need not occur in the same episode of therapy.

The following elements may be included at some point during the course of the brief treatment of developmental dysynchronies:

1. Specifying and describing the developmental dysynchrony in question.

  2. Clarifying the patient's personal narrative to this point.

  3. Helping the patient move actively toward achieving his or her developmental goal(s).

  4. On some occasions, helping the patient accept the likelihood that he or she may not be able to achieve a sense of being "on time."

  5. Frequently, treating the developmental dysynchrony in an interpersonal context (i.e., in a group therapy situation or with significant friends or relatives actively involved at some points in the treatment).

Specifying and Describing the Developmental Dysynchrony

For all of the reasons stated in regard to the focal area of losses (see Chapter 4), clarifying the issue or issues in question is a very important first step in the treatment of developmental dysynchrony. That is, giving the patient's problem a name, as well as indicating to the patient why this difficulty may be particularly relevant to him or her at the present time, helps the person focus in on what is "wrong" and why. In addition, emphasizing the developmental aspects of the problem can also help the patient see that now (perhaps more than ever before in his or her life), the opportunity and desire for change may be maximal.

  As a first example, we return to Victor, the 35-year-old photographer who had never had a long-term relationship with a woman. During the initial session, the therapist framed Victor's problems in developmental terms. He indicated that Victor probably felt "left behind" by the fact that most of his friends were married or had had numerous long-term relationships. The therapist also stated that despite his fears of women and his self-consciousness with them, Victor appeared to feel strongly motivated to address this problem: "You seem to be at an important choice point in your life. You feel like you've been lonely and isolated from women for too long. You seem to be more willing to take some risks and to try to make the significant changes you feel you need to in order to get on with your life." The therapist proceeded to use the patient's quitting smoking as another example of an extremely difficult developmentally related change at which the patient had succeeded ("You felt like you were getting older and that the smoking was ultimately going to kill you if you didn't stop now"). If Victor could use his developmental–existential *angst* to overcome his cigarette addiction, the therapist implied, he could use this same energy to change his relationship patterns with women.

  In a similar vein, Clarissa was a 29-year-old woman who presented with extreme anxiety and fear about the impending breakup of a 6-month romantic relationship. The more she described this relationship, the clearer it became that in many ways the patient *wanted* this relationship to end. Her boyfriend, Rudi, nearly 20 years older than she, was a hostile and emotionally ungiving man. Clarissa's relationships with men had been typified by extreme promiscuity and shallow interaction. Although she came from a wealthy, "high-society" family and had graduated from an Ivy League school, at points in her life Clarissa had "sold" her body and had been addicted to drugs and alcohol. She had had numerous venereal diseases, suffered from frequent outbreaks of genital herpes, and was frightened that she might have been exposed to AIDS by a bisexual lover. Clarissa also had a variety of vague physical complaints (arm and back pains) and felt as though her body were "giving out" on her. The therapist emphasized to her that now that she was rapidly approaching her 30th birthday, she seemed "very strongly motivated to change." He continued: "You feel like time is running out for you. You're burning the candle at both ends. You feel like you are old before your time. If you don't change soon perhaps you'll not even make it to 40." Clarissa agreed that although she had visited therapists before, she had never put much into treatment. She could clearly understand her situation when it was placed in a sharper developmental context. The strong support of the therapist for the part of her that felt an urgent need to change provided significant leverage in this direction.

It is central that three messages be conveyed to the patient in specifying a developmental dysynchrony as a focus for brief therapy. One message is that the therapist understands the patient's pain and lack of cohesion and integration in feeling "off time." Another is that the patient's acute distress represents a unique opportunity to overcome the developmental difficulty with which he or she is confronted. Third, it is also helpful for the patient to understand that developmental dysynchronies are not uncommon and that many people experience discomfort when they feel "out of time" with their peers. As we have mentioned earlier, we are not in total agreement with the adult developmentalist position (the "ordered-change account"). However, it is a perspective that is readily understood by patients and conveys a sense of the significance of developmental factors over the life course. Therefore, when such books appear relevant, we may ask a patient to read *Passages* (Sheehy, 1976), *Adaptation to Life* (Vaillant, 1977), or *In a Different Voice* (Gilligan, 1982).

Clarifying the Patient's Personal Narrative

In part, the patient's feelings of coherence and integration are threatened by his or her being "off time" because the developmental dysynchrony appears to make no sense: "Why have all of my friends been able to form intimate relationships, while I have been so disabled in this area?" "I have been in my job for 25 years and have hated it for all that time. How could this have happened? Why did I let it happen?"

In fact, those dealing with a developmental dysynchrony often have a life history that can help to explain why such a difficulty has arisen. In collaborating with the patient to make some sense of those experiences, events, and fortuitous circumstances that have contributed to his or her current state of affairs, the therapist can also strengthen the working alliance. This is particularly true if the therapist is empathic to those contributing factors that have been most painful and sensitive to the patient, and in regard to which the therapist can convey a strong sense of understanding.

As the patient is helped to make sense of his or her life to this point, what has happened and why it has happened are brought into clearer focus. Although the existing situation may not have changed, a greater sense of integration and coherence exists when the patient can better organize his or her own life story.

It is important for the clinician to note that this aspect of the therapy need not take many sessions. Psychoanalytically trained therapists may associate clarifying a patient's life history with years of protracted therapy on a weekly or biweekly basis. In fact, the type of clarification being discussed here can be achieved by a perceptive clinician in relatively few meetings (between one and four sessions). It is *not* an attempt to get a fine-grained or detailed description of the patient's life. Rather, the therapist hopes to understand enough about the patient's life to date that he or she can elucidate the major trends or themes contributing to the current developmental difficulties.

We again return to Victor, the photographer, so that some of the material described above can be further clarified. When he was in his 20s, Victor had anticipated that by 35 years of age he would be "settled down" with a woman and possibly have a family. It was hard for him to imagine how he could find himself in his current (lonely and basically celibate) state. However, as he and the therapist discussed his life history, several things emerged. For one, Victor had been "designated" by his parents as the child who would "take care of them" in their later years. While his two younger sisters had done poorly in school and in regard to career, Victor had always done well in these areas. His sisters, however, had each been able to form solid, long-term relationships, and both had been married for a number of years. His father, a cold, critical, and chauvinistic man, had been chronically ill since his early 30s (i.e., since Victor's childhood). An implied (and sometimes direct) message from Victor's father was "Your sisters and mother are just women. They can't do much. Some day you will grow up and be the man of this household." Consequently, Victor attended a nearby college, visited home several times a week, and devoted his life to his work and his family. Although he had some good friendships with men and women, very little would interfere with his pilgrimages to his parents' home (and his sisters' homes as well) to rake leaves, put up storm windows, mow lawns, and so on.

In addition, it became clear that Victor came to view relationships between men and women with some fear and trepidation. His father's difficult and hostile nature, paired with his mother's passivity and withdrawal, left him with a sense of isolation and dread in regard to such "intimate relationships."

In helping Victor to understand how his narrative "fit" with his current life situation, the therapist attempted to assist the patient in making sense of his present in light of his past. It was emphasized that Victor's achieving a better understanding of his life story might be useful in and of itself.

It should be noted that the therapist, while working with Victor in clarifying his life narrative, allowed Victor to use his favorite medium, photography, in service of this clarification. The patient was asked to bring in some of his portfolio, tracing his artistic career. His photos showed cold-looking, angular people or distant, isolated family groupings. These pictures were stimuli for an animated session about Victor's fearful response when he was with a woman to whom he was attracted, and also about his father's bullying attitude toward his mother. A clinician with whom Victor had had several visits 2 years prior to the current therapy had refused to allow him to bring in any of his work. He had felt that "it would have detracted from the treatment." This seemed to have impaired the alliance, and Victor quit that treatment shortly afterward.

Many patients have concrete objects (photographs, paintings, diaries, letters, audiotapes, etc.) that may be helpful to them in presenting their life narrative. The use of any such material should be supported and encouraged, rather than thwarted, especially when its possible use is initiated by the patient. In sharing such material with the therapist, the patient often reveals important aspects of himself or herself that contribute to a deeper understanding of the experiences leading to the current problematic situation. In addition, the alliance is enhanced by the therapist's willingness and interest in accepting the patient on his or her own terms.

At times, a developmental dysynchrony makes no sense to the patient because it has occurred as a function of chance or bad luck, rather than occurring through his or her own volition or in some way more clearly related to the patient's life history. This is especially true if the dysynchrony relates to an illness or loss. Should this be the case, the therapist may choose to emphasize either the loss or the dysynchrony. At times the therapist may decide to emphasize a "mixed focus," examining two or more foci simultaneously. It can be stated, however, that under most circumstances briefly discussing the patient's narrative may help place his or her reaction to the dysynchrony into a clearer context, even if it has occurred totally because of misfortune.

As an illustration, Tony, an athletic man in his late 30s, became severely depressed after a serious heart attack that was quickly followed by coronary bypass surgery. A year after his operation, he was still very anxious and had difficulty concentrating at work, with periods of over-whelming sadness. Tony, who had run numerous marathons, said that he now felt like "an old man." His return to his previous state of fitness was slowed considerably because of numerous orthopedic injuries that he sus-tained while attempting to "come back" too quickly from his illness. In discussing his family history, the therapist found that Tony's father had had a number of myocardial infarctions, beginning when Tony was 10 years old. Although his father had lived until Tony was in his 30s, he was perceived by Tony as "having died after his first MI." That is, his father became de-pressed, passive, and immobilized by his illness. It was Tony's fear that although he had also physically survived his heart attack, he would "die" psychologically, like his father. The therapist's insight regarding this issue helped Tony to understand his fear more clearly, and to move more effec-tively out of his immobilization.

Helping the Patient Move Actively toward Achieving the Developmental Goal(s)

In the third phase of the treatment, we believe that the emphasis should be upon helping the patient test active strategies for achieving his or her developmental goal or goals. In many (certainly not all) cases, part of the patient's being "off time" is related to a fear (which may be better under-stood when his or her narrative is clarified) of trying out particular behav-iors that could move the patient closer to his or her stated developmental goal. For example, the 25-year-old who cannot separate from parents to live alone or with roommates, the young woman who has no options for meeting men who might be eligible partners, and the man in midlife who has held the same job unhappily for 30 years have all usually been inhibited by their fears in attempting to take active steps that might help them to achieve their developmental goals.

It should be remembered here that some developmental dysynchronies occur not mainly because the patient has been fearful or reluctant to test out new behaviors, but because of external circumstances or genuinely bad fortune.

For instance, Dawn, a 29-year-old woman, had dated her boyfriend Toby from her last year of high school until her first year of graduate school, when both were 22 years of age. At that point they were engaged, planning to marry a year later. One month before the wedding, Toby was killed in an auto accident. Six years later, when she was first seen by the therapist, Dawn felt that she had mourned his death. However, she also felt that it was extremely difficult to meet men and that she was very lonely, strongly feeling the lack of an intimate relationship.

Whatever the reason for the developmental difficulty, there may be particular, active interventions that can assist the patient in overcoming the dysynchrony. These interventions may take the form of role playing, specific advice or directives for gradual behavior change outside the therapy, career counseling, and so forth.

To illustrate, Shirley, a 40-year-old school teacher, had been involved with teaching for most of her adult life. Although she enjoyed working with children, she had for years felt a growing sense of dissatisfaction with her job. Shirley began to sense that unless she soon moved into something else, she would be in teaching "forever." Shortly after she began to feel this, Shirley came to see a therapist. He referred her for career counseling so that she could clarify her professional interests. During this counseling, Shirley decided that she wanted to enter business. She had tremendous anxiety about going back into the job market. Shirley was asked by the therapist to mail him a resumé and a cover letter as if their next session were a job interview. During this visit the therapist and Shirley role-played several different types of job interviews, and discussed her thoughts and reactions to them. This meeting proved very helpful to her in the subsequent months as she went about seeking (and ultimately finding) a good position in her new career.

For Claudia, a single, 26-year-old woman who complained about being depressed and lonely, a somewhat different active strategy was used. She had not had a romantic relationship for many years. Claudia felt that she had no real opportunities to meet appropriate men. She was first asked to "find out as much as possible about how people you know have met romantic partners." The next session she came in with a list of possibilities: going to dances or single bars; using dating services; placing personal ads; and asking friends about setting up a blind date with someone they know. Claudia was then asked to actively pursue two or three of the stated options. As the therapist anticipated, she was anxious and objected to trying that many things at the same time. It was finally agreed that she would choose one of the options. Claudia decided that she would write and place a personal ad. The therapist asked that she get as much input as possible from her friends about what should go into the ad. The following session, she returned with a very funny and interesting advertisement which she had written with substantial input from friends. Once the ad was placed and Claudia began to get (many) responses, she and the therapist had extensive opportunities to discuss the men with whom she went out, as well as some of her fears about being in a relationship. (Had there not been this "live" opportunity to go out with numerous people, the therapy might have entailed much more abstract discussions about Claudia's concerns regarding intimate relationships.) Ultimately, she became involved with a man to whom she was introduced by a close friend (with whom she had previously discussed her ad).

Victor, the photographer, was encouraged to approach and ask out a woman for coffee whom he had known and been attracted to for many years. After weeks of ruminating, avoidance, and excuse making, it became clear that this was too big and too frightening a step for Victor to take at the time. The therapist, reassessing his strategy, felt that a time-limited developmentally oriented group (see Chapter 10) might be a useful "action step" for Victor. His response to the offer of the group was again to become anxious, worried, and ruminative. He came up with a variety of reasons (schedule, vacation, and cost) that would preclude his attendance. The therapist tried to deal with the excuses as they arose and to draw a parallel between how Victor was dealing with taking the action of joining the group and how he had dealt over the years with women. It was emphasized to Victor that joining the group "in and of itself would be a tremendous step toward achieving your goals." At the same time, the therapist kept in mind that the patient's ruminative style could not be simply sidestepped in encouraging his change. Therefore, he was encouraged to "be sure you think very, very carefully before you make the commitment to join the group." Victor was also given Yalom's (1975) book on group therapy so he could have as much data as possible before making his decision. He ultimately decided to enter the group and had an excellent outcome.

This phase of helping the patient move toward a definite action is central, in that it empowers the patient and helps him or her gain a sense of control. It is frequent to hear from patients that they feel as though "I am finally doing something about this issue."

As we have often stated previously in this volume, everything need not be addressed at the same time. Also, if a patient cannot take a particular type of action at one point, it may happen that such action can be taken at some other time, when he or she feels a greater sense of strength and/or desire for a particular change. Just as is the case with stopping smoking (i.e., the more attempts that a smoker makes, the more likely it is that he or she will ultimately quit), numerous unsuccessful attempts to modify a developmental dysynchrony usually portend that a person will eventually be able to make the change.

In this context, Cindy, a 40-year-old executive, visited a therapist intermittently over a 5-year period in regard to an "empty, loveless marriage." At first she and her husband were treated in couples therapy for about 3 months. During this time it became clear that Alvin, her husband of 15 years, a prominent physician/researcher, could not see the value of affect and emotion in any relationship, including his marriage. Alvin was a stony, rigid, and obsessional man who was almost totally consumed by his work. At night and on weekends (when he was not in his lab or out of town lecturing), he would read journals and drink heavily, often passing out on the couch. The couple rarely had sex. Several months prior to Cindy's initial visit to the therapist, Alvin had discovered that Cindy was having an affair with one of her colleagues. He had been angry and upset. Cindy had ended this affair, believing that her husband finally felt that there was a problem between them to be worked on. However, the couples' treatment seemed to underline the fact that Alvin could not or would not change, and that for Cindy the situation was really "take it or leave it."

Over the next 5 years, Cindy visited the therapist eight times (once for three consecutive bimonthly sessions, once for four bimonthly sessions, and once for one session). In these visits she spoke about her continued unhappiness with Alvin, her desire to leave him, and the two men with whom she became sexually involved over that time. Cindy thought constantly about leaving Alvin and "finally searching out a good relationship before I'm too old." During each of these series of visits, the therapist encouraged Cindy to talk with Alvin about her dissatisfaction and to think about (in concrete terms) what she would need to do in order to leave him. Each time Cindy "chickened out": "I'm too scared to leave him," "He's all I've known since I was 18 years old," "All of my single friends are lonely," "His family is wonderful to me," and so on. A litany of reasons to stay would invariably emerge whenever Cindy seriously approached the possibility of separating. Finally, nearly 5 years after she first sought treatment, Cindy came in once to tell the therapist (and to get some confirmation that what she was doing was "OK") that she had indeed made an irrevocable decision to separate from and divorce her husband. She had secured an apartment, had told Alvin of her plans, and would "find some way to make it as a single person, even if I can't find someone else." Over the previous 5 years (and more) Cindy had been changing internally, preparing herself to take this dramatic step. The therapist's support, and a developmental imperative (coming out of a sense of dwindling time to change), ultimately allowed her to get out of a hollow and unhappy marriage.

Helping the Patient Accept Limitations When Necessary

Because life is short, and because "you can't always get what you want," there are circumstances in which a patient may have to come to terms with the painful realization that a particular desired developmental event or set of events may never come to pass. Although there are a variety of ways in which this issue may come into play, it not infrequently emerges when the developmental goal that is "off time" is one that cannot be completed because of aging or because of physiological or physical limitations, or both. For example, a woman approaching menopause who wishes to have a child, but who has been unable to do so because of problems with infertility or lack of an appropriate relationship, may have to accept the fact that she will never have a child.

Often, this issue of coming to terms with the harsh realities of the limitations of one's life is a particularly vivid concern for those in their 40s and 50s. Usually, if a person has been "off time" during his or her 20s and 30s, there is still a sense that time remains for the person to get back on course. If a man or woman has done poorly in his or her chosen career, or has not ever been able to become involved in a career, there is always a belief when one is younger that the time will come when things may "turn around." In one's 40s or 50s, such a remarkable change (although it always remains possible) becomes far less likely.

Glenn, a part-time, perennial graduate student aged 45, illustrates such a confrontation with the limitations in one's life. He had completed all of his PhD course work more than 10 years before, but could not finish his dissertation. Although his university had given him numerous extensions, it appeared that if he could not hand in a completed dissertation within 3 months, he would be beyond the statute of limitations and unable to get his degree. Glenn, who had a family and held a middle-level position in a field tangentially related to his PhD area, simply could not bring himself to take the time necessary to complete his degree. The course of the therapy focused mainly upon helping Glenn to accept the fact that it was likely that he would never get his doctorate.

For Sidney, the situation was in many ways similar. He was a 57-year-old architect who, 3 years before seeking therapy, had been pushed out of a top-level position at a major architectural firm. Sidney had been completely unsuccessful in finding a new position: "No one will hire someone my age." He also felt that it was simply too late for him to change careers. He was forced to try to get free-lance work, and lived on an income that was a fraction of what he had made in his previous job situation. In part, the therapy with Sidney focused upon helping him accept this sense of being "off time." Once he came to terms with the fact that in all likelihood he would never again achieve a position in architecture on the same level, nor would he have the same income, Sidney turned to other areas to give him satisfaction. His only brother had slowly died of cancer several years earlier, and this had affected him deeply. Sidney became a part-time volunteer at a local hospice, where he was very well liked and felt a deep sense of emotional gratification.

When a patient must confront a developmental dysynchrony that may never change, whether because of time limitations, biology, bad fortune, or other life circumstances, the same issues come into play that are significant in dealing with losses. That is, never to have a child, or never really to establish oneself in the career of one's choice, may mean having to deal with the loss of the "dream" (Levinson *et al.*, 1978) that one has had for the course of one's life. For some people, this loss is as palpable as the death of a loved one, the loss of friends, or the breakup of a marriage. Under such circumstances, the reader is referred back to Chapter 4 on dealing with losses for guidelines that may be useful in approaching this type of focal problem.

Developmental Dysynchrony and Treatment in the Social Context

Inclusion of Significant Others in the Treatment

As is true with most focal problems, including significant others may be of major benefit in the treatment of developmental dysynchronies. Such problems almost always occur within a significant social context, and there is great value in evaluating and treating them within this context. Often, therapy visits with family members, friends, and/or lovers can help to place into much clearer relief the patient's personal narrative and the reason for the developmental difficulties. Such visits can also help to ally the therapist with the patient's support network, rather than work in opposition to it.

In a fascinating article, Hatcher and Hatcher (1983) discuss the fantasies of spouses or parents not involved in treatment regarding their husbands', wives', or adult children's psychotherapist. The authors polled a number of persons whose spouses or children were in long-term individual treatment and who had never had any direct contact with the therapists of those in treatment. For the most part, they found that the "nonpatient" spouses or parents often felt angry, threatened, and/or uncertain about what was transpiring in the treatment. Nonpatient husbands frequently had fears about their wives' becoming romantically involved with their male therapists. In general, nonpatient spouses/parents did not appear to be supportive or encouraging of their husbands', wives', or children's treatment. Hatcher and Hatcher write:

> Our title ["Set a Place for Elijah"] comes from the tale of Elijah, the magician and prophet. During the Passover meal, a seat at the table and a full cup of wine [are] reserved for Elijah and the door to the outside is left ajar—for it is expected that sometime the elusive guest will sip wine and participate in the family gathering.
> When a spouse or a child sees a psychotherapist, an invisible Elijah joins the family, certainly to help, but often unwittingly to distress the spouse or parents of the patient. The new member of the family may significantly influ-

ence the relationship between the patient and the other family members. The patient becomes involved in the treatment, has strong feelings about the therapist, and changes during its course. No matter how helpful the treatment may be, no matter what promise of a happier life it may hold, therapy may drive a kind of wedge between the spouse or parent and family member in treatment. (1983, p. 75)

If we apply these findings in a more general way, it is probably true that a number of significant people in the patient's environment may be threatened by the patient's involvement with the therapist and/or changes in the patient's style of interacting. However, if the therapist can make effective use of the patient's support structure and can involve significant others over the course of the treatment process, these people may greatly enhance the therapy process. Bringing in significant others may also serve a useful function in regard to reducing the intensity of transference and the dependency that the patient feels upon the therapist. These are factors that, when managed correctly, make it more likely that therapy will be time-effective and cost-effective. Moreover, although many developmental dysynchronies can be viewed as the psychological "property" of individuals, such dysynchronies almost inevitably pose developmental impasses in marriages or family life. Thus, a primary focus on the marital or family context of such "off-time" difficulties is frequently called for.

A number of factors should be considered when the therapist plans to involve significant others in the treatment of developmental dysynchrony (or other focal areas):

1. The therapist should discuss this possibility with the patient very early in an episode of treatment. It should be presented as a "natural" aspect of therapy: for example, "When I see a patient in treatment, I believe that it is often useful to have someone who is very familiar with you come in for a session or two to give me a somewhat broader picture of how things are going in your life," or "It is frequently helpful to the therapy to have a person come in with another family member; in this way I can get a clearer perspective regarding the situation in which you grew up." Especially when the patient defines the problem as being entirely his or her "own," it is advisable not to describe such marital or family meetings as being "marital therapy" or "family therapy," but rather as "therapy consultations." Although such initial consultation sessions (or "family meetings") may eventually evolve into conjoint therapy, labeling them as such from the outset may arouse fears in the patient of "confrontations" with other family members, or may be heard by those other family members involved in such a consultation as implicitly blaming.

The inclusion of a significant other in the treatment should not be presented as an unusual event, representing an exceptionally difficult treatment. It should also not be viewed by the therapist or patient as occurring because the patient is an inadequate reporter of his or her current or past situation. Rather, it is done because it is beneficial in most circumstances and facilitates effective psychotherapy.

2. The therapist should conceptualize what his or her goal is in planning a session or sessions with a significant other and the patient. If, for example, the therapist's intentions are to learn more about the patient's interactions in his or her family of origin and/or to clarify the patient's personal narrative further, a brother, sister, parent, or other available relative should be included. The therapist might also hope to modify some aspects of the patient's interaction within his or her family of origin. This may be particularly true under circumstances in which this problematic interaction has been contributing to the developmental dysynchrony.

As an illustration, we describe the case of Joyce, a 29-year-old writer. Joyce had had numerous very short-lived relationships with men until she met Frank, who was a college professor the same age as she. When the relationship with Frank began, a number of the issues that had plagued Joyce in previous relationships with men again became prominent. She became extraordinarily jealous (with little real basis in fact) and fearful that Frank was beginning to see other women. Also, she would have fits of anger directed toward Frank. At times minor conflicts might lead to explosive battles, with objects being thrown around; on a few occasions, even physical violence took place. Several months into this relationship, Joyce returned to see the therapist by whom she had been treated briefly some years before. By the time that Joyce had had her first individual session in this second course of treatment, Frank had decided to put their relationship "on hold" for a few months because the level of conflict was so great. The individual treatment with Joyce focused on what made an intimate relationship with a man so tense, anxiety-provoking, and conflictual. Joyce was seen in this course of treatment for a total of six biweekly visits. (She had previously had eight sessions with the same therapist spread over 2 years.)

The fourth visit in the course of treatment being described was planned to include Joyce's mother and father, who had come from a distant city for a Christmas visit. In previous visits Joyce had spoken at length about her father, an unsuccessful businessman who throughout her childhood had been "a terrible alcoholic." After Joyce left home, her father had "found AA" and had been sober for many years. Her mother she described as a "weak, denying, and manipulative woman," who could never confront her husband about his alcoholism, neglect of his children, or blatant womanizing. The session with Joyce and her parents proved to be extremely powerful and valuable for all concerned. Joyce was, for the first time in her life, able to speak directly with her parents about the pain and anger she felt in regard to her father's distance and neglect, and her mother's obfuscation of the problems in the family. Remarkably, her father, who felt enormous shame regarding his past transgressions, was able to ask his daughter and wife to forgive him. The therapist was also able to discuss with Joyce during this visit, and in subsequent sessions, how her family dynamics were relevant to her relationships with Frank and with other men. This session proved to be a significant turning point for her. When she and Frank again began to see each other, Joyce was far more effective in keeping her anger and jealousy in check. Approximately a year after the family visit, Joyce and Frank returned for a course of couples treatment. They were seen for eight sessions conjointly. About 2 years later they were married.

If, on the other hand, the therapist's goal in bringing in a significant other is to broaden his or her understanding of the patient's social support system, to learn how the patient interacts with significant peers, and/or to form an alliance with important people in the patient's support system, then the focus should be upon bringing in someone who the patient believes knows him or her well and is currently significant in an ongoing way. The treatment of Ezra, a 33-year-old gay man, exemplifies the use of a significant other in the manner just described.

Ezra entered treatment depressed and with various phobic symptoms. He had been unable to have close, intimate relationships with other gay men; he would quickly become distant in a relationship and would withdraw. Ezra also suffered from chronically low self-esteem. He viewed himself as "a wretch" whom no one could really love or care about. The therapist, after verifying that Ezra had some friends with whom he was very close, asked him to come in to their fifth visit with his very good friend Claire, who had known the patient since his first year in college. Claire's visit proved to be very beneficial to the course of the treatment. She indicated that although she and other good friends of Ezra realized his problems with insecurity and self-esteem, they viewed him very differently from the way he viewed himself. She and other people in their "crowd" perceived Ezra as being a caring, sensitive person who was known for his loyalty and helpfulness, especially in times of need. Two other events also proved to be very important to the course of Ezra's therapy. First, Claire strongly encouraged him to "hang in there" and not just leave treatment precipitously, as he had done with other therapists in the past. Coming from someone as close to him as Claire, this was a strong endorsement for sticking with therapy. Also, Claire reported that she believed that the patient had a fairly severe alcohol problem. Up until this point, Ezra had consistently denied such a difficulty. When Claire presented this problem, it was much harder for Ezra to continue his denial regarding this issue.

Obviously, if the goal of including family members in subsequent sessions is to address what appear from early meetings with the patient to be ongoing problematic interactions that directly involve the developmental dysynchrony, those family members who appear so involved should be included. At times, the family members most involved in a problematic way with the patient's dysynchrony are not identified as such by the patient, so the therapist needs to remain open and flexible as to who might be invited to future sessions.

3. The therapist should *always* clarify what has been told to the significant other about why he or she is being asked to participate in the session. A therapist who invites in a significant other without clarifying to that person why he or she is being invited is simply courting disaster. The quick assumption made by most people, especially spouses or lovers, is that "The therapist believes that *I* am to blame for Joe's problems," or "If Mary hadn't told the therapist so many bad things about me, he would have never asked that I come in." Often, the significant other comes in frightened and defensive. It is *always* very important to make clear just what has transpired regarding the visit between the patient and the significant other. The visit by the significant other should always begin with the question, "What has ──── told you about why I requested that you come in today?" After this is discussed, the therapist should then explain very clearly what he or she has anticipated in asking the person to participate, and what it is hoped will be accomplished.

Treatment of Developmental Dysynchronies in Short-Term Therapy Groups

Short-term group therapy based upon an adult developmental model (see Chapter 10; Budman, Bennett, & Wisneski, 1981) is an ideal modality for the treatment of developmental dysynchronies. The short-term group provides the patient with an environment in which other people are also struggling with the issue of being "off time." The cohesiveness and supportive atmosphere of a well-functioning short-term group allows members to test out new behaviors that may let them move closer to achieving their developmental goals. In addition, the time limit in these groups helps to emphasize the existential aspects of such developmental problems and to encourage active steps toward change, because, like the group, "life does not go on forever."

Time-limited group therapy based upon an adult developmental model is often incorporated into the treatment plan following a brief course of individual therapy. As with other foci addressed in this book, the treatment of developmental dysynchronies may have numerous components and various modalities may be used at different points in the treatment. None of these components is necessarily the *definitive* treatment, nor is one necessarily better than another. Rather, each aspect of the therapy may be seen as a part of the overall context of the therapeutic relationship; together, these aspects may have a cumulative effect.

THERAPIST PITFALLS IN DEALING WITH DEVELOPMENTAL DYSYNCHRONY

The major therapeutic error in the treatment of developmental dysynchrony is assuming a characterological rather than a developmental frame of reference. It is not difficult to view the problems that result when a patient is out of time with his or her peers as functions of an underlying characterological disorder. On some occasions, this view may be accurate, and the characterological problem may need to be addressed in order for any significant change to occur. (The area of characterological disturbances and their brief treatment is addressed in Chapter 9.) Often, however, whether or not an underlying character problem exists, a developmental perspective is effective in enabling the patient to achieve significant changes. In our view, it is most useful to *begin* with a developmental perspective, assuming that the patient is entering treatment ripe for change and hopes to get his or her life "on time."

6

Marital and Family Conflicts:
Early Treatment Issues and Assessment

In addition to the various developmental, symptom-focused, and characterological problems that individuals bring to psychotherapists, a very large proportion of patients' presenting problems, complaints, and concerns involve difficulties experienced within marital and family relationships. Although the various individual therapies as a group undoubtedly are called upon more often than marital and family therapy, any general practitioner of psychotherapy is well aware that consumers of mental health services routinely seek help because of relationship disturbances. For example, Gurin, Verof, and Feld's (1960) well-known survey of how Americans view mental health issues showed that 42% of all people who had sought professional help for psychological problems viewed the nature of their problems as marital, and another 17% viewed their problems as involving other family relationships. And Parad and Parad's survey of casework and therapeutic services (H. J. Parad & Parad, 1968; L. J. Parad & Parad, 1968) showed that over three-quarters of patients described their presenting problems as either "interactive" (37%) or "problem posed by another family member" (39%).

The emphasis of this chapter and the one that follows is on the brief therapeutic treatment of what Gurman and Jacobson (1986) call "relationally defined problems" in marriage and family life. While all "individual" psychiatric disorders can be viewed in a systemic context (Gurman & Kniskern, 1981), and while the burgeoning field of family therapy has spawned an impressive array of family-oriented treatments for many of these disorders (e.g., schizophrenia—C. M. Anderson *et al.*, 1986; depression—I. D. Glick & Clarkin, 1985; anxiety disorders—Hafner, 1986; substance abuse—Stanton, Todd, & Associates, 1982; and eating disorders—Harkaway, 1986), the general practitioner of psychotherapy most often encounters in his or her work problems that are either explicitly defined as relational and interactional or that are most parsimoniously viewed in this way. Indeed, such problems constitute the standard fare of much of psychotherapy, even for clinicians who do not identify themselves professionally as "family therapists" or "marital therapists/counselors."

THE LONG TRADITION OF BRIEF MARITAL AND FAMILY THERAPY

The majority of techniques, strategies, and methods of marital and family therapy are inherently consonant with the major principles of individual treatment discussed in this book. Indeed, in sharp contrast to the sorts of philosophical and technical controversies that have characterized the brief therapy movement in traditional individual psychotherapy, marital and family therapists have rarely had to struggle with ways to shorten the treatment process. By the usual standards of traditional individual therapy, marital and family therapy has been overwhelmingly brief, and some family therapy methods are explicitly time-limited (e.g., Stuart, 1980; Weakland, Fisch, Watzlawick, & Bodin, 1974). We have documented in Chapter 1 that most individual therapy is brief; the same is true of most marital and family therapy, with treatment of from 5 or 6 to fewer than 20 sessions accounting for more than two-thirds of the courses of treatment, even in private practice (Gurman, 1981). A key difference has been that while long-term, intensive treatment models exist among family therapists (Gurman & Kniskern, 1981), they have never set the dominant standards for practice, and no major method of family therapy has ever originated in long-term practice.

In addition to the fact that the *field* of family therapy has often eschewed the practices of the traditional mental health disciplines (social work, psychology, and especially psychiatry), other, more immediate factors make the probability of brief intervention high in working with marital and family problems (Gurman, 1981). For example, therapy focused on interpersonal difficulties predictably centers on the "between" of relationships as much or more that the "within" of individuals, leading to more emphasis on the immediate determinants of behavior (Pinsof, 1983). In addition, the sources of distress are not merely talked about in family therapy, but are present in the treatment setting, so that defenses are more readily identifiable and problem-focused behavior is more accessible for direct modification. Moreover, termination with couples and families is rarely as symbolically and affectively loaded as it is with individuals, since the major interpersonal attachments of patients in marital and family therapy are other family members, not the therapist (Gurman, 1981). Finally, family therapy is likely to induce therapeutic crises by its orientation toward action. Since most couples and families enter therapy in a crisis, "once that is over, its members typically want to back off from the enforced togetherness of the therapeutic session" (Brewster & Montie, 1987, p. 34).

VALUES OF THE BRIEF THERAPIST TREATING
MARITAL AND FAMILY PROBLEMS

Switching from working directly only with an individual to doing face-to-face work with a couple or family does not require the brief therapist to adopt a different set of values about his or her work. Indeed, all the values and attitudes of the brief therapist that we have discussed in Chapter 1 are appropriate for and facilitative of therapy with families. Some of these brief therapy values, however, take on a particular emphasis when a therapist is working with family systems:

1. Rather than focusing on the developmental–interpersonal character of individuals, the brief therapist emphasizes change in the family's characteristic style of problem solving. In particular, the brief therapist is concerned with helping the family to enhance its problem-solving capacities in the area of its life in which the presenting problem is embedded. The "character" with which the therapist is concerned is primarily the "character" of the couple's or family's interaction.

2. When working with couples and families, the brief therapist takes it as axiomatic that the healing power of relationships between and among family members always exceeds the healing power of the therapist–patient relationship. While the brief therapist is no less concerned with the quality of the therapeutic relationship than is the long-term therapist, the importance of the therapeutic alliance is seen as lying primarily in its power to facilitate bonding, adaptive functioning, and the like within the marriage or family.

3. The brief therapist not only sees individuals as constantly changing over time, but also sees intimate relationships, such as those of marriage and the family, as in an evolving flux. The brief therapist, then, always "maps" the developmental blocks, regressions, and status not only of each individual family member, but also of the family as a unit and of its central subunits (e.g., the marriage).

4. In adopting a health orientation rather than an illness orientation, the brief therapist assumes that spouses or family members are always going about life together in the best way they currently can. The couple or family is assumed to be capable of resolving its problems with minimal therapist input, until and unless overwhelming evidence to the contrary accumulates (Pinsof, 1983).

In addition to these different "twists" of the brief therapist's values as applied to working with couples and families, the brief therapist working with families also needs to feel personally congruent with several other values that are rather particular to working with ongoing, intimate relationships:

1. The brief therapist believes not only that changes in one area of relationship functioning may have "ripple effects" (Spiegel & Linn, 1969) in

other areas, but also that apparently small changes in a couple or family's characteristic style of interacting and problem solving may constitute the beginning of a shift in its basic relationship "paradigm" (Constantine, 1986), or way of experiencing itself. The brief therapist, then, is often content with small changes in relationships if these signify that a couple or family has gotten back on its developmental track and has established some adaptive new rules for its operation, even though these new rules may remain somewhat implicit and are not discussed in great detail or at great length.

2. When working with couples and families, the brief therapist values behavioral change as much as cognitive and affective change. The thoughts and feelings of family members need to be understood and respected, and may often themselves constitute the targets of therapeutic change. Still, interactional change cannot be maintained merely by family members' having new thoughts and feelings, but must be reinforced by overt action (Gurman, 1978).

3. While prizing behavior change in working with couples and families, the brief therapist also attends to the intrapsychic issues of individual family members, but usually in a manner quite different from that of his or her long-term therapy colleagues. The brief therapist assumes that since people shape each other's personalities, marital and family therapy can lead to profound individual change, and that behavior change can change the inner schemas people have of themselves and others in intimate relationships (Gurman, 1985c).

4. The work of the brief therapist with couples and families should be preventative as well as ameliorative. Thus, there should be an emphasis on resolving presenting problems in such a way that while changes are observable, a high value also is placed on patients' conscious learning of more effective methods and techniques of problem solving. It is important that people be able to generalize from what they have learned during therapy to other difficulties they may face after therapy. This value emphasizes that what should result from therapy should include not only change in the presenting problem and insight about relational dynamics, but also an enhanced capacity to solve at least some of the inevitable difficulties that confront couples and families, with minimal professional help.

INITIATING BRIEF MARITAL AND FAMILY THERAPY

Sources of Referral to Marital and Family Therapy

Except for the relatively small proportion of cases in which psychotherapy is mandated by someone other than the help seeker (e.g., court-ordered treatment), the lion's share of people who receive individual psychotherapy are self-referred. The route to the therapist's office is most often set down by one individual's desire for help because of the presence of unacceptable feelings or thoughts, undesired behaviors, and so forth.

The routes taken by people who ultimately receive marital and family therapy, however, are much more varied and often more complex (Gurman & Kniskern, 1979). There are three major sources or categories of referrals for marital and family therapy: self-referrals, referrals by agents outside the family, and therapist referrals. Although common images of "family therapy" usually conjure up a picture of Mom, Dad, and their children (and perhaps other relatives) meeting together with a therapist, most "family therapy," in fact, is conjoint therapy with the husband–wife dyad (Gurman, 1985a), typically referred to as "marital therapy" or "marriage counseling."

Self-Referrals

While referrals for marital therapy are regularly made by third parties (a wife's gynecologist; the couple's minister, priest, or rabbi; one partner's attorney; etc.), most couples in therapy are self-referred. That is to say, at least one of the partners initiates the first contact with the therapist.

However, considering cases in which one spouse calls for a first appointment (without an earlier intervention by clergy, physicians, etc). as "self-referred" may be, and often is, misleading in some very important ways. While we know of no published data on the matter, it is very clear to any therapist who regularly treats couples that (1) only in a small proportion of cases are both spouses equally and highly motivated to participate; (2) in many cases, one spouse is nearly dragged, psychologically speaking, to the first session; and (3) except with the most highly motivated and psychologically minded couples (and even with these, too), it is routine to find that at least one spouse (and often both) is convinced that the marital difficulty is caused by the *other's* behavior, irrationality, neurosis, or the like. Thus, although no agent external to the couple is usually involved in the couple's referral to a therapist, the differential motivation between the spouses for conjoint treatment is often sufficiently great as to render the notion of "self-referral" naive, if not at times quite absurd.

If the brief therapist first fails to acknowledge these observations in principle and then fails to inquire about such common differential motivation, a major tactical error may have been committed to one that is likely to lengthen the course of treatment significantly (or shorten it inappropriately by leading to premature termination). This error, of course, has to do with the need to establish a working therapeutic alliance very early in therapy. Spouses who begin therapy with different degrees of commitment to treatment alliance will make it very difficult (if not impossible) for the therapist and the marital partners to agree upon the central focus of their work, which is the cornerstone of all brief therapy. This issue is important in all cases of "self-referral" to family therapy, which are not limited to a marital focus, but may also include such varied problems as the interaction between stepparents and stepchildren; childhood or adolescent conduct disorders; and the "individual" disorders of children, adolescents, or adults. We have more to say about the therapeutic alliance in brief marital and family therapy later in the chapter.

Referrals by Agents Outside the Family

The second major source of referral to marital and family therapy is the broad array of public servants (teachers and other school personnel; police and the courts) and professional helpgivers (physicians, attorneys, clergy) with whom the family interacts as a group, or through its individual members or subsystems. When marital or family therapy is initiated by such external agents, there is not only a good chance of differential motivation for therapy among family members, but also an increased likelihood that *no* family member will assume much responsibility for the family's or couple's presence in the therapist's office. Certainly, many families and couples who enter treatment at the initiative of such external agents are relieved by and pleased with the referral, and quickly become as involved in treatment as do "self-referred" patients. But a significant number of these couples and families themselves see little if any reason to talk to a psychotherapist, and while they may be suffering, in a very real sense they are not the "patients" as we usually think of that term. The "patient" (or, more accurately, the complainant) is the external referral agent.

When dealing with couples and families, the brief therapist should always inquire carefully and in detail about how (through whom) each couple or family comes to be in his or her office. (In many clinic settings the opportunity for this inquiry will not appear until the first face-to-face contact, whereas in private practice it presumably appears with the first phone call to the therapist.) If the "patient"/complainant really is someone outside the family, and this goes unrecognized by the therapist, either of two unpleasant processes may quickly unfold. First, since the spouses or family members really do not want to be in a therapist's office, establishing a working alliance may be impossible. A second possible outcome is that the couple or family and the therapist will simply engage in a muddled search for a focus within the family, when, in fact, the family's focus is not about itself, but about why they are with the therapist in the first place. Sometimes the appropriate focus for the brief therapist is to deal directly with the referring agent, rather than the couple or family, after the initial assessment meeting.

For example, a colleague in internal medicine referred the A family to one of us because of the family's recent trauma of learning that Mrs. A was suffering from terminal liver cancer that could not be resected. She was expected to live no longer than 6–12 months. Present at the initial meeting were Mr. A, a highly successful local businessman, and the two A children— Kristin, age 17, a high school senior, and Mark, her 20-year-old brother, a junior at the local university. When asked why the family had come to see the therapist, Mr. A replied, "We just found out about 3 weeks ago that my wife has terminal liver cancer, and so Dr. Marcus thought it would be a good idea for all three of us to talk to someone." The therapist asked, "What did he think you should talk about?" "Everything that's been going on lately," was the response. With that, Mr. A described in detail his wife's early symptoms, the numerous tests she had gone through in the hospital, the initial uncertainty of her doctors about her diagnosis, and so on. And what had been happening in the family since Mrs. A's hospitalization? At first, Mr. A had stayed away from his job, but was now back at work "operating at about 70%, I'd say." The children's schoolwork had been temporarily disrupted, but now seemed "back on track—they're both very good students," he offered.

In addition to continuing to function rather well in their major work and academic roles, the three of them had spent a good deal more time together than usual, talking about everything from how to divide up and share household responsibilities to their deepest feelings of grief. They were not only working together quite well, but also had been grieving together. Both as a group and individually, they had also been spending "all our spare moments, plus some" at the hospital with Mrs. A. "We've always been a pretty close family, but I think we've been even closer since all this happened," Mark volunteered. They had also been able both to call upon friends and some members of their church congregation, and to accept unsolicited help with "practical sorts of things as well as emotional support." While they all agreed that "this is the worst thing that could ever happen to any of us," they felt they were "doing quite well, considering," and had not really understood why Dr. Marcus thought they should see a family therapist. "He's not really like other doctors," Kristin said, "he really cares about his patients, and not just about the medical stuff." "Sometimes, I think he thinks he's really a psychiatrist or something," Mr. A added.

The therapist discussed openly and directly with the family whether or not any of them thought there was any kind of help that he (or another therapist) might be able to offer to the family at this time. Mr. A said he appreciated the opportunity to talk to the therapist, but did not think the family had "a problem we need to see a therapist about." Kristin and Mark agreed: "Who knows how we'll feel [about needing a therapist's help] a few months from now? If we can't handle things ourselves, or with help from our friends, I think maybe we'd come back to talk to you again." A phone conversation with Dr. Marcus a few hours later confirmed that, indeed, he had not referred the family "because of any real pathology, like major depression or anything." Being sensitive to families' emotional as well as physical needs, he had talked to Mr. A about their traumatic situation, and "thought they were coping pretty well, but I just wanted to get a second opinion from someone who works with families all the time."

The presenting problem—Dr. Marcus's concern that "perhaps I'd over-looked something important in the situation"—had been addressed, and Dr. Marcus was reassured; the family's trusting relationship with their primary physician had been reinforced by their having a good experience in their meeting with the therapist; and the door had been opened, should any of them feel the need to consult the therapist in the future.

At other times, external agents refer family members to a therapist with the family's clear understanding of and agreement with the reason for referral, even though the reason is not for psychotherapy. As in all brief therapy, the therapist must identify this reason as soon as possible. In addition to the fundamental question of "Why now?", the brief therapist needs to understand "For whom now?" and "For what now?" The "what" may not be psychotherapy, but may be some service only a mental health professional can provide. For example, in the state in which one of us (Alan Gurman) practices, state law requires that before a married couple can be granted a final divorce hearing, the spouse petitioning for divorce must have had at least a single interview with a professional psychotherapist to explore the possibility of reconciliation, to prepare for the new unmarried status, and to plan for the needs of minor children. Although only the divorce petitioner needs to take part in the interview, it is fairly common for attorneys to refer both spouses to a therapist for this mandatory experience. The purpose of the law is not so much to establish expert opinion about the viability of a given marriage as it is to punctuate the separation–divorce process for the couple in such a way that should reconciliation be possible, a therapeutic avenue is provided to allow that possibility to be addressed.

Although it is tempting for marital therapists to be "marriage savers" (Weiner-Davis, 1987), this is not an appropriate role for the therapist (Gurman, 1985b, 1987; see our discussion below about dealing with separa-tion and divorce issues). If the therapist fails to acknowledge and accept that the couple (or one spouse) may be unswerving in their (or his or her) decision to divorce, and the consultation takes place merely in response to a legal requirement, a very distorted discussion of the couple's purpose and central focus in having the interview may ensue.

Therapist-Initiated "Reframing Referrals"

While many courses of marital and family therapy are initiated by patients themselves and by agents external to the family, a great deal of therapy with couples and families follows from a therapist's reframing of a patient's (or patients') problem, and a related recasting of what is likely to be the optimal treatment for that problem. In a narrow sense, this then constitutes a particular subtype of therapy initiated by an agent external to the family, and is not literally a "referral" (in the sense of sending someone on to another clinician). But this type of "reframing referral" is so common, and involves strategic matters that are so specific to this treatment context, that it requires consideration in its own right. How skillfully "reframing referrals" are handled by the therapist will have a major and often enduring impact on the quality of the therapist alliance that is initially established, as well as on the clarity and acceptability of the central focus of ongoing therapy itself.

There are two major types of therapist-initiated "reframing referrals": attribution-oriented reframing and intervention-oriented reframing.

Attribution-Oriented Reframing. The first kind of reframing occurs when the therapist presents to the patient(s) a formulation of the patient's problem that defines the problem as being different from the patient's formulation in terms of its substance, valence, maintenance and/or locus.

The "substance" of the problem simply refers to a person's perception of "what the problem is," and involves making distinctions among the cognitive, affective, and behavioral realms of the patient's experience. Reframing the substance of a problem usually calls upon interventions that are familiar to psychodynamically oriented therapists and behavior therapists. For example, a wife complains to her therapist in their first meeting about her despair in regard to her husband's lack of emotional involvement with her and their children, seeing the problem as his repeated distancing behavior. The therapist "hears" the problem differently, and tells the wife that perhaps her husband is distant not because he "is a cold person" who prefers to be alone, but because he finds emotional involvement to be very anxiety-arousing. The problem is primarily affective, and secondarily behavioral. Or, a mother brings her 13-year-old son to the therapist, concerned about his social isolation from his peers, which she attributes to his "shyness." In taking a social and developmental history, the therapist learns that the family has moved to this urban area from a rural farming community just within the last several months. Because of the family's struggle to keep their farm afloat financially the last several years, the children have spent almost all their time away from school doing farm chores and rarely playing with friends. The therapist suggests to the mother that the son's problem is not primarily his "shyness" (an affective attribution), but his lack of social skills (a behavioral, and perhaps cognitive, attribution).

The "valence" of the presenting problem refers to a person's perception of the (un)desirability of the problem. Attempting to shift a patient's thinking about the (un)desirability of a problem is a strategy that has been well developed and promulgated by so-called "paradoxical" family therapists (e.g., Madanes, 1981; Papp, 1983; Selvini-Palazzoli *et al.*, 1978). Revalencing a presenting problem most often involves the therapist's identifying for the patient the previously unrecognized positive consequences of the problem and/or the previously unanticipated possible negative consequences of resolving the problem.

For example, Mrs. M, a 34-year-old single mother, brought her 15-year-old son, Michael, to the therapist because of the increasing frequency of arguments between them and Michael's repeated rule breaking (curfews, TV time, household chores, etc.) over the previous several months. Mrs. M had divorced her alcoholic, ne'er-do-well husband when Michael, her only child, was 5 years old. Since that time, she had done virtually no dating (despite being very physically attractive and socially skilled), and rarely spent time with female friends outside her job. She denied being troubled by this state of affairs, and insisted that "as a single parent, I feel like I have to be a father *and* a mother to Michael—besides, I'll have plenty of time to date if I want to when Michael graduates [from high school]." About 3 years after the divorce, Mrs. M's widowed mother had begun to experience what was now a series of recurrent major depressions, and she called upon Mrs. M many times a week "to help her take care of things she can't do for herself." She did most of these things dutifully, despite her long-standing resentment of her mother for what she felt was the severe neglect she had undergone during her childhood.

In an early brief interview with Michael alone, the therapist saw that, contrary to Mrs. M's description of Michael as being insensitive to her needs, stresses, and the like, Michael was very concerned about his mother. He felt that she "watches over me too much and doesn't do enough for herself. Maybe if she had a boyfriend or something she'd think about something besides me. I think she has some sort of hangup about men since my dad was such a jerk." He also thought it was "ridiculous how much she helps her mother, since she really can't stand her!"

In the three-way meeting held immediately after the interview with Michael, the therapist suggested to Mrs. M that her son was not at all indifferent to her needs. In fact, he was very concerned about why she had never taken up dating since her divorce and why she continued to be so helpful to her mother, who demanded a great deal of Mrs. M, yet gave little in return (she did not even thank Mrs. M for all her helpfulness). The therapist reframed Michael's misbehavior as "not only not insensitive to you, but, in fact, extremely sensitive to your needs. Michael seems to believe that if you don't have him to worry about and complain about so much, you may have to face head-on whatever hangups still hang over your head about men since your marriage. I think he's also concerned that if you really develop a life of your own, you'll feel inclined to set some tougher limits with your mother, and that that could lead to a real blowout with her because of all the anger you've had stored up toward her for so long." At the same time, the therapist explained, Michael was deeply grateful for how

much Mrs. M had given up for him as a single parent. Perhaps his misbehavior, then, was his way of thanking her for all she had done for him: She
had limited her life so much to being a mother that he would feel guilty if he
took all that away from her (which she would surely feel had happened if
Michael were acting more responsibly and "needed" much less supervision
from her). Michael's misbehavior, then, expressed his ultimate loyalty to his
mother by keeping her in the job she had learned to do so well, by giving her
a good reason to avoid dealing with men, and by helping to prevent her
having a "dangerous confrontation" with her own mother. The "problem"
Mrs. M had presented was, in fact, the therapist suggested, "not only a
problem itself, but a solution to what sounds like much more frightening
problems." The "problem" unfortunately thus had very positive, though
unrecognized, consequences, and its immediate resolution might well lead to
some very unpleasant experiences.

As it did in this case, revalencing the presenting problem may lead to a
major refocusing of the aims of subsequent therapy. At first, Mrs. M
thought the therapist's reattribution about the problem seemed "kind of far-
fetched." The therapist reassured her that her reaction was quite understandable, even predictable, since "Michael's misbehaving out of loyalty to
you isn't done very consciously, if it's done consciously at all." At the session
the following week, Mrs. M said she had thought a great deal about what
the therapist had said, and had decided that, *if* the therapist was right,
Michael was "worrying about me much more than any 15-year-old should
have to." She added that her "problems with men aren't something I think
we should discuss in family therapy," and requested some time alone with
the therapist to deal with those issues. In individual therapy, Mrs. M and the
therapist maintained a focus on her fears of having to go through the pain of
another divorce, and her fear that "maybe there's something about me that
attracts losers and alcoholics like my first husband." Three biweekly follow-
up sessions with mother and son together focused on Michael's steadily
improving behavior at home. Michael was starting to see that what he was
doing out of loyalty to his mother might not, in fact, be in her best long-term
interests; now, he understood, he could "be loyal to her by not giving her
such excuses not to grow up herself," as Michael put it.

Since, the aim in brief therapy is to educate patients as well as to
ameliorate problems, such revalenced attributions about presenting problems are not offered as ploys; rather, as Skynner (1981) has said, they are
put forth "as expressions of the most essential truth, which subtly break the
rule that fantasy and reality must be kept apart, by relating the two in a
disguised, seemingly innocent fashion which expresses only the positive
aspects" (p. 76). Such "paradoxical commentary" (Gurman, 1981) (which
identifies the function of an individual's symptom or the dominant interaction pattern of two or more people, and provides a positive connotation of

the recurrent behaviors of concern) aims to make explicit the covert interactions that produce symptoms or relationship distress, so that they may be better understood, and so that the conflicts they reflect may be handled overtly.

The "maintenance" of the presenting problem indicates an observer's (including the patient's) explanation of how a particular problem is kept going. It is similar to what behavior therapists refer to as a "functional analysis of behavior" (Ferster & Perrott, 1968; Kanfer & Saslow, 1969), in which the problem behavior is examined in the context of its possible controlling factors. Whereas behavior therapists' functional analyses traditionally emphasize explicit environmental events that can be objectively identified, effective brief therapy with couples and families, as well as with individuals, requires that the therapist cast a broader net in trying to formulate clinically useful hypotheses about why a given problem persists. To arrive at a workable focus for treatment, the brief therapist working with couples and families needs to maintain a balance between interactional and psychodynamic perspectives. While the behavioral emphasis on tracking the antecedents and consequences of a problematic behavior is maintained, it is extended to include covert events (i.e., thoughts, feelings) as well as overt events.

In what often seems to be a bewildering array of problems, feelings, and apparently disconnected interaction patterns that are revealed in sessions with more than one family member, it may be quite tempting for the brief therapist to seize upon a central treatment focus at once, if only to reduce his or her own confusion and anxiety. The interactions between and among family members, and each member's interaction with the therapist and responses to the therapist's observations, interpretations, and questions, usually provide the "data" for numerous possible appropriate treatment foci and choices of interventions, and for as many hypotheses about what factor or factors maintain the major presenting problem.

The key ingredient in identifying the major factors that control the presenting problem is the therapist's "mapping" of the relationship between the presenting problem and *both* (1) the interactional sequences within which the problem behavior (or recurrent feelings or thoughts) is embedded, and (2) the thoughts and feelings of family members in response to the problem. While the trend in many contemporary methods of family therapy has been decidedly in the direction of the therapist's attempting to influence patterns of overt interaction among family members (Gurman & Kniskern, 1981), the brief therapist needs to keep in mind at all times that the private, covert experiences of family members (i.e., their thoughts and feelings) may be perfectly appropriate major targets of therapeutic change (Bogdan, 1984; Feldman & Pinsof, 1982).

The importance of the interconnectness between thoughts and feelings on the one hand, and observable behavior on the other, cannot be overemphasized. It is made especially clear when the therapist recognizes that often in brief therapy, the most efficient and time-sensitive way of influencing patients' thoughts and feelings is to change the characteristic ways of behaving that reinforce maladaptive thinking and unwanted feelings (Gurman, 1981, 1985c). In addition to attending to the fundamental brief therapy issue of "Why now?", the therapist must be concerned with "*What* now?" questions in terms of both problem identification (the "substance" of the problem) and problem maintenance. Regardless of his or her theoretical allegiance, the brief therapist must adopt an attitude of "If it doesn't matter now, it doesn't matter." The importance of this issue cannot be overemphasized. Behaviorally oriented (e.g., Jacobson & Margolin, 1979), structurally oriented (e.g., Minuchin & Fishman, 1981), and interactionally oriented (e.g., Fisch, Weakland, & Segal, 1982) family therapists all assume this stance as a matter of course, but it is equally relevant to therapists of psychodynamic persuasions (e.g., Nadelson, 1978; Sager, 1981) who practice brief therapy. There is something that is almost inherently intellectually satisfying in speculating about the historical origins of patients' difficulties, and doing so is often necessary to create a sense of coherence about problems. But dwelling on history—except as a way of constructing such coherence for the therapist, and as a strategy for establishing a similar developmental–existential coherence for patients as a staging ground from which change can be induced—is intrinsically contrary to the aims of brief therapy. It is especially contrary to the aims of brief marital and family therapy, given the numerous (and obviously overlapping) personal stories that exist in any marriage or family.

The "locus" of the presenting problem from the patient's view is the fourth aspect of the presenting problem that the therapist may try to influence in initiating a shift or reframing of the patient's complaints or concerns. In this type of "therapist referral," the essential question is "*Where* is the problem?" The therapist may at times "relocate" the problem within an individual, even when the patient or patients locate it between family members.

For example, Joan and Larry presented their major concerns as their recently increased fighting and "power struggles." Although the content of their arguments varied somewhat, it was most often, and most intensely, focused on the issue of whether the couple would move to the East Coast from the Midwest after Larry finished his studies for a Ph.D. While this issue had been "sort of hanging around in the background for quite a while," as Joan put it, it had now become a "hot" issue since Larry had completed his required coursework about 4 months earlier; he now expected to finish his dissertation research within 4 or 5 more months, and had begun applying for university teaching positions in the Northeast. Although the couple, married for 6 years, had many common interests and friends, and although

Larry, hard-working and ambitious though he was, had almost always been able (in Joan's words) to "keep a reasonable balance between his academic life and his family life," she now complained that "if he takes a job at one of those high-powered, supercompetitive Eastern schools, he'll get so caught up in his work, I'll never see him!" Larry acknowledged that certainly being a junior faculty member at a prestigious university would be very demanding of him, but tried to reassure Joan of his intention to maintain the "reasonable balance" between career and home by reminding her of the "countless" occasions when he had put aside his work on weekends and for couple vacations, even during very pressured times, "because I *wanted* to be with you!"

Further discussion, carried on into the second interview, made it increasingly clear to the therapist that Joan's worries about Larry's future involvement with her were an "emotional decoy." Raised in a rather small Midwestern town, Joan's life experience had rarely taken her beyond the borders of the state in which she was born. At the age of 27, although she had a master's degree in a "moderately marketable field," Joan felt intimidated by what she expected "life in the real world" would be like. She had always done well in school and on the job by working hard to use her considerable aptitudes, but was convinced she would not "be able to measure up [in the 'big city,' so to speak] against other people [in her chosen field], when selling *yourself* is just as important as selling your abilities." Further discussion of her fears in the third session led to her referral to a combination therapy–support group for professional women. She also contracted with the therapist for the next 4 months for cognitive therapy to center on her self-defeating beliefs about her ability to deal with "the real world," and assertiveness training to center on experimenting with "being less anonymous at work, and trying to take more initiative with people at work, just like you usually take the initiative with tasks and responsibilities." The therapist met with Joan and Larry together only two more times—once in midtherapy, and once just after therapy with Joan—mostly to stay apprised of how the work Joan was doing in therapy was affecting Larry and the couple's relationship.

At other times, the therapist may "relocate" the presenting problem between family members other than those between whom the patient or patients locate the problem.

For comparative purposes, we may consider the case of Craig and Susan, who presented to the therapist with complaints that at first seemed to echo those of Joan and Larry. Susan was a fast-rising 31-year-old "star" in the computer software industry who had produced such a flurry of innovations in her field over the last 3 years that several major computer companies had sought her out for very lucrative research and development positions in their firms. The job that was especially attractive to Susan was one in the "Silicon Valley" area of California, not far from where she had grown up and where her parents, brother, and sister still lived. Craig, unlike Joan, had no concerns about his work competence or social skills, and was himself an accomplished computer expert at the age of 30. He was confident that he would be able to find a good job in California and said he liked the idea of "not having to live through 30 or 40 more Wisconsin winters!" But he could not "just forget my mother," who had become quite socially isolated, at least in part because of "not wanting to make waves with my father," who was "downright paranoid about where she goes and who she's with." Both members of the couple agreed that they got along quite well "except for Craig's preoccupation with his parents," as Susan described it.

Craig was the eldest of the three children in his family of origin, which included his alcoholic father and his "very dependent" mother. At the age of about 10, "when Dad really hit the skids," Craig's mother began to work outside the home, and Craig soon emerged as the overresponsible, parentified child ("Our family had three parents, except one of them wasn't," he quipped sarcastically). In addition to being a kind of "junior father" to his younger siblings, as a teenager he also often took the role of marital mediator, trying to "appear to stay neutral in their fights, but really I got involved in that stuff because I was afraid of what Dad might do to Mom. For some reason, Dad usually treated me OK even when he was stinking drunk and on the rampage against Mom, and I knew he would never lay a hand on me. I was on Mom's side all the time, but I had to act like I wasn't."

The "preoccupation with his parents" that Susan referred to involved frequent phone calls to his mother and visits to their home nearby, "to kind of check up on things" and (primarily in the last couple of years) to listen to his mother's complaints of desperation about his father. While his father's alcoholism has waxed and waned over the years, he was now a "more or less dry drunk" who had always refused to seek professional help for his alcohol abuse or for any other problems.

After two meetings with Susan and Craig, the therapist told them that he was impressed by the many strengths in their relationship. He continued, "Maybe if you two were going to stay on here in Wisconsin, you'd be able to struggle along with all this stuff about your mother, Craig. But eventually, what's coming up now would probably come up anyway—maybe when you two had kids, or if you went back to school to get your master's [degree]." The therapist said he thought the couple's marital problems could only be resolved if Craig could "stop feeling so responsible for your mother's welfare." The therapist added, "I don't think you'll be able to do this by just stopping being your mother's 'therapist'—you'd feel too guilty. You're going to have to believe that your mother can take care of herself better, that she can handle your father better, that she can have friends of her own, and so on." The therapist proposed that he and Craig work together, and that he would be a "kind of coach" for him to help him find some new ways to empower his mother.

Craig met with the therapist every week for 6 months. During that time, with the therapist's support, Craig had several "heart-to-heart" conversations with his mother, in which he told his mother he was worried about her, but that he had to let her take care of her own needs more, "for both our sakes." Predictably, his mother resisted this idea and tried to draw Craig back into her marital struggles. After about 3 months, Craig began to realize that he had to "get tough" with his mother and "draw the line somewhere." He managed to coax and cajole his mother to join a local Al-Anon group—at first accompanying her to meetings, and later insisting she go by herself. He also arranged a meeting between his mother and the minister of the local church that his mother attended irregularly, in a moderately successful effort to get his mother reinvolved with the church community, help her to develop some friendships, and so forth. At the time therapy ended, Craig was still feeling "sort of ambivalent" about moving to California, but also sufficiently encouraged about his mother's "progress" that he thought he and Susan could move "without me losing sleep about this—at least not *every* night!" In the last session, Craig said he was surprised that his father had not been nearly as vengeful to his mother for doing things for herself "as I thought he'd be. I should have gotten tougher with her a long time ago."

The first two types of "relocations" of presenting problems, discussed above, involve "reducing" the unit of treatment, as in the cases of Larry and Joan and of Susan and Craig (although had Craig's parents, or just his mother, been willing to participate in therapy, the treatment unit might have been shifted rather than reduced). In the general practice of psychotherapy, the third and probably most common therapist "relocation" of the presenting problem involves "expanding" the unit of treatment. Most often, this expansion follows one person's appearing by himself or herself at the initial interview.

There are three major variations on this theme of expanding the treatment unit. First, a patient may present with symptoms that readily lead the therapist to a diagnosis of a major psychiatric disorder, particularly common Axis I diagnoses such as depression, anxiety disorders (e.g., agoraphobia), alcoholism, or eating disorders. Since the courses of such disorders, including the rate of recovery and the probability of relapse, are known to be influenced positively by the inclusion in treatment of patients' family members (e.g., depression—Coyne, 1987; anxiety disorders—Barlow, O'Brien, & Last, 1984; Hafner, 1986; alcoholism—McCrady et al., 1986; O'Farrell, Cutter, & Floyd, 1985; Stanton et al., 1982; and eating disorders—Minuchin, Rosman, & Baker, 1978; Schwartz, Barrett, & Saba, 1983), it is essential that the brief therapist include the spouses of adult patients with such disorders in therapy as soon as possible, in order for an appropriate distribution of the therapeutic focus (on intrapersonal and/or physiological vs. interpersonal factors) to be arrived at. *By the time most patients with psychiatric disorders have their first session with a therapist, they have been struggling with the common interpersonal consequences of such problems in families—frustration, sadness, anger—so much that they are relieved when their therapist suggests including other involved and affected family members. Even those patients who do not see any way in which their problem is "caused" by relationship difficulties know intuitively that their interactions with family members concerning their symptoms affect the continuation and resolution of their problems. With those patients who deny or simply do not "see" the interaction between symptom maintenance and interpersonal behavior, one or two symptom-focused, yet systemically aware, assessment interviews usually generate enough "evidence" of the relationship between the two to allow the therapist to be convincing about the need for at least "an extended evaluation that includes your [spouse/other family member]."

The second common variation on the theme of expanding the treatment unit beyond one individual occurs when the presenting patient identifies relationship matters as central, yet is inclined to take on the problem as if it were his or her own. For example, James Framo (personal communication, 1981) tells the story of a woman who called for an initial appointment with him, describing in some detail her conflicts with her husband. When Framo asked, "OK, when might you and your husband be able to come in together?", the wife made it clear that she wanted to come by herself: "I don't want *him* to know we're having marital problems!" she replied.

Most patients who are inclined to "take too much credit" for their relationship problems when seen alone are motivated to do so either by something personal about themselves, or by something they attribute to other family members. One or more of the following may be true of the patient who seems to "prefer" to take on a relationship problem as if it were his or her own:

  1. The patient may have a secret (e.g., an extramarital affair) that has not yet been revealed to the therapist, and that he or she fears would be revealed under the pressure of the other family member's presence—or, more likely, that he or she intends to tell the therapist about soon.

*When children or adolescents are diagnosed as having a major psychiatric disorder, there usually is no issue of at least one parent's presence at the start of therapy, since children never, and adolescents almost never, seek help for and by themselves. Expanding the unit of treatment (e.g., drawing in a reluctant father) or involving parents as copatients when a child has a discernible disorder is usually achieved much more readily than when an adult has a major psychiatric disorder.

2. The patient may feel excessively guilty about or overly responsible for the relationship difficulties. Such a person may feel and be this way because of an enduring personality style marked by inordinate self-criticism, inhibition of anger, or a maladaptive assumption of traditional gender roles in close relationships (e.g., "The woman has the responsibility to make things go right in a marriage").

3. The patient may insist that the other family member in question doesn't believe in "shrinks," in talking to anyone outside the family about family matters, and so on; or the patient may say that the other person "thinks it's all my problem [or my doing], anyway."

4. The patient may express concern that involving the other person would "upset" him or her too much; this may be an accurate prediction, but it is at least as likely to be a projection of the patient's own fear of dealing with the other family member.

In each of these situations, the therapist needs to communicate empathically but without hesitation that while the patient's reasons for not wanting the other family members involved are very important and may need to be discussed further, it will probably be best if these concerns are dealt with together with the other persons and the therapist, or at least after the therapist has had a chance to meet the others. If the therapist takes such a position, but does so too gingerly, the patient will pick up on the therapist's tentativeness and balk at the idea. Undoubtedly, some therapists may not believe that problem situations of the sort we are discussing here (i.e., acknowledged relationship problems require conjoint treatment. But if the brief therapist does believe that the interpersonal aspects of the presenting problem require conjoint treatment (of whatever theoretical orientation), yet (perhaps out of his or her own anxiety about pressing the matter) backs off from this position, the focus of the "individual therapy by default" will almost certainly be variable and unclear, and the course of therapy will be unduly and unnecessarily lengthened.

The third very common scenario of expanding the unit of treatment occurs when the patient identifies a distressing relationship problem from the outset and acknowledges that the relevant "other" family member or members also see the problem as relational. Except in those few situations in which another person does not or cannot appear at the first interview because of genuine extenuating circumstances (patients sometimes really do get flat tires, have children with ear infections, etc.), the therapist might wonder, aloud or privately, about the meaning of that person's absence. It is useful to do this in order to anticipate what sorts of alliance-building issues may be particularly important when this other person does appear. Expanding the therapeutic unit in situations of this sort, of course, usually progresses without a hitch, or at least with very few. Sometimes, little more is at issue then (usually) the couple's joint decision for one of them to "scout out" the therapist and the therapy situation (i.e., to see whether the therapist seems trustworthy and safe). While this task division may say a lot about the couple, it usually does not portend poorly for engaging with the other person.

In summary, then, therapist-initiated, attribution-oriented "reframing referrals" address these questions: "What is the problem?"; "Is the problem just 'bad,' or does it have 'desirable' consequences?"; "What keeps the problem going/prevents it from being resolved?"; and "Where is the problem? That is, who else is significantly involved in the problem, and in what ways?"

Intervention-Oriented Reframing. The second type of "reframing referral" addresses the all-important matter not of what the problem is or where it is (since therapists of different theoretical persuasions might agree on the answers to these questions, but disagree about what to do next), but *who should be included in ongoing therapy*—both in terms of maximizing the likelihood of a positive outcome, and in terms of establishing and maintaining a clear therapeutic focus in order not to extend the therapy longer than is necessary.

In considering the matter of who should be included in treatment, it is essential to note that the therapist may "relocate" the presenting problem for either or both of two main reasons: (1) The initial clinical assessment may make it clear that the factors controlling the presenting problem are very different from the patient's (or patients') beliefs about what and who maintain the problem; or (2) the therapist may judge that some choices about who continues in therapy are more likely to lead to change than others. Thus, for example, even though there may clearly be a marital problem, conjoint treatment of the husband and wife may not be the arrangement of choice, and working with one spouse alone (or each spouse alone) may be more effective. Likewise, even though one patient may carry the symptoms, it is often helpful to work with more than just the "identified patient," as we have pointed out earlier. A crucial consideration in the therapist's decision about whom to include in ongoing treatment is each possibly relevant family member's readiness for change, as we have discussed in other chapters. This notion is very similar to Fisch *et al.*'s (1982) emphasis that treatment of relational problems does not automatically require all involved family members, but does require that participation of the family member who is most motivated for change. In our experience, nonetheless, we have found that for most relationship problems, inclusion of more than one person is usually the optimal treatment format, though again (as in all brief therapy), the therapist's flexibility is essential.

The central question the therapist must consider regarding whom to include in treatment is whether to expand or reduce the unit of treatment, relative to who is present at the initial session. In general, careful consideration of the substance, valence, maintenance, and locus of the presenting problem will contribute a great deal to making this decision, and may even be sufficient for doing so. But in addition to this general orienting framework, two other specific guidelines are very useful.

As we have emphasized throughout this book, adults seen in brief therapy, with few exceptions, should be seen as part of the initial evaluation process with their "significant others." Typically, this means all those people with whom the identified patient lives over time. But this statement requires some essential qualifications. First, the identified patient may not literally (i.e., geographically) live with his or her "significant others," though he or she may emotionally live with them, as in the cases of college students who are away at school, married couples involved in a "commuter marriage," or adults whose parents live at some distance. Despite the idealized notion some therapists maintain of having all family members present at the outset of therapy (if not all the way through therapy), practical considerations often preclude practicing therapy in such a fantasy world. But aiming for this fantasy, while accepting reality, is justifiable, because it is usually much easier to "discharge" from ongoing treatment those persons who do not appear essential to resolving the problem at hand (or who may seriously interfere with or slow down the process of doing so) that to try to entice people into ongoing treatment long after it has begun with other family members. If an adequate alliance is established with all those present in, say, the first one to three evaluation sessions, bringing those who have been "discharged" back into treatment at a later stage is usually not problematic.

On the other hand, trying to introduce new participants into ongoing therapy often raises serious strategic problems. For example, the therapist by then may have established such a strong alliance with the ongoing participants that it will require a great deal of effort to balance his or her alliance among all those included in therapy at later stages. It may also require a (preventable) expenditure of time to do so—for example, by holding individual sessions with the newly arrived participants, so that they feel they are being attended to equitably and are being provided enough "air time" for their thoughts and feelings to be understood. The dangers of arbitrarily excluding potentially important family members before therapy is under way have been dramatically described and illustrated by Hurvitz (1967) in his discussion of treating marital problems by seeing one partner alone. Hurvitz notes several recurrent problems in such a practice: (1) transferential complications of the marital relationship; (2) an implicit message that the couple's own efforts to work out their problems are less important than the efforts of the therapist; (3) provision of a setting in which the other spouse is disparaged by the patient, thus reinforcing negative attitudes toward that person; (4) the nonparticipating spouse's increasing feelings of inadequacy as the patient spouse achieves personal gains from therapy; and (5) increasing the absent spouse's resistance to the patient's efforts to change the couple's patterns of relating to each other. Such unfortunate by-products of the arbitrary exclusion of the spouse may not only add unnecessarily to the length of therapy by adding "iatrogenic" problems to the clinical problems of concern, but may even be associated with destructive negative outcomes (Gurman & Kniskern, 1978a). Moreover, as Kohl (1962) has illustrated, treating one marital partner "successfully" may precipitate a pathological reaction or major psychiatric disturbance in the nonparticipating spouse. Such an occurrence is particularly likely when the core structure and most basic implicit "rules" of the marriage have been organized for an extended period of time around the treated patient's symptoms.

A second qualification about the inclusion of significant others is that the "significant others" relative to a given individual's problem may not be limited to members of that person's family. Especially in cases of childhood and adolescent difficulties, people outside the "live-in" family are likely to be massively involved in the problem, as the major complainants and/or maintaining forces of the problem.

Third, while we believe that the initial evaluation in brief therapy should begin whenever possible with these variously defined "significant others," the flexibility required of the brief therapist must also include the possibility of including different family members, or combinations of family members, in treatment at different points in therapy. For example, although in "mainstream" marital and family therapy there has been prejudice against the use of individual interviews in both the assessment and ongoing phases of therapy, there are numerous situations in which such meetings are indicated (Berman, 1982; Feldman & Pinsof, 1982). Some reasons for individual sessions are as follows: (1) to aid a failing or poorly established therapist–patient rapport and alliance, or to aid working on severe transference or countertransference impediments to change; (2) to minimize reinforcement of family members' views of one person as "the sick one"; (3) to assess a marital partner's commitment to his or her marriage when that person is evasive about his or her commitment in conjoint sessions; (4) to confront a family member about "missing links" of information that the therapist suspects are being withheld, and the withholding of which may be stalemating the therapy; and (5) to make it possible to go on with therapy when the verbal (and less frequently, physical) hostility between family members in conjoint sessions is so high and unmanageable that useful therapeutic work cannot continue in that context. Brewster and Montie (1987) emphasize that in the real world of family therapy and of treating relationship problems, variations in who is actually treated, and deviations from the idealized standard of working with whole family units (e.g., individual sessions), are commonplace and need not imply abandonment of a systemic–interpersonal perspective.

The second guideline we find to be especially valuable in decisions about whom to include on therapy and when derives from Skynner's (1976, 1981) notion of the "minimum sufficient network" for therapeutic change. Skynner's notion overlaps with Fisch *et al*'s. (1982) idea, based on interactional therapy of working with the most motivated family member or members (who may be the complainants, but may not be the "patients"); it also overlaps with Stanton's (1981) idea, based on structural–strategic therapy, of including the "systems of import" (i.e., those persons involved in the maintenance of the problem). Skynner (1981) operationalizes the notion of the minimum sufficient network as follows: "[N]ot only the *problem*, but the *motivation* to do something about the problem and the *capacity* to do something about it must all be brought together, if these functions reside in different persons" (p. 58; italics in original).

Thus consider, for example, two similar-sounding and common clinical situations. In both situations, the wife initiates therapy, complaining about her increasing disenchantment with her marriage and emphasizing her husband's emotional distance. In the first case, the wife has "reached her limit" and is very seriously considering a divorce, and has already taken some preliminary steps in that direction. She cannot yet muster the courage to leave and is feeling quite guilty about wanting to leave, aware that doing so will meet with tremendous disapproval from her family and her husband's family. Assuming that divorce is an economically viable possibility for her, that she has a reasonably supportive social network available, and so on, she has both the capacity to do something about her feeling of emptiness in her marriage and the potential for reducing her feelings of guilt. Her presence in therapy clearly contains both the problem (her dissatisfaction) and the motivation to resolve the problem. In the second case, the wife has not yet taken any steps toward separation or divorce. Though her complaints about her husband sound nearly identical to those of the first wife, she presents the problem of how to get her husband to be more intimate with her. In this situation, the problem (marital dissatisfaction) and the motivation for change are present in the wife, but it is most likely that she does not have the capacity to bring about the change she desires by herself. Indeed, her seeking the help of a therapist probably constitutes a conscious recognition that she has tried everything she could to bring about the changes she wants. It is her husband who may have the capacity to bring about the changes she wants. While her inclusion in therapy will probably be essential, it will probably not be sufficient. In contrast, the wife in the first case may be quite capable, in terms of both personal and social resources, to resolve her problem as stated, in therapy that does not include her husband.

Skynner's three-component guide for deciding who should be included in therapy lends an extremely important elaboration to the traditional notion of who are the "significant others" for a given patient. The significance of "others" is defined not in terms of sociological roles, but in terms of who has the problem, who has the motivation to resolve the problem, and who may have the power to do so. Thus, from the perspectives of both systemic assessment and the functional analysis of behavior (Ferster & Perrott, 1968), a therapist should not assume who may be "significant" people for resolving a clinical problem, but must *assess* their significance. Beginning therapy whenever possible with as many of the cast of characters who may be significant is almost always a more reliable and efficient route for making this fundamental clinical decision.

Early Intervention and the Establishment of Therapeutic Alliances

The brief therapist treating marital and family problems in a conjoint format faces numerous challenges throughout his or her time with the family. One of the most central challenges arises at the very outset of their work together, and is fundamental not only to the eventual outcome of treatment, but also to the question of whether treatment will follow the briefest course possible. The brief therapist aims to help induce change as soon as possible; yet a working alliance with the couple or family must be established for the anxiety-arousing process of change to begin. Thus, the therapist may feel pulled in what seem to be competing directions.

The Types of Therapeutic Alliances

At the same time, the brief therapist working with a couple or family faces the challenge of having to attend to multiple therapeutic alliances simultaneously (Gurman, 1981). Unlike the situation in one-on-one therapy, in which the therapist needs to build an alliance with only one person, the therapist treating couples and families needs to attend to three sets of alliances: the therapist–patient alliance, the therapist–couple or therapist–family alliance, and the family–family alliance, each of which is considered below. Thus, the brief therapist is attending to the establishment of complex therapeutic alliances and attempting to begin the process of change, all at the same time. Since many cases of marital or family therapy will flounder if therapeutic alliances are not attended to adequately, especially at the outset of treatment, all early interventions directed toward producing change within the marriage or family should ideally facilitate the patient–therapist alliance, or at least should be carried out with sufficient awareness of this alliance that its development is not impeded. Likewise, early interventions should aim to facilitate working alliances between and working among family members. Let us briefly consider each of the three sets of alliances that need to be developed early.

The therapist–patient alliance is that needing to be established between the therapist and each individual family member present. Each family member should find something of personal value in the first session; this may be achieved in different ways for different people, and for different people within the same family. For some (e.g., young children), receiving the therapist's empathy and warmth is sufficient. Others may require some sense of increased cognitive understanding of the presenting problem—its etiology, maintenance, or relationship to treatment options—or some sense of initial direction for behavior change outside the consultation room. In all therapy, the therapist–patient alliance is critical; in brief family therapy, it is initially fragile as well. Repairs to breaks in the therapist–patient alliance in individual therapy are more easily achieved than in marital and family therapy, where one person's refusal to continue treatment may seriously compromise the treatment endeavor. Naturally, it is incumbent upon the therapist to establish at least a minimal alliance with those family members most likely to constitute the "minimum sufficient network" for change discussed earlier. But since failure to establish an initial alliance with each family member may impede an adequate assessment of whom constitutes this minimal unit, alliance building must be multidirected.

The therapist–couple or therapist–family alliance differs from the therapist–patient alliance, inasmuch as it is the sense of alliance established with the couple or family as a dynamically related and irreducible unit. This alliance is usually fostered well in early sessions by listening for and speaking in the family's vernacular. In mirroring (and thus showing awareness of and respect for) the family's characteristic ways of handling tension, its characteristic ways of communicating caring, its rituals, its heritage, its history, and its connections with the world outside its biological boundaries, the therapist conveys an appreciation of what goes into this family's uniqueness. Just as no two individuals are identical, so no two families are identical, despite their commonalities. It is this quality the therapist needs to see and hear and reflect back to the couple or family. In so doing, the therapist helps to establish a bond with the couple or family group that transcends his or her responsiveness to the individual members of the family.

The building of the family–family alliance—or, more accurately, the family member–family member alliance—refers to the therapist's fostering of an empathic and collaborative set (Jacobson & Margolin, 1979) between and among spouses or family members. Couples in crises and families in distress can be predicted with confidence to detail and even exaggerate their differences in everything from styles of relating to personal tastes. While some or many of these differences may be quite real, it is essential in all family therapy, and especialy in brief family therapy, that the therapist recognize the similarities (if not commonalities) among family members. Straightforward inquiry about what family members value in each other individually and in their family (or marriage) as a whole, combined with the therapist's reflecting information and observations about unspoken alliances and loyalties, is crucial to the therapist's initial efforts to foster a sufficient sense of collaboration among family members to allow them to confront what is often a painful process of change.

Another central element in fostering this sense of common purpose (in addition, of course, to more individual, idiosyncratic purposes) is the way in which treatment goals are formulated and negotiated with the couple or family early in therapy. It is usually helpful for the enhancement of family collaboration for the therapist (1) to acknowledge and empathically summarize each person's major complaints, fears, and wishes; and (2) to suggest or illustrate to the family how the achievement of these apparently disparate aims may be linked. In so doing, of course, the therapist simultaneously strengthens the family's internal working alliance and his or her alliance with each family member.

Special Considerations in Altering the Unit of Treatment

While these considerations on establishing the three types of treatment alliances needed in brief family therapy apply to all contexts in couples and family treatment, some special alliance-building considerations apply when the therapist decides to expand or reduce the unit of treatment. When introducing new family members into therapy after first meeting with other family members (and presumably having established the beginnings of a working alliance with them), it is essential that the new participant's presence receive special recognition. Because the new participant will usually have been brought into the therapy at the therapist's initiative and urging, the therapist must assume the responsibility for orienting the new family member to therapy. This can generally be accomplished by summarizing the major themes that have emerged from previous sessions and by explicitly identifying the therapist's reasons for desiring the new person's presence. New arrivals to the therapy are often quite anxious about why they have been invited in (and frequently assume or fear that they have already been identified by their relatives or by the therapist as the villain, the cause of others' symptoms or distress, etc.), irrespective of what others in the family may have told them. A commonly helpful way of dealing with such anticipated anxiety is for the therapist to present his or her reason for wanting the new arrival's participation in terms of how it may be helpful to the *therapist* to understand more fully what has already been discussed in previous meetings. That is, the new arrival has been invited in as a sort of consultant to the therapist. Defining the relationship between the new arrival and the therapist in this way, or some variation of it, temporarily elevates the status of this person and tends to counterbalance both other family members' faulty attributions about this person and the person's one-down position.

When a new family member is introduced into a therapy that is clearly focused on interpersonal conflict, that person usually becomes absorbed into the process in quite a natural way, since the issues at hand inherently involve and include that person. On the other hand, involving the new arrival in a situation in which there has been a clearly identified "patient" (e.g., a depression, phobia, etc., is present) is often more difficult. While later in the treatment the new arrival may participate as a genuine copatient, nonsymptomatic family members often have genuine confusion and uncertainty at first about the need for their involvement in treatment They see the "patient" family member as "containing" the problem, and may question the need for their own presence. Even if the therapist has some well-formulated ideas about how the new arrival may be involved in the maintenance of the "patient's" problem, such thoughts are often best kept to oneself in the initial meeting that includes the new arrival. If the new arrival is sufficiently nondefensive that his or her problem-maintaining involvement can be identified and discussed overtly, such an opportunity should not, of course, be passed up. But if this is not the case, the therapist must strive for and be satisfied with a less ambitious aim for this meeting. If the therapist believes that the new arrival's continuing treatment participation is necessary, it is the therapist's task to help that person find something of potential personal gain to be realized by the elimination or reduction of the "patient's" symptoms. With family members who are more hesitant to continue, a tack that often generates motivation to return involves both the therapist's and the family's anticipating and speculating about the consequences of symptomatic change for particular family relationships (e.g., the marriage). While such an inquiry is almost always useful, it is particularly pertinent when the symptomatic family member has been symptomatic for a relatively long period. A "long period" may be usefully defined operationally and simply to families as any period of time in which the marital or family life of this couple or family has become significantly and regularly organized around the symptoms of the "patient" family member. The therapist may advise the couple or family that the nonsymptomatic member(s) should remain in treatment in order to deal with the important ways in which the family life will inevitably need to reorganize as the "patient" member's symptoms improve.

Patty, a 41-year-old married mother of two teenage children, was referred to one of us for "behavioral treatment" of her long-standing agoraphobia and generalized anxiety. Her referring pysician, an internist who had been a student of the therapist while in medical school, had been treating her intermittently with general support and moderate doses of antianxiety drugs for almost a year. Patty had been in individual behavior therapy with another therapist for almost a year about 3 years earlier, and felt that his work with her had been "moderately helpful." Patty had found her counseling with her internist to be useful in helping her maintain some of the gains she had achieved with her previous psychotherapist. She had recently stopped her intermittent sessions with her physician at the insistence of her husband, Mike. Mike, a very successful local land developer, had recently become irate with Patty because of her "refusal" (i.e., fear) to accompany him on an out-of-state business trip for which Mike thought "it was very important that I go with him for the social parts of the meeting." Mike demanded that Patty see a "real therapist who really knew about phobias." Patty's internist, apparently made to feel quite uncomfortable by being challenged in this way, quickly acceded to Patty's request for such a referral.

Patty attended the first session alone. From her description, it was clear that Mike had been excluded from both her counseling with her internist and her earlier behavior therapy experience. Though Mike had complained on occasion about not being invited into those treatments, these complaints sounded quite perfunctory. In fact, he was apparently enraged at the degree to which Patty's anxieties and agoraphobia had interfered with both their married life and his professional life; by Patty's report, he seemed clearly to view himself as a sort of victim of/bystander to what he sarcastically called "Patty's peculiarities" (i.e., her phobia).

In addition to conducting a detailed behavioral analysis of Patty's agoraphobic behavior and related anxiety (which appeared to load heavily on social anxiety, with concerns about others' evaluation and approval of her), and discussing the precise nature of her previous behavioral treatment, Patty and the therapist also addressed her husband's responses to her expressions of anxiety and to her demonstrably avoidant behavior. The therapist's impressions were that while Mike had shown a moderate degree of effort to be supportive, reassuring, or otherwise helpful to Patty several years earlier when her agoraphobia had first manifested itself, in recent years he had largely been angry at her and critical of her waxing and waning evidence of symptomatic improvement. Therefore, anticipating that Mike might actually slow Patty's progress in therapy if it were less than very rapid (even though, or perhaps, because she was now seeing a "real" therapist), the clinician asked Patty to invite Mike to join her for the second session. She was to tell her husband that "Dr._____ said he thinks he has a pretty good understanding of my problem and has some ideas how to go about treating it, but he's found in case after case that a phobic person's husband or wife almost always has some ideas about this kind of problem and how to solve it that are very valuable to him." Thus, Mike was to be invited in not to be castigated for his less-than-optimal emotional support of his wife (of which she often complained), but to serve as a quasi-consultant to the therapist. The therapist added that if Mike refused to accompany her or seemed hesitant, Patty should not argue the issue with him at all, but simply say, "Dr._____ also said that if you weren't sure you wanted to go with me, but would like to talk to him about the idea first, you could just call him, and he'd be glad to talk it over with you."

Given the degree to which Patty's phobia had become a sort of central organizing dimension of the couple's life, it was not surprising that Mike consented to attend the second session. In that session, the therapist first reviewed that he had learned about "Patty's problem" and tentatively outlined some possible behavioral treatment strategies he was considering, which seemed not to have formed a part of her earlier behavioral treatment. Approximately the first half of the session also involved detailed discussion with Mike about "Patty's problem"—its history, the form it took, when it was most severe, and so forth. Given both Mike's view that the problem was Patty's, not his, and his negative feelings about not having been included in his wife's previous treatments, the therapist thought it was essential in establishing an early alliance with Mike to be consistent with his implicit message about Mike's role in the therapy ("You can be my expert consultant"). Although Mike's demeanor for the first few minutes was cautious bordering on suspicious, by about the end of the first half of the session, he seemed to have relaxed quite a bit and to be fully engaged. (In an initial session with a couple like this, paying such consistent attention to one spouse might be a potentially major technical error, but it was essential to reduce Mike's defensiveness and facilitate his involvement. Moreover, the therapist felt confident that he and Patty had connected well in their first session, and that this early alliance with her was strong enough to allow such a focus on her husband's perceptions, ideas, feelings, etc.)

At about the middle of the session, the therapist switched the focus. He summarized the major patterns of behavior and feelings of which he was aware that demonstrated how central "Patty's problem" had become in the couple's lives. He then pointed out that while he firmly believed that both members of the couple wanted "Patty's problem" to be solved, "people often get themselves into 'habits' in how they live with each other. Even though they don't like them, these habits have a way of continuing anyway." He then invited both Mike and Patty to speculate about the many possible consequences of change in "Patty's problem". "People sometimes think that when a problem gets solved, it's solved, and that's it. It's as if they think that nothing else will change along the way. I know this may sound like an odd question, but—let your imagination fly just a bit—can you imagine any kind of undesirable consequences to Patty's getting over her problem? After all, even that good old silver lining might have a few clouds around it!"

This issue was presented in such a way as to address a very serious matter, but in a moderately playful way. Patty and Mike both were able to describe some genuinely worrisome possibilities that could follow her improvement (e.g., "I suppose she might start running around on me"; "I might go to business school myself and be better at making money than he is"), as well as some lighter possibilities (e.g., "Maybe she'll get so sure of herself she"ll run for President!"). With such an approach, the therapist helped to broaden the couple's view of the problem (i.e., helped them see that the "problem" also contained its current consequences and the consequences of its changing), connected it to "new" aspects of their lives together (thus making the problem more of an active than a possive concept), and demonstrated to Mike that while he could not solve "Patty's problem" (though he could, and eventually would, assist her in exposure therapy), there were "some potentially difficult aspects of 'Patty's problem' that really could become as much your problem as hers, so you have more to gain by being involved in the behavior therapy than just, hopefully, having a wife who's not anxious so much of the time."

By way of contrast, when the therapist chooses to "discharge" certain family members from ongoing treatment, it is incumbent upon the therapist to do so in a way that does not imply disregard for their feelings or concerns, or in a way that attributes to them malevolence or lack of caring about the problems at hand. Leaving "discharged" family members with the sense that they are appreicated for having contributed something of real importance to the therapist's understanding of the problem, and/or the therapist's chances of being helpful in its resolution, is what is necessary. It is very important in all family therapy, and especially in brief therapy, that the therapist try to avoid taking actions that are likely to compromise his or her chances of reinvolving "discharged" family members at a later time. The therapist's maintenance of a position of "maneuverability" (Fisch *et al.*, 1982) is fundamental in brief treatment. As Fisch *et al.* note, "A therapist needs to keep his options open as therapy progresses, shifting as needed during the course of treatment" (1982, p. 22).

MARITAL AND FAMILY ASSESSMENT

Two fundamental and major issues involved in the initiation of marital and family therapy have now been considered: "What is the problem?" and "Who is the patient?" We have seen that specifying and defining the problem in situations of marital and family conflict inherently and simultaneously require the therapist to consider who is most significantly involved in the maintenance of the problem, at what system level the problem is located, and who is to be involved in the resolution of the problem. In addition to these assessment considerations, which are necessary ones for the therapist's collaborative organizing of the purposes and goals of therapy, there are particular dimensions of marital and family relationships that also require the therapist's attention in order to formulate a plan for intervention.

In this section, we suggest a number of assessment parameters that we believe are essential in the planning and conduct of therapy with couples and families, regardless of the presenting problem, and irrespective of who is ultimately included in ongoing treatment. Very often, presenting problems are posed that fall immediately under one or more of these dimensions of overall relationship functioning. At other times, the problem or problems that bring the couple or family to therapy are not described in terms of any of these dimensions. Even in the latter type of situation, the therapist's assessment on these domains of family life will usually prove crucial to a fuller understanding of the nature and meaning of the problem; the scope of impact of the problem; and the interpersonal forces, patterns, and areas of difficulty within the marriage or family that maintain the problem. Attending to these dimensions will also increase the therapist's awareness of the strengths and resources a couple or family can bring to bear on problem resolution—a consideration often overlooked and underused in psychotherapy generally and within family therapy as well (Karpel, 1986). As emphasized numerous times and in numerous ways in this book, the brief therapist must place a high value on a health orientation rather than an illness orientation; must emphasize being in the world rather than being in therapy, as well as patients' taking the initiative outside the consulting room; and should use the least radical or invasive intervention possible in each case. To further these ends and implement these values, taking a comprehensive view of the couple or family, while still working toward a clear focus for treatment, is necessary.

The dimensions of couple and family assessment emphasized here are drawn from several methods of family therapy and models of family functioning, particularly structural (e.g., Jacobson & Margolin, 1979), psychodynamic (e.g., Sager, 1976, 1981) and problem-centered (Epstein & Bishop, 1981; Pinsof, 1983). As Liddle (1983) has emphasized, "It is insufficient to think of family diagnosis without understanding the corresponding and overarching model of therapy . . . the therapist's diagnostic findings and conclusions are woven into the fabric of the practical model of therapy, since the lens of the therapy model inevitably affects his or her diagnosis and assessment" (p. 3). Though our assessment schema derives from several approaches to therapy, some of which have been argued to be incompatible with one another, it does not reflect a random hodge-podge of elements. Rather, it reflects both the values and the technical aspects of our overall philosophy of brief treatment, with its emphases on (1) the recursive, reciprocal interplay between the interpersonal and the intrapersonal, and among the behavioral, affective, and cognitive realms of human experience; (2) current life experience and difficulties seen both in contemporary and in evolutionary, developmental perspectives, with change of both individuals and relationship systems assumed to be inevitable; (3) resolution of the presenting problem(s) for which treatment is sought; and (4) the potential healing capacities that exist both within and between people.

Dimensions of Assessment

In considering how the therapist goes about his or her assessment of a couple or family in brief therapy, some guidelines are in order. First, it is not advisable to view these assessment dimensions as all requiring detailed review and investigation in the first family session, as, for example, one might expect to do in a mental status exam with an individual. In our experience, a truly comprehensive family assessment typically requires at least two and sometimes three or four visits of about an hour each. How many areas of the family assessment the therapist will be able to address depends on several factors. A therapist who is comfortable with and skilled at taking charge of the direction, depth, and flow of early sessions will, of course, gain greater access to multiple aspects of family relationships. With families and couples who present in an acute emergency or in an intense crisis, comprehenisve assessment may well need to take a back seat to management considerations, short-term problem solving, and anxiety reduction. Even in the absence of an acute crisis, some families' characteristic styles of interacting will be so chaotic or hostile—or, at the other extreme, cautious—that the therapist's containment of chaos, modulation of strong negative feelings, or eliciting of active participation in the interview will be sufficiently challenging to preclude anything approaching a broad-scale assessment in the first session. Conversely, some couples and families will be so well focused and articulate about their problems and themselves, and so easily engaged affectively, that they will launch into rather profound and at times quite moving change-inducing dialogue with each other and with the therapist within the first session. In such (admittedly infrequent, yet quite real) situations, it is certainly best to facilitate the change process that is visibly under way, and it is certainly unwise to interrupt it because of the therapist's agenda (e.g., an insistence on a wide-ranging assessment). Most initial and early interviews will have a flavor of coherence and collaboration somewhere in between these extremes, and even in these modal circumstances, more than one session will be needed for an adequate assessment of the couple's or family's overall functioning. As emphasized earlier in this chapter in considering the multiple strands of treatment alliances that need to be attended to early in brief couples and family work, the therapist's need to understand the family or couple must not take precedence over his or her need to connect with family members.

A second important guideline for the conduct of the family assessment is that the various assessment dimensions are not all tapped in the same way. Some are dealt with via family members' self-report; others are dealt with only by means of the therapist's direct observation of behavior; and still others are dealt with only by means of the therapist's inferences. To state this another way, only parts of the therapist's assessment are conducted explicitly. In parallel fashion, not everything the therapist comes to understand about the family needs to be shared with them (if this were, indeed, even possible). In a related vein, as Haley (1976) has argued, it is probably not especially helpful to tell patients what they already know about themselves.

Finally, in any therapeutic assessment situation, but especially in brief therapy, all dimensions of assessment do not require equal emphasis. In most cases, a few areas of assessment will clearly stand out as especially pertinent to the therapist's understanding of the nature and maintenance of the problem(s) at hand, and some will rapidly be revealed to be of little (or even no) functional significance or relevance to the matters at hand. For example, some areas that pertain to the husband–wife relationship may be of limited or no concern in dealing with parent–child problems; conversely, some aspects of parent–child interaction may be quite irrelevant to problems presented in the marital domain.

Dimensions That Apply Both to Families and to Couples

Presenting Problems, Attempted Solutions, and the Consequences of Change. Taking seriously a couple or family's presenting problem(s), whether stated as interpersonal conflict or as psychiatric symptoms, is, of course, axiomatic in brief therapy, and we have discussed this matter in detail throughout this book. As others (e.g., Fisch *et al.*, 1982) have stressed, eliciting clear descriptions of the varied (and usually manifold) solutions of the problem that have been tried by individuals in the family, or by pairs or even larger subgroups of family members, is of equal practical value. Attempted but unsuccessful solutions to problems are as much a part of the problem as the unwanted thoughts, behaviors, and feelings themselves. This is particularly the case when the same class of unsuccessful solution efforts have been chronically applied to the problem at issue (e.g., futile attempts to "cheer up" a depressed person; demanding "spontaneous" shows of affection; etc.). No therapist wants to, and no brief therapist can afford to, recreate the family problem by repeating efforts at inducing change that have failed.

Of enormous importance is learning via family members' reports and direct observation, about the typical sequence(s) of interaction (and associated thoughts and feelings) that accompany displays of the problem. An often-overlooked attempted solution involves previous unsuccessful experiences in psychotherapy, which, of course, should not be replicated.

Problem-maintaining behavior—in particular, the repeated use of unsuccessful "solutions"—itself may be maintained by avoidance of the consequences of change. As Papp (1983) has emphasized, individual symptoms are often maintained by family-system-wide behavior that prevents the full-scale emergence of problems elsewhere in the family. Interactional "symptoms" or problems may be maintained in the same manner, as illustrated earlier in this chapter in our description of the case of the M family. In the brief therapy of marital and family conflict, it is essential that the therapist not limit his or her assessment focus to "the problem" as defined by the couple or family, but also anticipate and attempt to predict the likely consequences of the "successful" resolution of the presenting problem. The "successful" resolution of an individual's symptoms or of a particular inter-actional difficulty may carry significant negative ramifications for the func-tioning of *other* individuals or for other relationships within the family system, including extended-family subsystems not participating in treat-ment. While never losing sight of the presenting problem of the family or dismissing its importance, the brief therapist must consider the possibility that the focus of treatment may need to include the unacknowledged conse-quences of change as much as, or more than, the more obvious difficulty for which help is being sought.

Individual and Family/Couple Assets and Strengths. No matter how disorganized, disengaged, or enraged a couple or family may be, each family has knowable assets and strengths in each of its members and in its unity as a system. It is important that the brief therapist discover these assets and strengths, for two reasons. First, they may be called upon directly to aid the process of change (e.g., an emotionally distant father with great skill as a musician may be urged to share his musical knowledge and appreciation with his children). Second, simply identifying such positive characteristics may be crucial in the formation of the therapeutic alliance. While it is possible to do effective brief therapy with people toward whom one lacks positive feelings, it is easier to do so when a therapist finds *some* aspect of each family member attractive. For example, one of us had met for several sessions with a couple in which the husband was extraordinarily arrogant, controlling, and apparently insensitive to everyone. Arriving a few minutes late for the next session, the therapist, an avid gardener, found the husband eagerly studying a flower catalog from the coffee table in his office. The therapist and the husband got into an enthusiastic conversation about perennial borders. Not only had the therapist found something in common with the husband; he had also discovered a nurturant side of this usually abrasive man.

Just as individuals have assets and strengths, so, too, do couples and families, and it is valuable for the therapist–family or therapist–couple alliance that such characteristics be acknowledged and appreciated. For example, the members of a family that had experienced more than its share of emotional, medical, and financial tragedies were complimented on their "incredible perseverance and refusal to give up on life," even though these family qualities had little to do with (the content of) the problem they brought to therapy.

Communication and Problem-Solving Skills and Styles. Although some influential family therapists prefer to work quite indirectly in facilitat-ing change (e.g., Fisch *et al.*, 1982; Halen, 1976; Selvini-Palazzoli *et al.*, 1978), there is overwhelming research evidence that family members' com-munication skills and problem-solving skills are predictive of treatment outcome (Gurman *et al.*, 1986). Indeed, they may constitute the single most important class of behavior change with both couples (Jacobson, 1978) and families (Robin & Foster, in press). Where such interpersonal skills appear not to exist to a sufficient degree, they must be prompted, modeled, and coached by the therapist. Indirection cannot draw forth skills that have never been learned adequately.

In assessing individuals' communication and problem-solving skills, however, it is of paramount importance to distinguish between problems of acquisition and problems of performance. Some people simply have never learned the kinds of interpersonal skills that help to foster effective marital and family functioning, and can be said to face the challenge of acquiring these skills. Many other people, however, demonstrate that they have in fact learned such skills, but do not show them within the family. They are "good listeners" with colleagues and co-workers; they are sometimes even recognized as leaders because of their problem-solving capacities. Their difficulty in the marriage or family, then, is not one of acquisition, but of performance. They do not "use" their learned skills because doing so evokes too much anxiety (e.g., empathy may lead to too much closeness and/or vulnerability), or because not using them comes to be an effective means of controlling others, or for various other reasons. The therapist's challenge is to understand and help modify what blocks the usage of these skills—quite a different matter from teaching them anew.

The kinds of component skills the therapist assesses involve the family's competence in defining problems, generating possible solutions, making decisions about these possibilities, implementing the chosen plan, and evaluating the implementation. Commonly emphasized communication skills include empathic listening, pinpointing via specific and concrete problem identification, speaking for oneself rather than for others, and assuming responsibility for one's own thoughts and feelings.

Since in brief therapy one does not aim for reconstructing the "personality" of the family or couple, it is often sufficient to emphasize the assessment of communication and problem-solving skills as they are manifested in the one or two central areas of marriage or family life that seem to contain the presenting problem.

Styles of Influence. A closely related area is the characteristic style of interpersonal influence occurring in the family. It has been demonstrated by family researchers that people in distressed relationships typically call upon punishment and negative reinforcement (e.g., verbal threats, demands, physical assault, withholding via emotional withdrawal) rather than positive influence strategies (e.g., acknowledging and showing appreciation for the receipt of desired behavior) (Jacobson, 1981; G. R. Patterson & Hops, 1972). With all couples and families, but especially those who begin therapy with intense anger, resentment, and the like, the therapist's fostering the learning of a new style of requesting and maintaining behavior change is important. Indeed, inculcation of an attitude favoring positive styles of influence in families is frequently necessary just to maintain the family's continuing participation in treatment. Therapist passivity, lack of structuring, and inadequate focusing of sessions, especially in the face of high levels of coercive marital or family interaction, is likely to lead to termination of therapy long before it is called for.

Boundaries: Internal and External. The brief therapist, always concerned with individual patients' and families' capacities for successfully responding and adapting to normative developmental requirements and transitions, needs to be able to formulate a mental mapping of the family's internal structure and its interaction with the world outside. The concept of "boundaries" that is, "the rules defining who participates and how" (Minuchin, 1974, p. 53)—is central to this dimension of assessment. Family structure is "the sum of the rules of interaction patterns" (Liddle, 1983, p. 11). Families often experience stress and conflict, whether manifested in struggles between its members or in the symptoms of a single member, when their characteristic structure impedes the developmental needs of individuals (e.g., an emotionally disengaged couple is overinvolved with an autonomy-seeking adolescent) or of subgroups (e.g., a physically disabled child requires such a degree of attention from the parents that the marital couple has little mutual involvement as an intimate adult dyad). In order for healthy developmental processes to occur, each subsystem must be clear and differentiated (as they are not in the well-known case of the "parentified child" who has responsibilities toward siblings that are in the proper domain of parenthood). At the same time, for effective family functioning, subsystem boundaries need to be sufficiently permeable and flexible that interdependence among family members is not precluded. Often, clinically significant changes in symptoms or interpersonal conflict can be brought about in rather short order by modification of core structural arrangements that contain and impede effective subsystem functioning.

Life Cycle Status and Accomplishment. Just as individuals face normative developmental challenges and tasks, lags, and dysynchronies, so too do families and couples. It is so common for individual symptoms and interpersonal conflict to arise in the context of developmental impasses of the family as a system that it is incumbent upon the brief therapist to be thoroughly familiar with the emotional and interactional processes faced by families at different life cycle stages. Often, directing therapeutic attention to helping a couple or family get "back on track" by successfully negotiating its current developmental blocks is sufficient for resolution of the couple's or family's major presenting problem, although the couple or family certainly may not describe or experience the difficulty in systemic developmental terms. McGoldrick and Carter (1982) have detailed an outline of predictable developmental stages of contemporary middle-class families that we find unusually effective in helping therapists to organize a coherent sense of family evolution. Their accompanying discussion of this schema of family development is especially valuable to clinicians because of its elucidation of common clinical issues encountered by families at each stage. Here, we briefly summarize their schema and illustrate the kinds of relatively predictable tasks that need to be successfully dealt with at each stage:

• *The unattached young adult*: Differentiation from family of origin; development of peer relationships.

• *The newly married couple*: Realignment of relationships with family of origin and friends.

• *The family with young children*: Further realignments of family-of-origin relationship; modifying marital relationship to incorporate new family member(s).

• *The family with adolescents*: Changing parent–child interaction to allow appropriate degree of adolescent independence; increased attention to midlife marital and work/career issues.

• *Launching children*: Renegotiation of marital needs and expectations between parents and adult children.

• *The family in later life*: Dealing with losses via death, illness, or social and occupational roles; further modification of marital expectations and needs.

A life cycle schema such as this is not intended to be used prescriptively or as a fixed standard of family health and adaptation. Cultural, religious, ethnic, and other variations among families may significantly change the configuration or even the sequencing of such adaptive developmental challenges (McGoldrick, Pearce, & Giordano, 1982). It does, however, provide a general framework within which to organize a general developmental understanding of families.

As part of the brief therapist's concern with developmental matters, he or she also needs to understand and appreciate the developmental history of each family—for example, their locations and relocations; the absence or presence (and effects) of early-childhood developmental delays, injury, or illness; any marital separations that have taken place; the significance, meaning, and role of work and career in the life of the marriage and the family; economic stresses and successes; and so forth.

Affection and Attachment. Marital and family relationships are not merely social structures in which people try to receive rewards while minimizing costs, as some social-psychological theories, such as the exchange theory of Thibaut and Kelley (1959), posit. Marital and family relationships are fundamentally different from other relationships such as friendships, in that they are expected to provide the most intimate, trusting, and emotionally safe relationships in life. While it is generally accepted that infants, children, and adolescents need to experience successful bonding and attachment to their parents for proper developmental adaptation (e.g., Bowlby,

1969, 1973), the healthy adult's need for such attachments and sense of security is often overlooked or downplayed (cf. S. Johnson, 1986; Wile, 1981), even though there is empirical evidence that positive attachments lower the risk of psychological and physical symptoms (e.g., Myers, Lindenthal, Pepper, & Ostrander, 1972), and that severance of such attachments, as in divorce, predictably leads to increases in depression, psychosomatic illness, and so on (Bloom *et al.*, 1978).

As S. Johnson (1986) has clarified the matter, the key factors involved in both parent–child and adult–adult attachment are accessibility for emotional contact and responsiveness to emotional contact. "Accessibility" refers to "the availability of the attachment figure, the ease with which this figure may be contacted when needed" (S. Johnson, 1986, p. 262), while "responsiveness" refers to "the willingness to be affected or influenced by the other and to recognize the other's needs or desires" (p. 262).

Whereas many marital and family conflicts can be treated successfully by dealing exclusively or primarily with instrumental and structural issues and problems, others require an emphasis on family members' feelings of security, deprivation, and isolation among or between them. Indeed, often therapy will not be able to proceed, or will languish, if instrumental and structural problems receive the therapist's major attention in the absence of adequate bonding in the family or marriage. Family members' capacities for showing *and* probabilities of showing nurturance, caring, affection, reassurance, and the like must occupy part of the therapist's assessment attention.

In the context of brief therapy, two considerations along these lines stand out. First, just as we have distinguished between problems of acquisition and problems of performance in discussing communication and problem-solving skills, we need to do likewise in the domain of assessing family members' emotional accessibility and responsiveness. For example, construing the absence of nurturing behavior in a given family as a response deficit rather than a set of interlocking defenses may lead to an unnecessary investment of time spent in trying to enhance such nurturant capacities, when in fact the capacities already exist, and what is needed is removing the blocks to their appearing.

Second, it is often the insufficiency of nurturance, affection, and so on (whether this is the result of genuine response deficits or of defensive inhibition) that itself must become the focus of therapy, rather than, or in addition to, more instrumental or structural concerns. At times, interventions that successfully enhance attachment and bonding preclude the need for more rational problem-solving work. For example, married couples who have been locked into patterns of chronic arguing, agonizing, and antagonizing in their attempts at problem solving about daily matters of living may suddenly do truly exemplary problem solving and joint decision making immediately after a mutual expression of forgiveness for past injuries to their self-esteem or mutual empathic acknowledgment of each other's pain.

Dimensions Peculiar to the Marital Couple

When therapy is to be focused on the marital pair, five other areas need to be assessed.

Marital Relationship History. With great regularity, the problems couples bring to therapists are readily understandable in light of the evolution of their relationships. While it is occasionally possible to get a "fix" on the core marital difficulty with a rather ahistorical style of initial interviewing, more often such an approach will fail to capture the central relationship dynamics that explain why a couple is experiencing *this* particular kind of problem, at *this* point in time.

Indeed, if there is a single most important task of marital assessment, and one that is most valuable in arriving at a focus for treatment, it is the identification of the developmental meaning of the current conflict, no matter what form that conflict takes. Not all areas of the marital relationship need to be dealt with clinically, since disharmony is usually determined and characterized by a few major issues (Gurman, 1981; Sager, 1981). Nor is it necessary or even appropriate to deal with all the identifiable areas of each spouse's individual conflicts that impinge on the marital interaction. Rather, the interlocking individual conflicts and their reciprocal interlocking defenses, and the recurrent patterns of behavior that reinforce and perpetuate these defenses and failures of the partners to experience themselves and each other as whole persons, are what demand the most focused evaluation (Bagarozzi & Giddings, 1984; Gurman, 1981, 1985c). Marital conflict is usefully understood as occurring when fundamental (though implicit) "rules" of the relationship, which are central to either partner's or both partners' sense of self, are violated. Since these marital "rules" do not evolve randomly, but begin with both the conscious and unconscious expectations of marriage and of the marital partner, and are inevitably (even when unconsciously) modified over time, exploration of certain dimensions of the couple's history are fundamental to the brief therapist's most important question: "Why now?"

Since marriage is a core domain of both individual and family development, the therapist needs to understand how the couple has come to be a couple, and how it has dealt with the inevitable developmental markers of an evolving intimate relationship. Appreciating the pain, significance, and meaning of the current problem is almost always enhanced by addressing such matters as the following:

1. How and when did the couple meet? Married couples' relationships may begin anywhere between adolescence and old age (some even in childhood), and the timing of the beginning of this continuing relationship in the lives and development of each partner may suggest important hints to the therapist of the needs each partner has hoped to fulfill in establishing and continuing this relationship.

2. What attracted each partner to the other partner? Very often, the very characteristics of one's mate that formed the basis of the initial attraction are highlighted as the focus of the current conflict; the therapist's understanding of the connection between the couple's early mutual attraction and their present discord is an enormous aid in developing a central focus for treatment.

3. How did the couple handle conflict, disagreement, and disappointment when it first appeared in their relationship? This inquiry may supply clues that are crucial to a deep understanding of the partners' relationship expectations, fantasies, and fears.

4. What important shifts, if any, in the emotional tone of the relationship occurred at nodal points of transition toward deepening commitment to the relationship (e.g., agreeing to an exclusive relationship, formal engagement, beginning to live together)?

5. What were the reactions of each partner's family of origin to his or her choice of a mate? What was the psychological role of each partner within his or her family of origin at the time this couple connected? What alliances, coalitions, or boundaries within each family changed noticeably when the couple connected? To what degree was each partner comfortably differentiated from his or her family of origin when this relationship began, and when the marriage itself took place?

6. How has the couple dealt with nodal events and potential stressors (e.g., death of a parent, birth of a child, disruption/completion/shifting of educational or career interests and tasks)?

7. Have there been separations during the relationship (including the courtship period) other than those occasioned by, for example, illness, military service, or other requirements generated outside the couple? What was the issue at those times, and how did the couple get back together?

8. Have the partners been involved in extramarital relationships of significant emotional involvement, even in the absence of sexual involvement? Have there been significant nonperson "affairs" (e.g., "affairs" with one's work, family of origin, political causes, etc.), which signify a primary attachment to a part of life other than one's partner?

The Marriage Contract. Many of these experiences in the history of a couple, combined with experiences in other intimate adult relationships and each partner's first vicarious exposure to marriage (that of their parents), may be expressed in condensed fashion in what Sager (1976, 1981) calls the "marriage contract." In choosing a treatment focus, it is helpful to understand both the couple's current contract and the way in which their contract has changed over time. Sager draws useful distinctions among three parts, or terms, of marital contracts that appear at different levels of awareness. "Conscious, verbalized" terms of the marital contract are those that are discussed and dealt with overtly; "conscious but not verbalized" terms are elements of one's own contract (expectations, needs, desires) that are in conscious awareness but remain unspoken out of fear or for other reasons; and the "unconscious" terms of the relationship contract are those that by definition are beyond awareness, and are inferred by the therapist.

Thinking of marital assessment in terms of levels of awareness of the "marital contract" is very helpful for the brief therapist, because it leads naturally to his or her thinking about levels of conflict as well. Not all successful brief therapy with couples requires attention to unconscious determinants of the couple's current conflict. When the problems a couple brings to the therapist seem to be maintained by deficits in communication and problem-solving skills and/or by readily identifiable fears of self-expression, and especially when there is an overriding and continuing commitment to the relationship and an absence of chronic or severe narcissistic injuries in the couple's life together, brief therapy is often enormously helpful even when little attention is paid to what Pinsof (1983) calls the "remote determinants" of problem maintenance.

Sexuality and Sexual Functioning. When sexual problems constitute a major portion of a couple's presenting concerns, a detailed discussion of their individual sexual histories and their joint sexual history, and of overt or more sexual dysfunctions, is obviously called for. When such difficulties are not compounded by chronic anger and resentment or by intrusive character pathology, brief, directive sex therapy (Kaplan, 1974) may be initiated.

But a more common scenario in the experience of the general practitioner of psychotherapy is one in which sexual dysfunctions or conflict over other aspects of the couple's sexual interaction are present but are not highlighted by the couple early in therapy, and perhaps are not even mentioned. Far too often, in our experience, therapists fail to inquire about this realm of the marital relationship early in treatment. While constituting an important oversight in couples therapy generally, such an avoidance may be especially unfortunate in brief therapy, since numerous, seemingly isolated marital complaints may be mere "admission ticket" masks for sexual conflict. If the sexual relationship in the marriage is not addressed directly by the therapist early in his or her work with the couple, a large degree of unnecessary and avoidable fumbling around for a treatment focus may ensue.

Commitment to the Marriage. When a couple requests "marital therapy," it is imperative that the brief therapist be as certain as conditions allow that the stated request is in fact the "real" request. As we discuss in more detail later regarding separation and divorce, a failure by the therapist to ascertain what kind of help is being sought will almost certainly lead to a rambling, unfocused therapy experience.

When a couple seeks the help of a therapist, the likelihood that separation and/or divorce has been recently, or is now, being considered seriously should be assumed. There is no danger in the therapist's making such an assumption and talking to the couple on that basis, whereas there is a great danger that follows from *not* making such an assumption, and thus not inquiring directly about each partner's commitment to the marriage.

In speaking of "commitment ot the marriage," we do not mean that the therapist needs to understand whether each partner is unswervingly sworn to maintain the relationship "till death us do part." Rather, what needs to be assessed is whether the marital partners have a sufficient desire to maintain the relationship *for now and the foreseeable future*, and thus to allow a useful therapy to be pursued. We have seen innumerable "marital" therapies flounder when one partner felt no continuing commitment to the marriage, but stayed in it (and, at least for a while, in therapy), because of guilt over leaving; concern that his or her mate would decompensate if he or she left; excessive loyalty to his or her family of origin; fears of being unable to establish new intimate relationships; and, of course, "the welfare of the children." Such "marital therapies" are rarely "therapeutic" until, in frustration over the lack of therapeutic focus, the partner who has already emotionally left the marriage bolts from treatment precipitously. It is far more humane for all concerned, as well as more time- and cost-effective, for the brief therapist to confront the matter of each partner's marital commitment early on.

While spouses can and do lose all sense of commitment to their marriage because of its adversiveness and painfulness, without either of them being involved in extramarital relationships, the presence of a "third person" will inevitably affect how committed the partners feel toward each other. Hence, just as inquiring about such "taboo" subjects as the couple's sexual relationship is important for focusing the therapy, open discussion of extramarital involvements is of at least equal importance.

Substance Abuse and Spouse Abuse. As we have emphasized in Chapter 3, whenever alcohol or other substance abuse is occurring, its treatment must take precedence over all other possible therapy foci. As with sexual dysfunction and extramarital relationships, substance abuse and marital violence are matters that very often are not highlighted or even explicitly identified by couples seeking therapy. Because they pose such potential dangers, singly or in combination, and because the presence of either in a marriage usually precludes a clear treatment focus for brief intervention, asking about both matters needs to be a routine part of the initial assessment process. The prevalence of marital violence is sufficiently high (Bassis, Gelles, & Levine, 1984; Strauss, Gelles, & Steinmetz, 1980) to justify the therapist's inquiry in this area, even in the complete absence of any obvious clues that might be suggestive of the presence of violence in a given marriage.

Pulling It All Together and Negotiating the Focus

Marital and family assessment is not done for the purpose of labeling families, but as a means for the therapist to construct a usable plan for the selection of a central focus, and to develop a plan of action designed to induce change. As treatment proceeds, modifications, revisions, and refinements of the initial focus may occur, but is imperative when such shifts of focus occur in brief therapy that the therapist and the couple or family know explicitly not only what the focus is shifting toward, but also what it is shifting from. Both in these situations, and in situations in which the initial focus is maintained throughout the treatment, then, it is of the utmost importance that the initial focus be clear, and that the therapist's rationale for the focus he or she suggests also be clear. Since in the first few marital or family interviews a great deal of ground may have been covered, some guidelines are in order for what and how the therapist pulls together all that has been discussed and presents this to the couple or family:

1. The therapist should acknowledge the importance of the major symptom(s) presented, and/or the most affect-laden relationship concerns; if different family members express different primary dissatisfactions or complaints, the therapist must be certain to acknowledge each of them.

2. Whenever possible, and in a language understandable to the couple or family, the therapist should link these concerns, complaints, and/or symptoms in such a way as to illustrate the reciprocal influence among them, and to estabish a treatment focus that includes (or at least is concretely responsive to) each person's concerns.

3. The therapist should summarize the overriding hopes and wishes each member of the couple or family has for the marriage/family, and, whenever possible, should point out the similarities among these positive strivings.

4. When this is appropriate to the problem(s) and situation at hand, the therapist should emphasize the need to deal with "first things first" (e.g., substance abuse, violence), and provide a succinct rationale for doing so.

5. The therapist should provide the couple/family with a developmental framework within which they can understand the appearance and significance of the major stated complaints and concerns.

6. When this is appropriate to the concerns at issue, the therapist may "normalize" the couple's or family's difficulties by briefly providing relevant information about families facing similar crises and conflicts.

7. Without exaggeration, the therapist should point out the most striking strengths and assets the couple or family has demonstrated, including characteristics and qualities that the spouse/family members themselves have not explicitly identified or have even downplayed, yet that are obvious to the therapist, as well as those they readily acknowledge.

8. The therapist should be explicit about which members of the family (or people outside the family) might be most important to include in subsequent sessions. When family members who are present are to be (at least for the time being) "discharged" from therapy, the therapist should briefly explain why this is his or her preference. Similarly, when the therapist feels that family members (or others) who are not present need to be included, a rationale should be provided for their inclusion.

9. The therapist should explain to the spouses/family members that their active participation and taking of the initiative will be needed if therapy is to be of maximal benefit, and that such participation may include time and activity outside the consulting room as well as within it. When one or more family members (especially adults) have had more than just a fléeting experience in previous individual psychotherapy, the therapist should point out that the kind of participation involved in marital/family therapy is likely to be quite different from what they have experienced in those therapies.

This style of "pulling things together" for and with the couple or family should clearly communicate, by its form as well as its substance, that assessment is not a static event frozen in time and space, but is itself a part of the process of change.

7

The Brief Therapy of Marital and Family Conflicts

As is evident from even a cursory examination of the professional literature on marital and family therapy, or a scanning of the titles of the numerous family therapy conferences and workshops that have become available in the last few years, marital and family intervention has been directed toward an extraordinary array of clinical problems. As we have noted at the beginning of Chapter 6, our major emphasis here is on the brief treatment of clinical problems that are explicitly relational in nature. In order to exemplify the developmental emphasis of our approach to brief therapy, we focus in this chapter on a cluster of clinical difficulties of couples and families that absolutely require the brief therapist to (1) attend to the developmental aspects of family conflicts; (2) sequence his or her interventions according to the real-life phenomenology of families facing these problems; (3) set clear and attainable goals; (4) make carefully considered decisions about whom to include in treatment at different points in time; and (5) anticipate both the short-term and longer-range implications of dealing with these difficulties. To this end, we address here the domain of problems spanning threats to the continuation of marriages, marital and family dissolution, and the re-establishment of family life via remarriage.

The processes of contemplating separation and divorce, possible experimenting with dissolution of the nuclear family, reaching a decision to divorce, living through the early postdivorce phase of life, and re-entering a subsequent marriage are replete with an enormous range of developmental challenges and difficulties. The disturbances experienced at both individual and system-wide levels are typically sufficient in number and intensity to create what often seems to the therapist a bewildering array of reasonable simultaneous foci. Yet order must be brought out of this usually very real turmoil and chaos—to help couples and families address their immediate suffering, to help them get "back on track" developmentally, and to establish a clear focus for the work of brief therapy. Of all the possible related "clusters" of problems of marital and family life a general practitioner of psychotherapy may face, there can be no doubt that those involving the potential and actual dissolution of marriage will account for more of the therapist's clinical time than any other (e.g., childhood or adolescent behavior problems, major psychiatric disturbances of adults, etc.).

While the occurrence of extramarital sexual affairs (ESAs) certainly does not per se constitute a phase of marital and family dissolution, it is also addressed here both because it is so often the initial stimulus to a couple's considering ending a marriage, and because it is so often involved in marital conflict even when divorce is not considered. Humphrey and Strong (1976), for example, surveyed a representative sample of the clinical members of the American Association of Marriage and Family Counselors, and found that approximately 50% of the cases they were treating involved conflict over ESAs. And Greene, Lee, and Lustig (1974) reported that while only 30% of couples in their sample reported ESAs at the beginning of therapy, the figure rose to 60% once a therapeutic alliance was established, roughly corroborating Humphrey and Strong's findings.

Several often-cited figures attest to the impact of marital dissolution in the United States, and hence its likelihood of being faced as a clinical issue:

1. There are approximately 1.2 million divorces each year in this country (P. C. Glick, 1979).
2. As of 1977, 40% of the couples married in that year would go on to divorce (P. C. Glick & Norton, 1977).
3. Among people born between 1946 and 1955, 49% are predicted to divorce in their first marriage (P. C. Glick, 1984).
4. At least 40% of first remarriages will also end in divorce in less than 4 years (P. C. Glick & Norton, 1976).

As a result of these marital outcomes and the subsequent evolution of these affected individuals' lives, it is estimated that about 40% of the children born between 1970 and 1979 will spend at least a part of their childhood or adolescence in a "binuclear family"—that is, a combination of one-parent households and stepfamily households (Crosbie-Burnett & Ahrons, 1985)—and that roughly half a million new stepfamilies (meaning 2 million or more people) are formed each year (Visher & Visher, 1979).

We are not aware of any reliable data on the proportion of couples who seek therapy for marital conflict or family therapy for parent–child problems, and who eventually divorce after treatment. But when one considers the number of couples who separate without eventual divorce, the number of couples who divorce without prior separation, and the number of couples who "merely" contemplate seriously the possibility of separating and divorcing without ever doing either (e.g., in the context of the revelation of an ESA), it is abundantly clear that no psychotherapist can avoid for very long dealing with individuals, couples, or families who have considered dissolution, are going through it, or have already gone through it.

BRIEF THERAPY OF EXTRAMARITAL AFFAIRS

Of all the problems that lead married couples to seek therapy together, we know of none that arouses such intensities of rage, narcissistic injury, self-doubt, and disorientation as the revelation of an ESA. And while spouses often complain of the distance-generating (or distance-regulating) meta-phorical "affairs" of husbands with their careers, wives with their mothers, and so on, no such "affair" is as relationally explosive as the ESA.

For most couples, the revelation of an affair—especially if it has not been a transient "one-night stand," but has been going on for some time, and with obvious emotional as well as sexual involvement—signals marital distress in unambiguous terms that are undeniable. Yet, in our experience, only a very small percentage of "third parties" to affairs (a.k.a. "victims") react with such a sense of affrontery and fundamental betrayal that they quickly and resolutely seek a divorce. While no married person "deserves" to take responsibility for his or her mate's choosing to have an ESA, it is generally acknowledged that ESAs do not arise from thin air, so every person who has been "cheated on" knows that he or she was somehow involved in creating the conditions in the marriage that led up to (not "caused") the ESA. More often, then, when an ESA leads to divorce (an ESA never "causes" divorce), it does not do so in a linear A-B fashion, but after a complex process of soul searching, expressions of anger, and efforts to develop insight into the need for the ESA. Like nothing else, ESAs signal marital distress and thus may provide the impetus to seeking professional help—either to improve the relationship, to determine whether the relation-ship can be tolerated without improvement, or to confirm a decision to move ahead toward separation and/or divorce.

ESAs carry an extraordinary variety of meanings and consequences for both the "unfaithful" spouse and his or her partner. And it is apparent that the power of feelings aroused in both under these circumstances can easily overwhelm a therapist if he or she does not have a plan (albeit a flexible one) for what to do first, next, and so on. The appropriate focus for ongoing therapy in any given case can only be determined by careful attention to several tasks and issues.

First, the brief therapist will usually need to emphasize calming both the spouses, who are probably caught up in either a mutual "if it weren't for you" harangue or an equally nonproductive, repetitive agreement that one person was to blame. Usually, the "unfaithful" partner's genuine agreement to end the ESA significantly reduces the immediate stress and distress. When he or she refuses to do so, conjoint therapy cannot proceed without being a sham. Couples therapy in the face of an ongoing ESA does not allow the issues that need examination and discussion (see below) to proceed; if it continues beyond a mere handful of interviews (during which the "unfaithful" spouse may be persuaded to remain in therapy—preferably by his or her spouse, not the therapist), it will predictably meander and be filled with little more than intellectualizations, denials, and self-recriminations. No brief therapist who genuinely values working toward agreed-upon aims, with a clear focus for change and a sensitivity to the rationing of treatment time, should participate in such a pseudotherapy.

While doing crisis intervention and trying to help re-establish some emotional order, the therapist will simultaneously be trying to assess the major immediate effects of the ESA revelation: the presence of retaliatory behavior; the potential for suicidal or other self-destructive acting-out behavior; the degree to which others (e.g., friends, relatives) have been recruited for emotional support and/or "ganging up" on the infidel; the extent to which the "faithful" spouse feels the basic fabric of marital trust has been severed; and so on. More or less at the same time, the therapist needs to assess the degree of continuing commitment to the marriage by each of the partners. Relatedly, the therapist needs to assess the degree of continuing commitment by the "unfaithful" spouse to his or her lover, even if that relationship has been nominally ended, but still exists in that spouse's heart and fantasies. An abrupt crisis-generated termination of an ESA in which there has been significant caring and nonsexual intimacy may well lead to a genuine reactive depression in the "unfaithful" partner, making some treatment goals temporarily unachievable.

The therapist should by now have begun to explore the motives and reasons for the ESA: an attempt to heat up a cool, distant marital relationship; an attempt to cool down a too-enmeshed marital relationship; a narcissistic indulgence designed to bolster a flagging sense of self-esteem; an "experimental testing" of one's attractiveness to the opposite sex preparatory to reaching a final decision whether or not to divorce one's mate; and so forth (Nichols, 1987; Williamson, 1977). This discussion will necessarily include the quality of the marital relationship before and during the ESA (Sprenkle & Weis, 1978).

If the couple maintains the marriage and continues in therapy, the most time-consuming phase of therapy will be that devoted to rebuilding the relationship and the gradual re-establishment of trust. Trust is rarely re-established quickly following an ESA, and herein lies some challenging and pivotal decision making for the brief therapist. While it is tempting to respond to the myriad of truly minor events that can be experienced as new crises or even catastrophes following an ESA (e.g., the "unfaithful" mate's late arrival for dinner; the "faithful" mate's fleeting urge to have a power-balancing retaliatory counteraffair following what would, under other conditions, have been a rather minor moment of conflict), the brief therapist must resist this understandable temptation, and encourage the couple to call upon its own conflict management resources (which, one hopes, have been worked on in therapy sessions). An overly enthusiastic therapist may aim for too much change too quickly, and rush ahead of what is reparatively appropriate for the couple. Thus, rather than trying to hasten the rebuilding of trust in an ESA-involved marriage, by, say, meeting weekly for 15 weeks, the brief therapist must consider having four or five consecutive weekly meetings, followed by biweekly or even triweekly sessions over an additional 5–8 months.

While the preponderance of interviews in the brief therapy for ESAs should be conjoint, infrequent individual sessions (held with full disclosure to, and with the approval of, the other spouse!) may be held for very specific reasons—for example, working through guilt in a nonpunitive relationship with the therapist. Children may also be seen infrequently (and will usually need to be seen only briefly), in order to have their parents' current marital status clarified; to receive reassurance; and, when appropriate, to be pulled from the center of the marital conflict, or to be relieved by the therapist of the job of being parental confidants.

Keith and Marge were in their early 40s and leading an apparently "charmed life," with two popular and successful high-school-age children, when Marge's affair with Don came to light. Keith's extraordinary success as a real estate developer had allowed the whole family opportunities for travel and cultural exposure well beyond what most people usually even fantasize about. Both spouses had come from stable, if rather controlled and undemonstrative, familes. They had met in college, when Keith was a prelaw student and Marge an elementary education student. Marge was especially attracted to Keith's "incredible persistence" and "reliability." For his part, Keith found Marge's "soothing and caring style" irresistible. Often when they dated, Marge would serve almost as a sort of untrained client-centered listener, reassuring Keith about his academic abilities when his confidence waned, and even going out of her way to gather together extra study materials for him when he was anxious about an upcoming exam. Though he not infrequently showed distress about his school work, "he never for a moment felt like throwing in the towel."

This pattern persisted through the end of college and through law school, until, in Keith's senior year, Brian was born. Always nurturant, Marge was a very loving, if rather doting, mother who almost instantly redirected almost all her energy into the couple's first child, all the while feeling quite guilty that she "couldn't be there for Keith enough."

By then, though, Keith had had enough professional successes that his confidence was bolstered tremendously, and he rarely felt a need for the kind of "soothing" Marge had provided early on in their relationship. This gradually acquired self-confidence, paired with unusual natural aptitude, found Keith several years later in the limelight among local business people and public officials. In a word, he was locally "famous" and highly respected. But for his "fame" he and Marge paid the price of his rare moments at home, Marge's increasing resentment toward his "love affair with money and work," and his (now two) children's emotional absence from his life.

Marge, who had taught third grade for only 1 year before Brian was born, had returned to school "to brush up on all the things I needed to know to get back into teaching, and maybe get a master's [degree]." Up to this point, she had self-sacrificially managed to repress her rage at Keith's virtual emotional abandonment. However, when Don, an ebulliently outgoing divorced midlevel university professor, found her enthusiasm for her work impressive and took a special interest in her academic progress, her pent-up anger toward Keith broke into her full conscious awareness.

She pleaded with Keith to go for marital therapy, and while he acceded to her request, business commitments always seemed to get in the way of even an initial appointment with a therapist. Marge spent more and more time with Don, and soon they became "really good friends," talking not only about their common professional interests, but also sharing trips to the museum together, feeding the ducks along the lake shore, and so on. Their deepening friendship of several months had evolved into an ongoing sexual relationship about 4 months before Marge and Keith first came to therapy. By chance, a neighbor of the couple, out for a stroll along the wooded path by the local lake, had come upon Marge and Don embracing.

Marge was overcome with guilt (or at least fear) for the first time during her ESA with Don, and revealed the ESA to Keith a few days later— "when the kids were at a basketball game, so they wouldn't be there when I told him what was going on." Keith became enraged and tearfully despondent at the same time, and "literally begged her to stop seeing Don." Marge was "actually touched" by "the first sign I'd seen that I mattered to him at all in years," but refused to end her ESA "unless he would come here for counseling and put his heart into it." And so therapy began 2 weeks later. Keith was visibly shaken by his wife's revelation and showed symptoms of a reactive depression and severe acute anxiety, for which mild anxiolytic medication was prescribed by the therapist's psychiatric colleague. After the third session, Marge agreed to put her relationship with Don "on hold for now, so we can do what we should have done 10 years ago"—namely, focus on her and Keith's disengaged parallel lives.

Though Keith showed occasional desperate, retaliatory flurries of threats to "see to it she won't be able to go on living [financially] like she's used to," these efforts at restoring some equitability of power were short-lived, and within a month or so he and Marge were able to settle down to the hard and painful work of beginning to "rediscover each other," as the therapist put it in the fifth session. The evolution of their disengagement was rather easily traced (in fact, more easily than with many couples), and Marge's motivations for her ESA were shared quite explicitly. Conjoint therapy was held at 2-week intervals over the next 4 months, later moving to monthly intervals for the last 3 months of treatment. As Keith began to take risks in revealing his "soft side," Marge felt renewed attraction to him, and "officially" ended her relationship with Don. Marge, for her part, became "less of a silently suffering martyr" and became more self-assured and less willing to back off from overt conflict with Keith. Though she had anticipated that such assertiveness would "drive him away, or at least turn him off," Keith reacted in neither of these ways. In the end, Keith had discovered that he could be "caring without being unmasculine," and Marge had discovered that she could be "strong without being insensitive."

STAGE THEORY AND MARITAL/FAMILY DISSOLUTION

Obviously, divorce is not an event punctuating life at a single point in time, but a complex unfolding process. Virtually every social scientist or clinician author who has dealt with divorce has underlined the importance of thinking about divorce as a series of stages. Salts (1985), among others, labels this body of thought "stage theory." But J. K. Rice and Rice (1986) somewhat iconoclastically and usefully point out that the many temporal sequencings of the dissolution process that have been offered are "less a theory, and more a description based on the sequence of events [that] categorize[s] common phases of divorce" (p. 62).

These various "stage theories" may emphasize either individual emotional processes, requisite tasks, interpersonal structural realignments, or some combinations thereof. "Stages" are argued to range from as few as two (Weiss, 1975) to as many as seven (Kessler, 1975). These numerous temporal mappings of the dissolution process suggest that the differentiation of the developmental phases of divorce is not empirically well validated. More importantly, however, the existence of so many "stage theories" implies both that the "stages" of family dissolution are not discrete but continuous phenomena, and that one does not "discover" such stages, but creates them by the maps and perspectives one uses. The clinical application of all this is that individuals, couples, and families do not experience clearly defined, nonoverlapping, highly predictable periods of events.

All these numerical and terminological variations aside, there is an emerging consensus (at least among clinical authors—e.g., Kaslow, 1981; Nichols, 1987; D. G. Rice & Rice, 1986; J. K. Rice & Rice, 1986; Salts, 1985) that dividing up the terrain of marital and family dissolution for treatment purposes, a simple (or, at least, simplifying) triphasic approach offers maximal practical utility. Hence, the first phase/stage is referred to as the "predivorce period," the "decision-making period," the "predivorce decision-making period," the "deliberation period," and so on; the second phase is variously dubbed the "separation/divorce stage," the "divorce/restructuring stage," the "litigation period," the "transition period," and so forth; and the third phase is referred to as, for example, the "recovery period," the "reequilibration stage," or simply the "postdivorce period."

Before we move to considering the brief treatment of couples and families in these various phases of dissolution, four practical clinical guidelines for the use of stage theories of whatever sort need to be underscored:

1. The therapist must clarify the current stage of marital dissolution. Since it takes two to marry (usually), but only one to divorce, the stage of dissolution that best describes a couple is the most "advanced" stage already reached by any individual spouse. Obviously, one partner cannot be in the postdivorce stage without the other partner also being there, at least legally speaking. On the other hand, it is very common in clinical practice to find that one partner is at a higher level of dissolution than the other in intent and fantasy.

2. Even if both spouses are at the same level or in the same "stage" of divorce structurally, they may be at very different "places" emotionally, and thus may require rather different kinds of help from the therapist. For example, a couple may be at the decision-making "divorce/restructuring" phase clearly enough; however, the husband, who has been in an intense and caring ongoing affair for 4 years and plans to marry his lover, is well past the individual psychological task of accepting the reality of the decision to divorce, and his wife, who has learned of his tryst only 2 months ago, may have barely entered the emotional phase of dealing with this reality.

3. Children (by which we mean adolescents as well) in the same family may be genuinely aware, whether consciously or unconsciously, of the degree to which their parents have progressed into the divorce process. However, they may be at widely different levels of understanding and information regarding this process. Therefore, they may be at quite different phases of dealing with the family dissolution themselves, and this will lead predictably to engagement with different emotional issues. The common shibboleth that "the kids always know what is really going on" is mere silliness in many cases. A not-unheard-of mistake in this realm (and one that has the potential to extend the length of therapy significantly beyond what is needed) is for the therapist to assume that since "the kids already know," it is fitting for the therapist and family to "jump right into" the most painful feelings of family members and talk about all manner of matters that are well beyond where particular children are in their own individual "stages" of dealing with their parents' divorce.

4. Just as different individuals, adults or children, may be at different "stages" emotionally in the divorce process, it is worthwhile to remember that the life cycle phase of the *family* at the time when divorce becomes inevitable must also be considered as a significant factor in planning and carrying out the work of therapy. For example, the divorce of young couples without children generally creates a good deal less pressure for the

involvement of the couple's own parents in therapy than when the couple has young children or adolescent children. Similarly, there is less pressure for the involvement of adult children when an older couple is divorcing, since as adults these children clearly have relatively free access to their parents, and vice versa (Beal, 1980).

The Predivorce Period

Therapy and the Decision-Making Process

Assessing the commitment of each marital partner to remaining in the marriage should be as "routine" a part of early work with any couple or family seeking treatment for any reason whatsoever as assessing suicide potential is in work with any depressed patient. In other words, all couples and families beginning therapy should be considered to be in a potential predivorce decision-making period until there is sufficient evidence to the contrary.

When both members of a couple entering therapy are firmly committed to the marriage, or when both are about equally undecided on the matter but cooperative in their efforts to struggle with the decision, no special treatment considerations regarding dissolution need to be given great weight in the early phases of their work with the therapist. Whether treatment is focused on marital dissatisfaction, parent–child conflict, or individual symptoms, therapy will emphasize working to resolve those problems. With couples who are either strongly committed to their marriage or undecided about their commitment, the therapy should have the same basic focus— namely, working to bring about whatever changes are desired and appropriate. This is self-evident in the case of committed couples. It is also probably the most viable approach with the questionably committed: We agree with Stuart (1980) that the aim, initially at least, with such couples should be to help them experience the possibilities of a more satisfying relationship before finally deciding whether to remain together. Of course, with some people (e.g., obsessives, those with very limited social skills, and those with dependent personality disorders), the therapist's suggesting a treatment plan in and of itself may merely constitute "more of the same." In our experience, setting an explicit time limit (or limit on the number of sessions) for the therapy is quite helpful with such couples. Such a limit, if its terms are reasonable (e.g., 8–10 sessions over 3–6 months), both allows for changes that may make a difference to the couple to occur *and* simultaneously insures that the decision of whether to stay together is never lost sight of. In some cases of mutual indecision, "structured separation with counseling" (Granvold, 1983; Granvold & Tarrant, 1983) is a method of intervening that may be useful, and this strategy is considered below.

Generally, this predivorce decision-making phase of therapy will be marked by major attention to the marital dyad in conjoint therapy (Storm &

Sprenkle, 1982). Even when couples present for therapy with a reasonable degree of cooperation, and certainly when they do not, it is always important for the therapist to inquire about the current status of the couple's children (e.g., academic performance, social relationships, general physical health). Preferably, a session (or even part of a session) with the children present may be held within the first four or five visits, so that the therapist can observe the children directly and interact with the family as a whole. During this phase of therapy, nonsymptomatic children usually should not be seen in therapy on a regular basis, except when some family structure conditions warrant their presence (e.g., when a child is nonsymptomatic but has clearly been put in the role of marital mediator, maternal or paternal ally, etc.).

When steps toward divorce begin after the couple has been in therapy for some time, it is unusual for the partners to present the therapist with a joint decision to divorce. Typically one partner has made the decision (Gurman, 1985b). Nichols (1987) notes that only about 15% of divorces in the United States are equally desired by both spouses. When a "diagnosis of irreversibility" (Bloch, 1980, p. 95) is put forward by one marital partner, the therapist's primary responsibility is no different in principle from his or her responsibility in therapy in general: It is to keep alive the couple's existing options, and to help to increase their range of possible options. This can be done in several ways, each of which allows new information into the system. First, since a person on the way out of a relationship always has more power than the person who wants to maintain it, the therapist's initial response should focus on the partner opting for divorce by clarifying and perhaps challenging his or her motivation: Is the decision a veiled way to express anger at or disappointment in the therapist for lack of therapeutic progress? Why has the decision been reached now? Is there a new lover? Have in-laws or friends been pushing for divorce? Is the divorce decision aimed at redistributing the power balance in the marriage? Did the decision follow closely on the opening up of treatment issues that seemed frightening? Did the decision occur right after a major marital argument?

Discussion of these and other possibilities brings up new information, and thus the therapist's and the couple's options are increased. If any of these possibilities, in fact, fit the decision situation at hand, the therapist can intervene accordingly to deal with the problems that underlie the decision to divorce. Of course, all these immediately preceding considerations and suggested inquiries and interventions apply as well to couples who begin therapy when one spouse has just recently announced his or her decision to divorce. Whenever this occurs, the therapist's major initial task is to treat the decision as real.

While we know of no data on the matter, it is our clear impression that when one marital partner reaches a firm decision to divorce, conjoint therapy ends or comes to a temporary standstill at least as often as not. While certainly many couples will remain in conjoint therapy for the therapist's help during the restructuring period, just as many will not. Either both partners leave therapy, angry that the therapist has failed to "save" their marriage, or quite the opposite occurs—the partners are thankful for the help they have received in reaching a decision, but feel in no need for additional help at that point in time. Even more commonly, one spouse will want to stay on in treatment, usually the partner who is being left (Nichols, 1987; J. K. Rice & Rice, 1986). Although the therapist may prefer for various reasons that both spouses stay in treatment, J. K. Rice and Rice (1986) underscore that "the format of the therapy sessions should mirror the reality of the relationship at any given point in the divorce process" (p. 284). Even when both partners wish to continue conjoint work at this juncture, the therapist is well advised to begin to split the sessions between conjoint meetings and individual meetings. The spouse wanting to maintain the marriage will understandably feel abandoned, narcissistically injured, and angry. If, as is usually true, the partner being left is likely to have to shoulder the enormous burdens of single parenthood, confusion and anxiety will also run high. The major goals of individual therapy at this time will be to help the patient (whether "leaver" or "leavee") accept the reality of the separation and divorce-to-be, and deal with the gamut of intense emotions occasioned by one of life's major stressors (Bloom *et al.*, 1978).

If the "leaver" spouse wishes to continue conjoint therapy at this point, it is vital that his or her reasons for wanting to do so be made clear. If the decision is motivated by guilt, this feeling is probably best dealt with in individual sessions. If the motivation is a caretaking one to "help" the mate, this task should properly be taken over by the therapist, the patient himself or herself, and other caring people in the life of the "leavee." While many "leavees" and a few "leavers" will want to meet conjointly to "review" the reasons for the leaver's decision, this is rarely useful; it is uncommon, indeed, for both partners to be able to engage in such a "review" with relative dispassion. By this point in therapy (not to mention this point in the couple's real daily life), the leaver's motivation to leave should be readily apparent to all concerned in the therapy. When denial, repression, or even suppression reigns supreme, reintroduction of the emotional "facts" behind the impending dissolution is better accomplished by the therapist than by the departing spouse, since the therapist is in a far better position to allow the "leavee" patient the freedom to feel angry, abandoned, and emotionally injured, while simultaneously keeping the patient reasonably open to examining his or her own contribution to the deterioration of the marriage. Continued conjoint work, at the point at which one partner is resolute in the decision to divorce, should shift its emphasis quite clearly to other matters, to be considered below in our discussion of the "restructuring" period of dissolution.

Bob and Marla entered couples therapy in their seventh year of marriage, prompted by Marla's renewed anger at Bob for returning to his periodic pattern of alcoholism. Marla, aged 29, in her first marriage, and Bob, aged 35, in his second marriage, lived together at the outset of therapy, with their 4-year-old son, Eric. Although Marla, a nurse, was aware of Bob's history of intermittent alcoholism during their courtship, he drank infrequently during that time, and usually only in moderate amounts during the first 2 years of their marriage. Until about 6 months before they sought therapy, Bob had, according to Marla, "really gotten plastered only maybe two or three times since we started dating." But even during these extended "dry" periods, Bob was short-tempered and critical with Marla "about even the pickiest things."

Bob, an experienced and apparently rather talented mechanical engineer, had "never quite made it" professionally. He spent an inordinate amount of time "living in a dream world" (according to Marla), trying to invent and patent an amazing array of devices and products, in the hope that he could own his own business and "not have to kowtow to some pseudoprofessional boss who doesn't know half as much as I do about engineering."

Marla, the eldest of three children, had been "parentified" as an early adolescent, taking on the major caretaking burdens of her almost crippled arthritic mother and her depressive father. While her inclination to be hyperresponsible for others had served her well as a nurse, it had not been adaptive in her marriage. Bob complained angrily and often that "she's always trying to reform me and make me perfect." Part of Marla's attempts at "reforming" Bob included trying to persuade him to "give up all these 'get rich quick' invention fantasies, and just keep a secure 9-to-5 kind of job." Bob had been laid off from his job 3 months before therapy began. In fact, he had been fired because of repeated conflicts with his boss over how much freedom he was allowed to be "creative" in his work.

During this unemployed period, Bob had begun to drink heavily and regularly, though he still spent several hours each day "working on some things in my office at home." He had become so "absorbed with himself" that he left little time to be with either Marla or Eric.

Marla focused her despair on "having to live like a single parent, but not having it even that easy!" She cared very deeply for Bob, but was "not willing to go on living like this indefinitely." Bob was angry at Marla for "threatening to abandon me at one of the worst times in my life." To the therapist, Marla did not appear to be "threatening" her husband. In the last year or so, she had increasingly come to recognize the self-destructiveness of her excessive taking of responsibility toward Bob; this recognition was due in no small measure to her short previous individual therapy with another therapist, which had focused on the repetition of patterns in her family of origin and in her marriage to Bob.

At the therapist's urging, Bob went to his first AA group meeting after the third couples session; Marla had already gotten involved in Al-Anon, in an effort to find support for her taking less responsibility for Bob's drinking, career, parental involvement, and so forth. Bob and Marla worked hard in conjoint therapy, and demonstrated their mutual caring often. After several sessions, Bob was no longer fleeing disagreements at home, and Marla was generally resisting her urges to take over for him.

But Bob refused to attend AA meetings regularly, pointing to his decreased drinking (from almost daily to two to three times a week) as evidence that he could "do it alone." Marla was profoundly disappointed when Bob firmly insisted he did not "need" AA, seeing his declaration as "another excuse not to grow up." Bob and Marla continued to work through their feelings about past grievances, made noticeable if not dramatic changes in their problem-solving and communication skills, and had become clearly more open with their feelings and willingness to take emotional risks with each other during the first 3 months of (mostly biweekly) therapy.

These changes, though certainly welcomed by Marla, led her to feel even more confused than she had been before therapy. While she now had reason for some optimism about Bob's capacity to deal with her more collaboratively in regard to various marital issues, she felt that she could not allow herself to "backslide" by once again putting herself in a caretaking position with Bob (whose drinking had improved only moderately, and who continued to seek "regular" employment); nor was she willing to "let him [Bob] pickle his brain in front of Eric day after day."

In the tearful 10th session, Marla told the therapist that a few days earlier, she had asked Bob to move out of their apartment and that she had contacted an attorney and was about to file for divorce. "I guess I'll never know if he really means it [i.e., intends to work on his alcoholism] and cares about it for himself as long as we're together, and he'll never know for sure if *I* really mean it [i.e., intend not to be so responsible for his successes and failures] unless we split up for a while," Marla said.

Bob was to move out a few days later, at the end of the month, and did so with resentment but no significant arguments. Over the next 3 months, the therapist saw Bob alone on two occasions, at his initiative. Bob's unspoken, yet transparent, purpose was to try to induce the therapist to persuade his wife to reconsider her decision by describing to the therapist all the "positive changes" he had made during the couple's separation. Marla was also seen individually on three occasions. She needed a "mirror" she could talk to "so I can listen to myself and see if I really believe what I think I do." She felt "renewed," she said, by not "having to worry about Bob all the time," and, even as the custodial parent, had begun to "get back to life the way I think it's supposed to be for someone my age, or at least the way I want it to be." By this, she meant that she had been exploring some potential new friendships ("I'm not interested in romance with anyone just yet, thank you") with work colleagues, and had decided to enroll in a short series of specialized weekend-long nurses' training workshops.

Over the following 4 months, Marla was seen once alone "to work through some of my guilt" (over initiating divorce proceedings), whereas Bob did not seek additional meetings with the therapist. The couple was seen together one more time, about 3 weeks before their final divorce hearing, for the therapist's help in negotiating certain details of Bob's visitation rights and parental responsibilities.

Structured Separation Therapy

Structured separation therapy (SST; Granvold, 1983; Granvold & Tarrant, 1983) is a marital treatment method that has been designed and refined (cf. Greene *et al.*, 1974; Toomin, 1972) specifically to facilitate a conflicted couple's decision whether to divorce or remain together. It is a time-limited approach to fostering such decision making, which can be extremely helpful whenever divorce indecision prevails. It is particularly useful when indecision is accompanied by extreme conflict (e.g., physical or emotional abuse, intense anger); when one partner exhibits intense jealousy and rigid controlling of the other partner; when there are midlife crises marked by disillusionment, self-doubt, and so forth; or, as noted earlier, when the dominant affect in the marriage may be desultory, depressive, and hopeless, but no perceptible action is being taken by the couple to move either closer together or further apart.

Decision making about whether to divorce is facilitated by SST in these ways: (1) It temporarily cools off intense conflict, if this is present; (2) it forces the obsessive, mutually fearful couple who have been stagnantly unhappy but immobile to confront the reality of their impasse, both together and as individuals; (3) it allows for the exploration of alternative relationships, if relevant (whether in fantasy or fact), and/or for other expressions of personal development; and (4) it allows—indeed, requires—more independent functioning by the partners.

The structure of SST involves a number of essential elements. The duration of the separation is negotiated between the therapist and the couple, and between the spouses. We generally find a month to 6 weeks to be too brief for maximum benefit from the experience, while a period approaching 6 months seems to dilute its intensification value too much, so that 3 months is most often the time frame in which we work. During this period, no final decision about dissolution or reconciliation is to be reached by the couple.

Treatment continues during the separation; although conjoint sessions predominate, individual sessions may be held as well, perhaps every second or third week. Additional agreed-upon separation periods may be renegotiated at the end of the couple's initial time apart, though there are clearly diminishing returns for continued extensions, and we find it most appropriate for subsequent separation periods to be briefer than the original period (e.g., 1–2 more months).

In arriving at a structured separation agreement, the couple needs to negotiate and come to terms about the following kinds of matters: what kind of contact is to take place between the partners, as well as the acceptable circumstances under which they are to be together; whether sexual contact between the partners is possible, who may initiate it, and so on; whether dating other people and having sexual contact with others are allowable for either or both partners; and what is to be done about child-related and financial/household management issues (e.g., the frequency and nature of time with the children for the parent living out of the home, as well as temporary maintenance and child care). The agreements reached by the couple in these matters may be written down, both to heighten the reality of the action being taken and to symbolize each partner's commitment to this phase of the treatment process.

Although the notion of a "trial separation" may be raised by a patient, and the idea of an SST may then be presented by the therapist, more often it is the therapist who initiates the discussion of the possibility. When the telltale signs of chronic indecision are present, it falls on the shoulders of the brief therapist to take the initiative to introduce or sharpen the focus of therapy by addressing the potential values, benefits, and implications of a time-limited SST. While some patients will respond to the idea of such a therapeutic separation with initial anxiety—fearing it will become "the first step in his inevitable way out the door," as one wife put it—the positive aspects of an SST must be emphasized, in that it provides a directive intervention and directed format in which both individual and shared marital developmental impasses can be confronted. While efforts toward behavior change within the marriage during an SST certainly should not be blocked by the therapist, and may help the couple arrive at a decision about dissolution versus reconciliation, the SST arrangement is primarily powerful by virtue of the parallel self-reflection that is allowed the marital partners, without undue pressure to decide what they want to do immediately, and by virtue of the element of choice that is reinjected into the marital relationship.

Finally, if one or both partners decide to go on to divorce at the end of the SST, the period of *structured* separation will *de facto* have provided a successive approximation of divorce. As a result, it will have somewhat eased the inevitable pain of divorce by exposing the partners and their children to some dimensions and elements of the divorced state gradually; by allowing opportunities for the enhancement of individual coping skills; and by permitting the expansion of and/or reconnection with alternative supportive social structures and individuals.

The Need to Work in Good Faith

Up to this point, we have considered intervention in predivorce situations in which the decision to divorce grows out of the therapy experience, whether unilaterally or even precipitously, or somewhat more collaboratively after a period of a structured separation. In both cases, we have assumed a rough equality of indecision between the spouses as to whether or not to divorce. Unfortunately, however, the psychotherapist in general practice will not infrequently find himself or herself sitting with a couple in which one partner is not working in good faith with either his or her mate (which is the mate's problem) or the therapist (which is the therapist's problem). Although this partner may appear for the therapy sessions, he or she will put little energy into the experience; or, if the partner seems reasonably involved in the therapist's presence, he or she will not engage in out-of-session homework tasks mutually agreed upon with the therapist; or, in some cases, both will occur. Certainly, some people who "engage" in the therapy in this manner do so because they are inordinately fearful of making any ripples, let alone waves, in their marriages; because they are too financially, emotionally, or otherwise dependent; because they are too fearful that if they take any action or show any real feeling, they will emotionally (or, at times, physically) destroy their mates; and so on. Still, characterological impasses and obstacles notwithstanding, when such a style of (non) involvement in the therapy is prominent, the brief therapist should at once begin to wonder whether this patient has already left the marriage mentally and emotionally but is not saying so. It is incumbent on the brief therapist to raise this possibility explicitly, yet supportively. A "marital" therapy that for one duplicitous partner is really unacknowledged divorce therapy will flounder and sputter; everyone except the deceiver will be utterly confused and disoriented, and either spouse may become angry at the therapist (with one not really caring, of course) for the ambiguities and contradictions that abound in the sessions. Brief therapy requires not only clarity and energy, but also honesty.

The Restructuring Period

Whether a couple or family enters the restructuring period of dissolution during therapy or preceding the start of the therapy, the same issues will need to be attended to, though the pain of dealing with them may have been lessened somewhat if the partners have been trying to work cooperatively on their difficulties in the relative emotional safety of the therapy. As already noted, couples (and their children) who have lived and struggled through a structured separation may have a "leg up" on coping with the profound emotional unheaval and loss of divorce, as well as the potent structural changes that need to be incorporated into everyday life. For those who have not been gradually exposed to the divorce process via SST, the reality of divorce often becomes undeniable, emotionally as well as geographically, for the first time.

This beginning of the transition period from intact to divorcing family now introduces a period of general stress, phenomenological as well as observable disorganization, and often eruption of diagnosable psychiatric disorders (e.g., depression, panic attacks, etc.). This state of affairs will typically continue in fits and starts for up to 2–3 years (Wallerstein & Kelly, 1980). The first year of this period is commonly the most tumultuous and upsetting time in the divorce process for children (Bloom *et al.*, 1978; Hetherington, Cox, & Cox, 1977; Sager *et al.*, 1983), especially younger children. Denial, grief, and fears of abandonment by the parent with whom a child still lives are common; feelings of guilt for having caused the marital breakup, as well as fantasies about reuniting the parents, are also commonly experienced. Perhaps nowhere else in the practice of psychotherapy is the relevance of our "general practitioner" model of brief therapy—in which time in treatment is rationed, often over very long intervals—illustrated more compellingly than in dealing with patients involved in the lengthy roller-coaster process of divorce and its aftermath.

In this "middle" period, not only must a host of conflicting feelings and urges be confronted and reconciled, but legal, financial, and housing modifications and arrangements, as well as social and parental realignments, must also be addressed. This is also often the period during which there is an intensification of grandparental reaction to and/or involvement in the divorce process. Friendship relationships often change dramatically during this time, especially for the husband and wife and at times for children (e.g., if they do not continue to live in their accustomed home).

Conjoint family therapy of the parents and their children, and perhaps intermittent grandparental involvement, is probably ideal throughout this phase of divorcing. Unfortunately, securing the regular involvement of all the adults who are likely to be saliently involved in the divorce is as often a therapist's dream as it is a clinical reality. If the therapist is to succeed at even intermittent, yet sustained, therapeutic participation by both spouses (soon to be ex-spouses), it is absolutely essential that he or she make it explicitly clear that the therapy is not "marital therapy" in any sense, but is intended to promote the good and welfare of the couple's children. Husband–wife conflict is dealt with only insofar as it impedes or precludes the couple's working together in their parental roles.

As noted earlier, it is rather common for one spouse to continue in individual therapy with the therapist who originally treated the couple (or family, depending on the presenting problem). Under this circumstance, the alliance between the therapist and the spouse who is not in individual therapy with that therapist may be severely strained, and will need particular attention and nurturance if the therapist is to help maintain that partner's ongoing therapeutic involvement.

Psychoeducational interventions during this period may also be both helpful and efficient. Predicting the wide swings of mood, feelings of parental involvement and distance, and so forth may help to "normalize" such experiences. In addition, encouraging children to read and discuss with their parents books about divorce written for them (e.g., Gardner, 1971, 1978) is usually well received and beneficial.

The Postdivorce Period

Phase 1: The Single-Parent Family

Ahrons (1979, 1981) has argued cogently (with supporting empirical evidence) that the notion of the "single-parent family" is a factual misnomer, in that divorced families typically consist of two one-parent households. Nonetheless, when the truncated family enters therapy, it is generally because the phenomenology of the "single-parent family" is real enough to the parent (usually the mother) who predominantly lives with the children. For this parent, an almost inevitable problem is what Beal (1980) refers to simply yet clearly as "task overload." Even if all the other changes in the initial postdivorce period are being handled relatively well, the task overload of the "living-with" parent itself is often sufficient to lead to significant depression, chronic anxiety, and the like. Even the "living-with" parent whose ex-spouse stays in regular contact with the children often feels as if she has to do the work of two parents, and this is often literally true. Typically, the last area of the "living-with" parent's life that is adequately considered and attended to is her need for time and space alone.

Often, the "living-with" single parent will seek therapy for herself as a means of creating a reliable refuge from the frenzy of single parenthood, and for general emotional support and consistent aid in problem solving. In some families, the "living-with" parent's mere entry into individual therapy will bring about a rapid reduction in her child's behavior problems or psychiatric symptoms. This is likely to happen when a single parent approaching "burnout" has a child who has become "parentified" and assumed parental functions and roles (including being the parent's amateur psychotherapist) that are inappropriate. At times, the parent's simply informing the parentified child that she is receiving professional help for her difficulties allows the child to become nonsymptomatic, in cases where the child's symptoms have been a sort of indirect protest against his or her precocious position in the family.

For both ex-spouses, the individual developmental tasks in the period following divorce are approximately the same: assuming increasing autonomy and independence in family functioning; continued mourning of the loss of the mate; establishing new social relationships, including, but not limited to, romantic relationships; renegotiating involvement with one's extended family, including one's ex-in-laws; providing support for the continuing adjustment crises of one's children; and so forth.

Obviously, mourning may be quite abbreviated and/or repressed by a divorced person who continues to be involved with a lover who entered his or her life while he or she was still married. Nonetheless, it is common for adults in the early postdivorce period to engage in what Weiss (1975) calls an "obsessive review" of why the divorce occurred, who was at fault, what could have been done differently to prevent the divorce, and the like. Working through such issues and correcting faulty attributions about the divorce experience are often major developmental tasks in this period, and thus regularly become the focus of individual therapy. As matters of these sorts are being dealt with, the patient is implicitly, as well as explicitly, addressing his or her preparation for (likely) remarriage.

Predictably, the postdivorce adjustment of children is a major concern to ex-spouses. In addition to those children and adolescents who become parentified and are for a time thereby blocked in their own development, others may find themselves in the middle of custody or visitation disputes or litigation, parental competition for "favorite-parent" status, and other conflicts. There is sufficient empirical evidence, and overwhelming clinical evidence, that the single best predictor of children's postdivorce adjustment is the quality of the ex-spouses' coparental relationship (Goldsmith, 1982). While this factor is clearly multidimensional, it involves such primary elements as the degree of mutual emotional support provided by the parents, and the degree of the parents' cooperation in child rearing.

In this context, Ahrons's (1979, 1981) notion of the "binuclear family" is especially pertinent. The "living-away" parent's reality and importance as a biological parent need to be acknowledged, despite possible mutual antagonism between the former mates. While the postdivorce adjustment dilemmas and difficulties of parents are usually best addressed in individual therapy, the emergence of emotional or behavioral problems in the children of divorce should always at least be assessed with the entire family present. Likewise, when grandparents appear to be significantly involved in the maintenance of children's problems, child–parent conflict, or parent–parent conflict, they also should be brought into the therapy. One common risk in such whole-family participation in therapy after divorce is that children (especially younger children) may see such meetings as offering hope for the reuniting of the parents. In order not to reinforce this fantasy, and in order to maintain a treatment focus, the therapist must see to it that the goals of therapy are as explicit and clearly delineated as possible, and that these aims will be restricted to issues of parenting and coparenting.

Six-year-old Danny was brought to therapy 2 months after the start of the new school year by his father, Ed, and his stepmother, Barbara. In his first-grade class, Danny had become labeled as a "problem child" and was in serious difficulty both socially and academically. He frequently attacked other children, without apparent provocation, and appeared to have most of his classmates frozen in fear of his outbursts (he was the largest and, by all reports, the strongest boy in his class). Although his IQ was estimated by school officials to be at about the 90th percentile, his concentration on academic tasks was minimal, and he appeared at times to be doing some of his work (such as math) incorrectly quite intentionally. At home, he would "fly into rages" against Barbara when Ed was not at home, telling her he hated her and was going to kill her or Becky, Barbara and Ed's 4-month-old daughter. Barbara, who felt she had "no power over him," actually feared for Becky's safety because of the intensity of Danny's "absolutely crazy-sounding 'fits'". Married to Ed for only a year and a half, Barbara said that Ed "is OK with me about the baby, but won't let me have any say whatsoever when it comes to Danny." Ed agreed that in large measure this was true. In his first marriage to Ellie, which had ended less than 2 years earlier, both he and Ellie had "screwed around with lots of people." He felt very guilty about all this in terms of its possibly damaging influence on Danny. In effect, he had vowed to himself to "make it up to Danny"; in trying to do so, he worked hard to limit the influence of all other adults on Danny, and spent almost all his time away from work with his son.

Danny's mother, Ellie, had gotten engaged late that summer to Bill, who was to become her third husband "between Thanksgiving and Christmas." Danny had spent his kindergarten year and the entire summer between kindergarten and first grade, except for occasional weekends, with Ellie (and, later, Bill). Ed was "horrified" by the "complete lack of discipline, or any other kind of time with him [Danny] that mattered" from Ellie, based on what Danny provocatively reported to Ed. Ed had confronted his ex-wife, accusing her of leaving Danny home alone for hours at a time, allowing him to watch "violent and downright pornographic movies" on their cable TV, etc. Ellie denied all of this. Barbara added, in a moment of angry side-taking with Ellie, that she didn't "think Ellie was *that* bad of a mother—I think Ed exaggerates a helluva lot about everything about her."

The therapist saw Danny as caught up in a web of unfinished divorce business and partially connected adult relationships: Ed and Ellie were still enraged at each other for their years of mutual narcissistic injuries and betrayals; Ed was overinvolved with Danny and excluding his new wife from that relationship; Barbara and Ed were on the verge of separating; and so on. But as caught up as Danny was in this multicharacter web of hostility and estrangement, he himself also pulled powerfully on the strands of the web. Angry at both his parents for having divorced, he felt devastated when his father and stepmother had a new baby just before he returned to live with them, his father's overinvolvement with him notwithstanding. Barbara wanted Danny to return to his mother, but rarely said so. Danny was not only threatening his half-sister and his stepmother; he was also expressing rage at Ellie and Bill for their impending marriage.

In a brief individual session with the therapist soon after therapy began, Danny said in no uncertain terms that he was "going to get my dad and Barbara divorced." "Then what would happen to your mom?" asked the therapist. "She'll get rid of Bill and marry Dad," he proclaimed with a feeling of anticipatory victory and vengeance. The therapist congratulated Danny for his honesty and directness.

The therapy with this family, which lasted for 6 months at 2-week intervals (after three consecutive weekly sessions at the outset), was multi-pronged. Danny's classroom teacher and his school psychologist, with input from the therapist, established a behavior modification program focused primarily on Danny's social behavior toward both peers and adults. This in-school program was coordinated with a parallel approach at home. Since Barbara and Danny's relationship was still tenuous at best, she was not allowed to participate with Ed in providing consequences for Danny's school behavior. On the other hand, she was empowered by the therapist to be "in charge, just like any other adult should be, when dealing with Danny alone." Both of these changes were very difficult for Ed, who, out of an undue sense of guilt, had taken to "giving in to him even when I know I shouldn't;" nonetheless, he "steeled" himself to follow the therapist's sugges-tions. These more direct matters of child management *cum* parental realign-ment were monitored regularly, but came to occupy less and less in-session time after about 2 months, as Danny's inappropriate behavior decreased noticeably both at home and in school.

At the same time, and throughout the course of therapy, therapeutic attention was paid to the adults as adults and to their conflicts. Two sessions were held with both biological parents and both stepparents (Ellie and Bill married, as planned, in early December) present, in order to sort out and negotiate the nature of each parental person's involvement with Danny; to establish adult consistency (while allowing for appropriate and necessary variations) toward Danny in terms of in-home limits, prerogatives, and the like; and to reach agreement about the kind of "conversations" with Danny that were acceptable in each household about the parental pair in Danny's other household. Although there remained some rough edges to these agreements, the therapist's explicit stance that Danny's "four parents" had a responsibility to leave him out of their struggles generally prevailed. Follow-ing these two sessions, Danny was brought in for two sessions with his "four parents." The adults' display of a relatively united front at first angered Danny visibly and quite dramatically; he thrashed about the therapist's office, kicking his mother and father and cursing them, each in turn. Ed (who was 6'3" tall and weighed about 220 pounds) set appropriate limits rather quickly by enveloping and restraining Danny in a sort of "bear hug," holding Danny's arms with his arms and Danny's legs with his legs. In a few minutes, Danny ceased this enraged megatantrum and began to weep quietly. He finally had begun to believe that Ed and Barbara's marriage was real, and that Ellie and Bill's was also real; he seemed to be in mourning for his grandiose fantasy, now dashed, that he could reunite his parents.

During the first 2 months of therapy, the continuing conflicts between Ed and Ellie had been "temporarily put on the back burner," in order to emphasize the needs to stabilize Danny's extended-family system in as many ways and as quickly as possible. Over the next 4 months, the therapist met with Ed and Ellie together several times (but without Barbara and Bill) to help them work through feelings of mutual betrayal that had never been adequately discussed, though they had been acted out numerous times. The therapist made it clear to Danny that his parents were not meeting with the therapist "to get back together again, as much as I know you still want that, and will for a long time. We're meeting so your mom and dad can finally *really* get divorced, so you won't have to get into trouble so much and be so unhappy." Danny understood.

Phase 2: The Remarried Family

Of the millions of divorced individuals in the United States, it is estimated that 75–80% will remarry (Baker, Druckman, & Flagle, 1980); as previously noted, it is also estimated that of these remarriages, about 40% will end in divorce within 5 years (Glick & Norton, 1976). Remarriages bring with them all the potential for conflicts and crises that exist for first marriages, plus certain cultural expectations (e.g., the "wicked stepmother" and the fantasy of "instant love") that are either misguided or unachievable. Moreover, the structural complexities of remarried families are enormous. (The reader should note here our preference for the term "remarried families" [Sager *et al.*, 1983] when referring to the entire larger family system resulting from remarriages, and our use of the traditional term "stepfamilies" [Visher & Visher, 1979] when referring to the subsystem of the remarried family system consisting of the new marital pair and any children from a previous marriage brought into that new marriage.)

While any psychological or psychiatric difficulty that can arise for children within any family structure can, of course, arise within remarried families, therapists whose work includes contact with remarried families (or, more likely, stepfamilies) can expect to see some predictable problems. These problems, which may exist in their own right or may co-occur with a variety of psychiatric diagnoses, may include the following: continuing problems over the loss of a parent; conflicted loyalties to both biological parents, or even grandparents; disorientation of a sense of belonging, related to a change of sibling position from family of origin to stepfamily;

practical as well as affective difficulties brought on by living in two house-holds; having to deal with unreasonable expectations of stepparents and/or having unreasonable expectations, both positive and negative, of steppar-ents; continuing fantasies of the biological parents' reuniting; and unjustifi-able guilt over having contributed to, or even "caused," the marital rift and breakup (Visher & Visher, 1979). In addition, a struggle often encountered in clinical practice involves the conflict between the push for developmen-tally appropriate cohesion in a newly formed stepfamily and the also devel-opmentally appropriate urgency for increasing adolescent autonomy.

Problems such as these, plus common parent–child conflicts (e.g., over discipline, adolescent sexuality, and sexual expression), derive in part from a stepfamily's unsuccessful negotiation of, management of, and coming to terms with one or more of several fundamental structural differences (de-scribed by Visher & Visher, 1979, and elaborated here) that exist between stepfamilies and biological nuclear families. First, stepfamilies are always born of loss, and this incontrovertible fact is not negated by even the most cooperative of postdivorce coparental relationships. Second, each "half" of a stepfamily by definition has its own past history, with its own traditions, rituals, "insider" language, and so on. Third, parent–child bonds, with all their biological voltage, predate and precede the new formed husband–wife bond. Fourth, except in the relatively less frequent cases of stepfamilies emerging out of the death of a parent, there is another biological parent living elsewhere whose reality has powerful effects on the stepfamily, whether that person remains deeply involved with his or her children or is largely cut off from them. Fifth, children in stepfamilies often live (albeit for unequal periods of time) in two households. Sixth, there is no legal relation-ship between a stepparent and his or her stepchildren, whatever the emo-tional relationship between them may be or become. Seventh, in contrast to the roles of biological parents, the roles of stepparents are unclear, and have little if any predictable grounding in terms of societal standards and expec-tations. Finally, as Sager *et al.*'s (1983) notion of the "remarried family suprasystem" conveys, a stepfamily may have three sets of grandparents, and, of course, additional second- and third-degree relatives. Thus, when a marital problem, child problem, "individual" adult problem, or adult–child problem is presented to a therapist by a stepfamily, the need for the sort of comprehensive systemic assessment detailed earlier in this chapter is brought home in full force.

In addition to using Visher and Visher's (1979, 1982) differential de-scriptions of biological versus stepfamily structures as a mental mapping entrée into defining what constitutes the problem for which help is sought and what maintains the problem, the brief therapist might also consider the developmental issues and tasks facing remarried families as described by McGoldrick and Carter (1980) in arriving at a clear focus for intervention. McGoldrick and Carter differentiate those developmental tasks that precede the literal formation of a remarried family from those that follow it. At the stage of conceptualizing and planning the new marriage and family, they identify the following sorts of developmental issues: (1) planning for the maintenance of cooperative coparental relationships with ex-spouses; (2) planning for helping children deal with fears about the new family, and with loyalty conflicts and membership uncertainties in two family systems; (3) planning for changes in relationships with extended families to include the new spouse and his or her children. Beginning at the point of the literal establishment of the new family system, major developmental challenges include (1) changing family boundaries to allow for adequate inclusion of the new spouse/stepparent (and his or her children, if any); (2) continuing ongoing access of children to their "living-away" biological parent(s), grandparents, and other blood relatives; and (3) sharing memories and histories of each "half" of the stepfamily as a way of fostering stepfamily integration.

The number of possible stepfamily configurations is enormous, with different combinations of the previous marital status of each spouse, as well as the presence or absence of custodial and/or noncustodial children (Sager *et al.*, 1983). Add to this the varieties of emotional and structural problems that regularly appear in clinical stepfamilies, and the seemingly endless bits of relevant data and impressions the therapist may pull together about any given stepfamily's current problem situation (e.g., L. Katz & Stein, 1983), and the therapist can easily become mired in a sea of possibilities for a useful treatment focus. As a practical guide through this morass for the brief therapist, we have found that two key concepts provide a helpful intrapsychic–interpersonal compass: "bonds" and "boundaries." These two concepts subsume the overwhelming majority of common individual, dyadic, triadic, and system-wide issues common to clinical stepfamilies. "Bonds" suggest emotional involvement (whether too close or too distant), loyalty dilemmas, and the like, while "boundaries" suggest issues of membership, space, time, and authority (McGoldrick & Carter, 1980), as well as alliances, coalitions, power, role diffusion–differentiation, and so on. Since no therapist, brief or otherwise, can keep in mind all the sorts of issues likely to be relevant to stepfamilies, asking "What are the most important/problematic bonding issues for this family?" and "What are the most important/problematic boundary issues for this family?" will help a good deal in arriving at a central focus for treatment.

Finally, as in all systemically sensitive therapy, there is the unusually vexing matter with stepfamilies of whom to include in treatment. L. Katz and Stein (1983) provide a very reasonable set of guidelines for such decision making:

> 1. Members of more than one household generally are seen together when a child develops symptoms that appear to be related to the presence of too-rigid boundaries between the households.

2. Members of more than one household generally are not seen together when a child develops symptoms in the context of permeable boundaries between the households.

3. Members of two households usually are not seen together when the known potential risks may outweigh the benefits.

4. Members of more than one household are usually not seen together when the children are not having problems that are generated by household boundaries.

5. Various subsystems (e.g., marital pair, stepsiblings) in the family may be seen apart from other subsystems when that subsystem has particular tasks to resolve apart from the rest of the stepfamily.

6. Everyone living in the stepfamily household should usually be seen together when the major presenting problem is one of stepfamily integration.

7. Individual members of the stepfamily may be seen alone when issues that are quite independent of the stepfamily are being dealt with.

In order to arrive at well-reasoned judgments about these sorts of parameters, it is preferable, as suggested earlier, that as many possibly relevant members of the family system be included for the initial assessment; from this group, the "minimum sufficient network" (Skynner, 1981) may then be drawn.

8

Symptomatic Presentations:
The Uses of Clinical Hypnosis

The mind is its own place, and in itself
Can make a Heav'n of Hell, a Hell of Heav'n.
 —John Milton, *Paradise Lost* (1667/1692)

Every experienced brief therapist finds that some (often a significant) percentage of patients present themselves for treatment with an exclusively (or nearly exclusively) symptomatic focus. For most of these patients, their central problems, such as pain, sleep disturbances, eating or habit disorders, or the like, may be comprehensible to the therapist in an I-D-E frame of reference. From the perspective of the patient, however, either the connection between his or her difficulties (e.g., severe insomnia) and the therapist's proposed focus (e.g., loss) may appear extremely obscure and of little value, or the symptomatology may be so acute and consuming that little else can be addressed prior to first treating the symptom itself.

For some of these patients, the successful treatment of their major symptom is sufficient and satisfactory therapy. For others, symptom improvement leads to an enhancement of the therapeutic alliance and allows them to address other areas. For yet another subgroup of patients, for whom the I-D-E focus, even if accepted and addressed, may not lead to rapid symptomatic change, a temporary focus on symptomatology may be necessary.

In any case, in order for a brief therapist to have the breadth and latitude to deal with a variety of common foci, he or she should have skills in psychosocial treatments that emphasize symptomatic improvement. Bennett and Feldstein (1986), in a long-term follow-up study of presenting problems and patient satisfaction in a large HMO mental health department offering mostly brief therapy, found that patients who sought treatment because of an "exclusively" symptomatic difficulty (e.g., a habit disorder, pain problem, or sleep disturbance) were the most highly dissatisfied group of patients surveyed. The authors believed that this occurred because most of the brief therapists in their study de-emphasized symptomatic approaches.

188

In our view, the brief therapist should have some facility in symptomatic approaches because, to paraphrase an old expression, "the customer is usually right." Someone who arrives insisting on symptomatic improvement with regard to a particular habit disorder will probably not be easily persuaded that what he or she really wants is to explore her overall personality style. Similarly, most chronic pain patients (at least initially) will be much more interested in reducing their pain than in learning about what in their history makes them so depressed when they are in pain.

Strupp and Binder (1984) cite an excellent example of such a symptom-oriented patient:

> Adam was in his late twenties when he sought hypnotherapy because he was unable to eat anything but an unusual sandwich made of strawberry jam and salami. He had read about hypnotherapy as a way of achieving greater self-control, and sought a therapist who could (paradoxically) *make* him control himself. Although Adam desired to eat other foods, he reported becoming nauseated whenever he attempted to consume anything but one of these sandwiches. Adam dreaded the experience of eating, and would typically go hungry until evening, when he would hastily construct three or four such sandwiches and would wolf them down in private, usually in the bathroom.
>
> In seeking the transactional significance of Adam's difficulties, the therapist began with inquiry about how his eating habits might affect his relationships with others. When the issue of relationships was raised (in the first session) Adam rather suddenly revealed that his main reason for seeking treatment was to improve his marital situation. The issue of idiosyncratic eating habits was important, in his view, only because it was the main topic about which he and his wife disagreed.
>
> Over the next three sessions the therapist discovered that Adam came from a family in which his father was helpless and ineffectual, and in which his mother was extremely intrusive, controlling, and domineering. Even as an adult, Adam feared getting a telephone call from his mother. Only one relative in the entire extended family showed any ability to stand up to Adam's mother. It was this relative who introduced Adam to strawberry jam and salami sandwiches (when Adam was in grammar school), and it was this relative who had helped Adam assert his wish to eat these sandwiches despite his mother's insistence that he join the family in eating food she had prepared. Transactionally, then, Adam learned to eat unusual sandwiches as a way of preserving his identity and self-respect against the influence of a tyrannical and overbearing parent. His eating habits were a kind of last stand, a way of saying to his mother, "I control what I put in my body. Your influence stops here!"
>
> Unfortunately, while the therapist was busily unearthing the details of Adam's history, he was neglecting the status of the therapeutic environment and relationship. Recall that Adam had originally requested hypnotherapy. Based on the emerging formulation of the transactional significance of his symptoms, the therapist had discouraged hypnotherapy as simply a further manifestation of Adam's preoccupation with issues of control and of his diffi-

culties relating assertively to women (his mother and his wife). *However, the therapist communicated this message somewhat categorically (that Adam's difficulties were embedded in ongoing patterns of interpersonal transaction and that hypnotherapy was inappropriate in this case).* Adam's response to the therapist's handling of this issue was, in retrospect, a predictable extension of the established pattern: he resisted the therapist's controlling stance and terminated therapy abruptly. (pp. 86–87, italics added)

It certainly may have been quite true that Adam's difficulties had far more to do with interactional problems than with a habit problem modifiable by hypnosis. However, it is probably necessary to treat many patients like Adam on their own terms. It is possible that focusing on a symptom may have a significant impact; even when it does not, the therapist has joined with the patient in trying to overcome the difficulty. To try to "argue" a patient out of a symptom focus is often ineffectual and unsatisfying therapy.

We have chosen clinical hypnosis as our favored approach to symptomatic difficulties. Although carefully controlled comparative clinical trials still remain to be done (Wadden & Anderton, 1982), indictions from meta-analyses that hypnosis can be a potent change technique for habit disorders such as smoking (Holroyd, 1980), obesity (Mott & Roberts, 1979), and pain problems (E. R. Hilgard & Hilgard, 1983) appear quite encouraging. Although the more subtle applications of hypnosis may require extensive study and training, the basic components are easily learned and practiced by the experienced clinician. Some aspects of the hypnotic approach, such as "pacing" the patient, can readily be applied more generally to brief and long-term psychotherapy (Grinder & Bandler, 1981).

In this chapter, we hope to give the reader a broad overview of clinical hypnosis, and particularly its uses with patients who present with a central focus upon symptom difficulties. As noted previously, on some occasions hypnosis may be a very useful tool, even if the major emphasis of treatment is not a symptom per se. Some of these situations are described in our examples.

A HISTORY OF CLINICAL HYPNOSIS

Centuries before Christ, the Egyptians, Greeks, and Babylonians built temples dedicated to the gods and goddesses of sleep. Individuals afflicted with pain or anxiety problems slept at the temple and were attended to by a priest or priestess. Appropriate prayers, poultices, foods, and ritual baths were provided to the pilgrims. At times the temple priests would use a hypnotic approach (which later came to be known as "fascination") in order to induce a sleep-like trance in the patient (Ellenberger, 1970). Suggestions were made to the supplicant that he or she would get well; some remarkable cures were thus achieved. In following centuries, the secrets of hypnosis and trance were repeatedly rediscovered and lost.

One of the most prominent actors in the history of hypnosis and hypnotherapy was an Austrian physician named Franz Anton Mesmer (1734–1815). He claimed that by passing magnets near the body of an afflicted person he could induce convulsions, which he called the "crisis." The patient would often lose consciousness during the crisis and awaken in a much improved state of functioning. Over time, Mesmer found that some patients would go into crisis just by his touching them. He came to believe that he and some of his followers possessed "animal magnetism," which could be transmitted to people and to inanimate objects.

Two French commissions (one of which included Benjamin Franklin as a member) investigated Mesmerism in 1784. These scientists concluded that animal magnetism was "merely" a function of the patient's "imagination" and not based upon scientific phenomena (Wolberg, 1982). In the years following Mesmer's death, magnetism continued to flourish in Europe and the United States but began to take on trappings of the occult, becoming associated with clairvoyance and paranormal phenomena.

In 1841 James Braid, a Scottish surgeon, became interested in the use of magnetism as an anesthesia for surgical operations. Braid coined the term "hypnotism," which came from the Greek word *hypnos* ("sleep"). At the same time, Esdaile, an English surgeon, began to use hypnosis for anesthesia in India. He claimed to have done hundreds of operations using trance as the major form of anesthetic. A number of clinicians and researchers experimented with the therapeutic uses of hypnosis throughout the 19th century. Liebeault, Bernheim, Charcot, and Janet all made important contributions in this area.

In the late 1800s, Sigmund Freud became familiar with the work of Liebeault and Bernheim and went to France to study with them. He and Josef Breuer made major modifications regarding the ways in which hypnosis was being used at the time. Rather than simply relaxing the patient and then making suggestions for improvement, they began to use hypnosis in order to explore the reasons for the particular symptoms in question. By the turn of the century, however, Freud had rejected hypnosis on the grounds (1) that many patients could not be hypnotized; (2) that hypnotic cures were often just temporary; and (3) that symptoms served a protective function for the patient, and thus simply removing a symptom was inevitably doomed to failure. Freud's hostility toward hypnosis had a pronounced effect upon the field: Hypnosis again became associated with superficiality and charlatanism. Although work continued in scattered settings, with such people as Erickson, Spiegel, the Hilgards, and Wolberg leading the way, it is just in the last several decades that interest in the therapeutic uses of hypnosis has again increased dramatically.

CONTROVERSIES IN HYPNOSIS

Because so little is clearly understood about the nature of hypnosis and hypnotic phenomena, and because the field has often been dominated by powerful and charismatic individuals, it is an area of much controversy and widely divergent opinions. We touch here upon two of the major controversies in hypnosis, because of their relevance to the practicing clinician:

   1. Hypnotizability: Can anyone be hypnotized, or must a patient have a susceptibility to hypnosis?
   2. Trance induction: Does one have to use "official" trance inductions in order to hypnotize a patient?

Hypnotizability

A major question in the hypnosis literature is whether hypnosis is useful for everyone, or just for that group of people who are "good" hypnotic subjects (i.e., highly susceptible to its effects). In the earliest days of clinical hypnosis, the emphasis was upon the power of the hypnotist. It slowly became clear that even for clinicians with outstanding hypnotic skills, some patients appeared refractory to a variety of trance induction approaches. In the late 1950s, Weitzenhoffer and Hilgard (E. R. Hilgard, 1965) introduced the Stanford Hypnotic Susceptibility Scales. This work was soon followed by other scales of hypnotizability (Barber & Wilson, 1977; Spiegel, 1974; S. C. Wilson & Barber, 1978).

   Studies of hypnotizability indicate that subjects with good hypnotic abilities generally have a high capacity for imaginative involvement (E. R. Hilgard, 1974; Tellegen & Atkinson, 1974). They also have the ability to form vivid images and the ability to control this imagery (Sheehan, 1979; Spanos, Valois, Ham, & Ham, 1973; Sutcliffe, Perry, & Sheehan, 1970).

   Work by J. R. Hilgard (1970, 1979), later confirmed and extended by S. C. Wilson and Barber (1981, 1983), indicates that good hypnotic subjects often have had a history throughout their lives of imaginative and fantasy-related behaviors, such as daydreaming, reading or hearing imaginative stories, enjoying science fiction, and acting in plays. These individuals also frequently had imaginary playmates in their childhoods.

   An interesting correlation discovered by J. R. Hilgard (1972) in her studies of hypnotizability was that between hypnotic susceptibility and the remembered severity of punishment received as a child. She writes: "Of the most severely punished, 41 of 62 subjects, or about two-thirds, fell in the upper half of hypnotic susceptibility scores. Of those least severely punished, only 21 of 58, or about one-third, had high hypnotic susceptibility scores" (1972, p. 396). These findings were later replicated with a second sample (J. R. Hilgard, 1974).

On one side of the hypnotizability controversy stand those authors such as the Spiegels (Spiegel & Spiegel, 1978) and Perry (1977), who view susceptibility to hypnosis as basically a trait, subject to little if any genuine modification or enhancement. The other side is represented by authors such as Diamond (1977), the Lanktons (Lankton & Lankton, 1983), Araoz (1985), and Erickson and Rossi (1979, 1981), who believe that hypnosis can be used by most people if a clinician is able to teach a patient adequately how he or she can best experience it.

J. R. Hilgard's (1972, 1974) data on hypnotic susceptibility and childhood punishment, cited above, may support a cognitive–behavioral (learning) model of hypnosis. In reviewing Hilgard's work on the relationship between punishment and hypnotizability, Bowers (1976) concludes:

> Since low-susceptible subjects were evidently not punished as severely as high-susceptible subjects, the availability of such fantasy escape routes was presumably less important to them. On the other hand, alternative "natural hazards," such as boredom, isolation, lack of playmates, and prolonged childhood sicknesses, may also serve to develop in childhood the fantasy skills necessary for adult susceptibility to hypnosis. Moreover, as we have already seen, there seem to be relatively "hazard-free" routes into the development of absorptive skills. So, although punishment may serve as one basis for high hypnotic susceptibility, it is probably not necessary for its development. (p. 122)

If hypnosis is a type of skill rather than an overriding personality trait, then perhaps with some training most people can profit from this approach. The review by Diamond (1977) strongly supports this learning position, as does N. W. Katz's (1979) study on this question. Although considerable controversy remains regarding the issue of modifiability (Kihlstrom, 1985), it is our belief that, within certain constraints, most people can experience and profitably use hypnosis. We are in agreement with Diamond (1977) that elements such as patient preparation, demystification of hypnosis, attitudinal factors, a good therapeutic context, and the teaching of cognitive strategies to enhance hypnosis can all contribute to a patient's ability to learn hypnosis if he or she does not begin with strong imaginative skills.

We would conclude that one's susceptibility to hypnosis is probably a learned coping style (Frankel, 1976). If an individual has had reason or opportunity to learn the skill of intense imagination while growing up, and is called upon to use it again by the therapist during hypnosis, he or she will probably prove to be a fine subject. However, for those people in whom this skill is less keenly developed, some training and teaching will probably be required. A comparison might be made with swimming: Some children appear to be "naturals" in the water and learn to swim with almost no lessons, while others need extensive coaching (and perhaps coaxing) in order to become decent swimmers. We presume that hypnotizability, like the readiness to swim, is not for the most part a genetically carried trait, but probably in the main a function of developmental patterns, family and environmental circumstances, temperament, and learning. With adequate motivation on the patient's part and adequate skill on the therapist's part, most people can presumably be taught hypnotic skill.

Trance Induction

A second important controversy in the area of hypnosis relates to the question of whether or not an "official" trance induction is necessary in order for a patient to be treated hypnotically. Prominent figures such as Wolberg (1982) and the Spiegels (Spiegel & Spiegel, 1978) assume that the trance induction itself is an important component of hypnotic treatment. All emphasize these procedures in their treatment approaches.

Barber (1984a), in contrast, believes that although trance inductions may impress the subject with the special qualities of the situation, they are for the most part irrelevant to the power of hypnosis. He defines hypnosis as "a situation in which individuals are purposefully guided by carefully chosen words and communications (suggestions) to 'let go' of extraneous concerns and to feel–remember–think–imagine–experience ideas or events that they are rarely asked to experience" (p. 69).

Barber (1984a) reviews an impressive study by Ikemi and Nakagawa (1962) examining the question of the necessity for hypnotic induction. In their research, Ikemi and Nakagwa first exposed five young men to standard hypnotic induction procedures. After this, the subjects were told that they were being touched on the arm by leaves from a poison ivy bush (actually, they were being touched by harmless leaves). Eight other subjects were assigned to a suggestion-only treatment (which included no induction procedures). The suggestion-only subjects with eyes closed were similarly told that they were being touched by poison ivy, when, in fact, they were feeling harmless leaves on their arms. All the subjects in this study had a history of reactivity to poison ivy.

The investigators found dramatic results. All of the subjects in either condition showed some degree of dermatitis in response to what Barber (1984) calls "the believed-in suggestions." In the second part of their study, the researchers revised their procedures: That is, the subjects receiving hypnotic induction and the subjects receiving the suggestion alone were touched by actual poison ivy leaves, which they believed to be leaves of a harmless plant. In this phase, four of the five hypnotic subjects and seven of the eight suggestion subjects did *not* react with any signs of contact dermatitis. From this and other similar investigations, Barber concludes that believed-in suggestions, in and of themselves, with subjects who are fantasy-prone are sufficient to reproduce hypnotic phenomena.

Although they have developed some intriguing induction techniques, Milton Erickson and his followers (Erickson, 1964) tend to de-emphasize the need for formal induction procedures. A variety of indirect approaches have been described (Zeig, 1980); these, by means of metaphors or long (at times confusing or boring) stories or tasks, put the subject into a trance or trance-like state.

Our position on the need for formal trance induction is similar to our position on the question of hypnotizability. It is probably the case that for some patients who are hypnotic virtuosos (and perhaps some hypnotherapists who are compelling and powerful in their suggestions), formal induction procedures are unnecessary. For others, induction, if done correctly, can be a form of imagination or fantasy training. The patient may be taught to concentrate on his or her internal imagery and sensations, as well as on "experiencing" therapist suggestions (e.g., hand levitation, heaviness, etc.). Thus, we would assume that for some patients and therapists, hypnotic induction per se is superfluous and an unnecessary part of the technique. For most people treated and for most clinicians using hypnosis, however, induction can be seen as an opportunity to teach skills that may then be applied in the hypnotic treatment. It is doubtful that hypnosis represents an altered state of consciousness, the door to which is magically opened by trance induction (Barber, Spanos, & Chaves, 1974; Sarbin & Coe, 1972).

PREPARING A PATIENT FOR HYPNOSIS

In order to be able to achieve maximum cooperation from a patient with whom hypnotherapy is to be used, the clinician should discuss common misconceptions and fallacies regarding hypnosis, in addition to providing useful information. It is frequently the case that patients have gotten most of what they believe about hypnosis from books, movies, or stage shows. Since popular beliefs about this approach are so often erroneous and unrealistic, it can be helpful to address some of the most prominent of these myths with the patient before doing anything else.

The "Stuck-in-Trance" Myth

Many people fear that hypnosis will place them into a state of deep trance from which it will be extremely difficult to rouse them. It is, in fact, most unusual for a subject to go so deeply into a trance that he or she cannot come out of it immediately at the suggestion of the therapist. If this does occur, it is almost always due to a loss of rapport between the hypnotist and the subject, leading to a passive–aggressive unwillingness to exit the trance (Barber *et al.*, 1974; Wolberg, 1982). Kleinhauz (1982) describes a case of emergency dehypnotization in which the 19-year-old female subject of a stage hypnosis went into a 7-day stuporous trance. Although the trance was brought on by her stage hypnosis experience, the subject was a very disturbed young woman who had had several other severe hysterical symptoms prior to the incident in question.

For the most part, if the subject fails to come out of trance rapidly (which, again, is highly unusual), he or she is probably in a state of physiological sleep, from which the patient can be awakened or allowed to sleep through.

The "Svengali" Myth

Research indicates that although some individuals may follow suggestions to commit antisocial acts while hypnotized, these individuals will also follow the same suggestions while not hypnotized (Conn, 1972). Orne (1972), in a review of legal cases, found no instances where hypnosis was used to induce antisocial or destructive acts without an intense or long-standing relationship between the hypnotist and patient. This relationship itself, he concluded, could account for the behavior in question.

Although over the years hypnosis has become associated with the image of the domineering hypnotist taking control of the subject, this myth has drawn to a great degree upon the model of the stage hypnotist. Those who have ever seen stage hypnosis have observed subjects behaving in exceptional ways: imitating ducks, lying flat as a board between two chairs, and responding "without free will" to posthypnotic suggestions. What is not generally understood is that the stage hypnotist's "success" is due to effective selection of subjects more than to any other factor (Barber *et al.*, 1974).

The "Weak-Minded Subject" Myth

Many people view those who can be readily hypnotized as "weak," "controllable," "easily dominated," and so on. As we have noted earlier in our discussion of hypnotizability, this is not the case. Good hypnotic subjects are highly imaginative, fantasy-prone people who have learned to develop and control vivid imagery. Indeed, there are indications that those who are psychotic and very severely disturbed may be the most difficult to hypnotize.

The "Superficial Effects" Myth

Another popular myth regarding hypnosis has been that its effects are superficial and insignificant. Along the same lines, it is often assumed that the changes that do occur are "all in the subject's head." In fact, a variety of clearly observable and persuasive effects have been documented:

- Alteration in allergic responsivity (Platonov, 1959)
- Beneficial treatment of congenital skin diseases, such as "fish skin" (Frost & Weinstein, 1971; Mason, 1952)
- Cure of warts (DePiano & Salzberg, 1979; Surman, Gottlieb, Hackett, & Silverberg, 1973)
- Breast enlargement caused by hypnosuggestive procedures (Willard, 1977)
- Inhibition of bleeding (Chaves, 1980)
- Minimization of the effects of burns (Ewin, 1978)

Dealing with Myths

We have found it useful to discuss with the patient all of the previously mentioned myths, and then to describe what hypnosis *is*. In our view, it is a technique for using strongly focused attention and imagery, which can lead to substantial cognitive and physiological changes and thereby to the alleviation of distressing symptomatology. We believe that where appropriate, it can be taught to and used by the majority of patients treated in outpatient psychotherapy.

It is also useful to tell the patient at this point that it may be helpful to him or her when working with hypnosis to try to "suspend reality concerns," to "let go of an analytic focus," and to "become as present-centered as possible" (Diamond, 1972; Gregory & Diamond, 1973).

HYPNOTIC INDUCTION

The Major Components

Once the therapist has presented the patient with information regarding hypnosis and has answered any questions the patient may have, the therapist may begin the induction. There are literally hundreds of induction approaches, and every experienced hypnotherapist develops several idiosyncratic ones as he or she goes along. The major components of many inductions, however, are as follows:

1. Relaxation (usually with eyes closed)
2. Focused attention on internal states, memories, or images
3. Use of "naturally" occurring phenomena
4. Failure-free "tests" of the trance state

As we have explained earlier, we view the induction as an opportunity to help the patient learn how to experience hypnosis, not as something that is done *to* the patient. Therefore, the emphasis is not upon trying to find some way to "put" the patient into trance, but rather upon the best way to teach the patient how to feel and imagine the associated phenomena. Indeed, E. R. Hilgard and Hilgard (1983) were told by highly responsive hypnotic subjects that they viewed the hypnotist as a "permissive guide" (p. 20).

Relaxation

In order to allow maximum concentration and focus, the patient should be encouraged to relax, with his or her eyes shut. Directions pertaining to comfort, a restful attitude, and freedom from tension are beneficial.

Focused Attention on Memories, Internal States, or Images

The hypnotherapist helps the patient focus inward on particularly vivid memories, images, or states. He or she can describe to the patient to what aspects of the internal experience to attend to most carefully.

Use of "Naturally" Occurring Phenomena

Many inductions use naturally occurring phenomena to enhance or verify the trance state or to emphasize the "specialness" of the hypnotic situation. As a simple example, suppose the therapist asks the patient to begin the hypnosis sitting in a chair, with eyes closed and one arm extended in front of him or her. The therapist then says, "As your hand feels heavier and heavier, it will slowly begin to fall toward the arm of the chair. As this occurs you will feel increasingly focused upon sensations in your arm and hand . . . and you will experience a pleasant sense of relaxation when your arm finally touches the fabric on the chair." The therapist is relying on "natural" events to take their course. Certainly the patient's hand and arm will feel heavier after a few minutes of being held forward. The therapist's suggestions of attention to sensations in the arm will make these more likely. Finally, the muscles in the patient's arm will be relaxed at the same time that the fabric of the chair is touched and the arm no longer needs to be elevated.

Failure-Free "Tests" of the Trance State

A good hypnotherapist does not challenge the patient to do something or not to do something during the trance induction. For example, it would be inappropriate in a trance induction for the therapist to indicate that the patient *must* or *will* experience hand levitation at a given point in the trance, or that the patient cannot open his or her eyes. Direct challenges of that type leave open the possibility of failure for both the patient and the therapist. Instead, the patient is presented with "no-fail," easy suggestions, many of which the patient can follow in a variety of ways. Suggestions for deep relaxation constitute an example of such "easy" directions that most subjects are able to follow (S. C. Wilson & Barber, 1978). Other, more difficult suggestions are presented in a way that indicates that any response (including no response) is a success. For example, hand levitation can be presented as follows:

> And now you *may* begin to feel an interesting sensation in your hand . . . and it may be your right hand . . . or it may be your left. Perhaps your hand will begin to feel light and buoyant . . . as if there were helium balloons attached. . . . And it may begin to rise slowly from your lap . . . or perhaps your hand will feel heavier . . . weighted down . . . as if there were a 5-pound weight on it. . . . In any case, your focus is upon your hands, and you wonder what you will feel.

These are directions that no subject can "fail" during the induction procedure.

Sample Inductions

Three sample hypnotic inductions with commentary are presented below. As we have indicated previously, the possible trance inductions that one can use are endless. The inductions described are just three possibilities. It may be helpful to tailor a particular induction to the interest and cognitive style of a given patient, to the degree that this can be done.

Therapist: Before you begin to go into a trance, I'd like you to get as comfortable as possible in your chair.

[The therapist sets an expectation that the patient *will* go into trance.]

You can simply let your eyes close, and let your whole body relax. . . . If you feel any tension or tightness anywhere in your body, you can let it melt away.

[The patient is encouraged to focus on body sensations.]

You will find that although it is necessary to concentrate on the sound of my voice to begin with . . . after a little while your unconscious will listen for you, while your conscious mind drifts wherever you wish.

[Most people will drift into other thoughts.]

And you may find that as you sit and relax, your blood pressure is going
   down, your pulse rate is slowing, and your breathing is becoming
   slower and slower.

["No-Fail" suggestions.]

You may let yourself feel a greater sense of comfort and relaxation as you
   become more and more deeply involved in a state of trance. . . . And
   your mind may wander. . . . You might picture a lovely beach scene.
   . . . Perhaps it is a beach you know, or maybe it is somewhere new. You
   wonder what you will see and hear and experience.

[The therapist helps the patient begin to develop imagery.]

You can let yourself see the scene with great clarity and vividness . . . where
   you are . . . what the sand feels like touching your feet . . . the colors of
   the water, and the sky, and the clouds. . . . Perhaps you hear people in
   the distance. . . . Maybe you can smell that salty fresh smell that you
   often find near ocean water. . . . You might even spy some gulls flying
   nearby . . . and hear them as they fight over some food.

Therapist: If you sit and relax comfortably in the chair, your eyelids may
   slowly shut. . . . And as you slowly and gently breathe through your
   nose, I would like you to silently count backward between 100 and 1.

**[This may be a good induction for someone who is oriented toward
numbers.]**

Each time that you exhale you can go down by 1. . . . As you feel more and
   more comfortable and relaxed, you may find that the numbers may be
   harder to keep straight.

**[Most people will have some difficulty keeping the numbers clear after a
short period.]**

Did you just count 87 or 78? You may find that your conscious mind wishes
   to go to other imagery and pictures. . . . [etc.]

Therapist: As you comfortably relax in the chair, you can allow your eyelids
   to feel heavier and to close. . . . As you move into a trance state, you
   might picture yourself riding an escalator in a large, spacious department store. . . . It is a very large place with many escalators going up
   and down. . . . As you ride the down escalator, you might allow
   yourself to feel increasingly relaxed with each floor you go down. . . .
   And you can hear the whirring sound that escalators make as they
   operate. . . . And you can feel the heavy black rubber on the moving

hand rail. . . . You can see all the people and the various departments that you pass. . . . But with each floor that you come to, you feel an increasing sense of comfort. . . . [etc.]

Trance Utilization

Once the induction is accomplished, what is called "trance utilization" begins. Just as assessment and treatment are probably inextricably bound, so too are trance induction and trance utilization. There are probably some benefits for many patients just in feeling relaxed and focused upon internal states (e.g., see Benson, Greenwood, & Klemchuck, 1975).

We have divided the uses of hypnosis as described below into various sections, according to the given problem. In these sections we elaborate more precisely on how hypnosis may be used for the given complaint in question. However, in general, we use trance in order to help the patient to develop clear and vivid imagery; to allow certain suggestions to be more distinctly remembered by the patient; to build an affect bridge (Edelstien, 1981) to the root of some particular problem; or to assist the patient to modify a psychophysiological state (such as pain). The specifics of these interventions are described later.

Exiting from the Trance State

At the completion of hypnotic work, the therapist generally says something like the following:

> In a few moments I will begin to count backward between 5 and 1. . . . When I reach 1, you will be able to open your eyes. . . . You'll feel awake, alert and aware. . . . You'll realize how you can use hypnosis for your own benefit. . . . When you work with self-hypnosis at home, you will be able to go into trance readily. . . . As you use trance more for yourself, you will be able to do it better and better. . . . You will probably see it as a very valuable and helpful tool. . . . 5 . . . 4 . . . 3 . . . 2 . . . 1.

As we have emphasized previously, it is the rare patient who does not readily open his or her eyes and exit from trance at this point.

Self-Hypnosis

There are those who contend that all hypnosis is self-hypnosis (Araoz, 1985). Although this point remains somewhat controversial (Kihlstrom, 1985), it does appear to us that hypnotic techniques learned in sessions with the therapist can be reinforced and used most efficiently if the patient practices these at home as well. Therefore, we often audiotape hypnotic sessions, or make self-hypnosis tapes for the patient that he or she can use outside the office.

SPECIFIC PROBLEM AREAS

The four problem areas that we describe here to illustrate the use of hypnotic techniques are insomnia, habit disorders (including smoking and obesity), anxiety problems, and pain.

Insomnia

It appears that more than any other single factor, psychological disruptions are the most frequent causes of insomnia (Coleman, 1983; Kales, Bixler, Tan, Scharf, & Kales, 1974; Roffwarg & Erman, 1985). In addition, survey data demonstrate that more drugs are used for sleep than for any other therapeutic purpose (Institute of Medicine, 1979). A study by Mellinger and Balter (1983) indicated that 11% of those taking sleeping pills were seemingly dependent upon them and had been taking them for a year or longer.

There are a variety of pharmacological and nonpharmacological treatments for sleep disorders (Hauri & Sateia, 1985; Mendelson, 1985; R. M. Turner, 1986). We have found, however, that a hypnotherapy approach can often be useful for people who seek treatment for a relatively acute sleep disorder related to anxiety and rumination (often around particularly stressful circumstances in the patient's life). These patients sometimes present with what has been called "dream anxiety attacks" (Roffwarg & Erman, 1985; Spielman, 1986). Fear of such "nightmares" may lead to terror at bedtime, and thus to even more insomnia.

After first establishing that the patient's insomnia is not a function of "sleep hygiene abuse" (Roffwarg & Erman, 1985) (i.e., sleeping too late in the morning, irregular arousal at bedtimes, daytime naps), the therapist should examine the patient's use of alcohol, tobacco, caffeine, and other drugs that disturb sleep. Once it has been established that none of these factors is the central problem, the patient should be asked to maintain a "sleep log" for 1 week. This log should contain details such as when the patient goes to bed, about how long it takes to fall asleep, and thoughts or ruminations at any points at which the patient awakens. Patients who have night anxiety attacks should describe the precise content of these nightmares fully.

Once the therapist and patient have established as clearly as possible what the precise nature of the insomnia is and when and how it occurs, and once they have determined that it is not a function of sleep hygiene abuse or abuse of any of the substances named above, hypnotherapy can be initiated. As we have emphasized earlier, hypnosis should first be explained to the patient. Part of the problem for many of those presenting with insomnia is that they fear that once they feel themselves awakening, they will not be able to go back to sleep. Therefore, in dealing with a sleep disturbance, the therapist should also explain briefly that everyone goes through stages of deeper and lighter sleep throughout the night (Karacan & Moore, 1985). The fact that the patient begins to awaken at different points through the night need not be a cause for alarm. Even if the hypnotherapy is successful, this cycle will continue.

The approach to hypnotherapy that we have found most useful for those with sleep problems is as follows:

First, the therapist should ask the patient prior to hypnosis what the most relaxing place the patient has ever been to is, or what activity he or she finds most restful and tension-free. Some people may describe a past vacation at a tropical beach resort; some may prefer an inn with snow coming down heavily outside; some may talk about running or swimming; and so forth. Whatever the relaxing scene described relates to, the therapist should encourage the patient to elaborate as much as possible. What does this inn look like? Where is the fireplace? What kind of music would be playing? What would the temperature be like? What might the patient smell? And so on.

The therapist should tape the trance and hypnotic induction so that the patient has this material to use at home. It should be recommended that the tape be played at bedtime and at any awakenings.

Once the trance is induced, the patient should again be told about the "normality" of periods of deeper and lighter sleep. Following this, the therapist can have the patient develop the imagery previously elicited regarding the restful and tension-free place or activity. Using many of the patient's own words, the therapist can have the patient vividly imagine the scene in question and the comfort and fatigue that might be felt in the given circumstance.

We have found that relatively few (two or three) office sessions, with regular practice at home, may have a dramatically beneficial impact on this problem; the following case example illustrates this.

Ken was a 32-year-old businessman who presented with severe problems in falling asleep and in staying asleep. Obtaining a history, the therapist learned that in the past 3 months Ken had suffered some significant reverses in his business. He had also been rejected by a woman with whom he had started going out. Although his problems were clearly interpretable in an I-D-E frame of reference, the patient had no interest in addressing anything other than his sleep difficulties. The second of three children, the patient had an older brother who was psychotic and had been in and out of hospitals. Ken was perceived by his parents as unintelligent and marginally competent. He had been able to overcome much of his insecurity regarding his intelligence and had done very well until recently as a small businessman. It appeared that Ken feared opening up any issue other than his sleeping because this would amount, in his mind, to an admission of incompetence.

The initial treatment sessions focused first on obtaining a history and then on having Ken keep a sleep log. In the second session, a sleep relaxation tape was made. In the third and final visit, the therapist elicited feedback on how the tape was working. Since Ken was a scuba diver, the therapist decided with him that this was the imagery to be used in the treatment. Below is a transcript of the sleep tape. The induction procedure is omitted.

> Ken, I'd like you to get as comfortable and relaxed as possible in your bed before using this tape. . . . Let your eyes close . . . and just allow yourself to feel a sense of tiredness . . . drowsiness . . . and fatigue. . . . And as you lie in your bed . . . feeling very comfortable and relaxed . . . you can let your mind begin to drift back to our session . . . in which we used hypnosis. . . . You can allow yourself to remember what it felt like . . . to become increasingly relaxed . . . to let go of your tension and anxiety . . . and to begin drifting deeper and deeper into a comfortable state of trance. . . .
>
> And you can allow your mind to begin to picture yourself . . . scuba diving in California . . . on a gorgeous, warm summer's day. . . . And you can imagine yourself wearing all of your equipment—your wet suit, your tank . . . your flippers, your mask . . . your watch . . . and preparing to go into the water. . . . And you have a buddy with you, as you know you should . . . and that can be anyone you like . . . anyone you feel comfortable with . . . anyone with whom you'd like to go. . . . It can be a real person whom you know . . . or a fantasized person. . . .
>
> You begin going into the water . . . and feel the waves breaking against your body . . . until you're finally at a depth where you're able to dive in and go under. . . . And as you begin swimming under the water . . . and feel what the wet suit feels like against your body . . . and what the mask feels like against your face . . . you realize that you feel extremely comfortable and extremely relaxed. . . . You can hear yourself breathing . . . you can hear the bubbles . . . and feel all your muscles as you swim along. . . . And you wonder about what you'll see . . . and what kind of experiences you'll have on this dive. . . . Your buddy is swimming near you. . . . You swim along and see various fish . . . and plants . . . and rocks . . . and it's all very interesting . . . and very enjoyable. . . . As you dive, you find yourself more and more engrossed . . . with things around you . . . and you think about how beautiful everything that you're seeing is . . . and how relaxing and pleasant and comfortable this dive is . . . and just how you feel completely at peace . . . as you do this dive. . . .
>
> And as you swim along . . . you realize that time is going by more quickly . . . than you were aware of . . . and that soon it will be time to come back up again. . . . And after a short period of time . . . both you and your buddy . . .

get ready to return to the surface. . . . And as you return to the surface . . . as it becomes lighter and lighter . . . with the sun shining through the water . . . you're thinking about how beautiful . . . and comfortable . . . and wonderful . . . this entire scene is. . . . And when you finally come to the surface . . . you slowly swim to the shore . . . and come up onto the beach . . . and you feel wonderful . . . exhausted, but wonderful. . . .

You've enjoyed yourself . . . you felt terrific . . . in doing the dive. . . . It's been a wonderful experience . . . and now you feel so fatigued . . . so pleasantly fatigued . . . that you decide to just take off your tank . . . and your flippers . . . and your wet suit . . . and just lie down on the beach . . . for a few moments . . . just to relax. . . . And you spread a blanket out on the sand. . . . Your swimming buddy has gone elswhere at this point . . . and you just lie down on the blanket yourself . . . in the warm, comfortable sun . . . in order to get a little bit of rest . . . before packing up your car to go home. . . . And just let your eyes close . . . and let that good feeling of fatigue . . . after a positive day's work . . . just overcome you. . . . And you feel so fatigued, so tired . . . and so sleepy . . . and so good . . . that your mind just drifts off . . . to a deeper . . . and deeper . . . state of warm, comfortable relaxation.

After Ken had used the sleep tape for a week, his sleep had improved significantly. When contacted 2 months later, he reported that he had continued to improve, and that he was now almost asymptomatic.

When developing relaxing imagery with a patient, the therapist should be sure to query the patient extensively prior to the trance about his or her likes and dislikes. If a therapist tries to use swimming imagery with a patient who is terrified of the water, or a comfortable scene in the country with a patient who has severe allergies to ragweed and pollen, the treatment will have little chance of success.

Habit Disorders

Smoking

The effectiveness of hypnosis as a treatment for habit disorders has been difficult to evaluate because of vague or insufficient data in many reports (N. W. Katz, 1980; Wadden & Anderton, 1982). In Holroyd's (1980) review of hypnosis as a treatment for smoking, however, she concludes that under favorable treatment circumstances, "at least half, and frequently more than two-thirds of the smokers who begin treatment stop smoking and remain abstinent at least six months. In comparison only 30% of people treated by nonhypnosis interventions remain abstinent after three months (89 studies summarized by Lichtenstein & Danaher, 1976)" (p. 353). Among the favorable treatment circumstances that Holroyd cites are these: at least several hours of hypnotic treatment; an intense interpersonal interaction with the therapist or group; the use of trance suggestions designed to capitalize on the specific motivations of the individual patients (such as health, cleanliness, or family pressures); and adjunctive follow-up contact.

The exact nature of the hypnotic suggestions in the studies reviewed by Holroyd varied greatly. Some, for example, involved covert sensitization (e.g., feelings of nausea), while others had the subject feel healthier and happier seeing himself or herself as a nonsmoker in the future. The major issue appeared to be, as Holroyd notes, that tailoring suggestions to a given patient's underlying motivation proved much more effective than giving the same suggestion to all patients regardless of their particular motivation.

Hector was 42 years old and had smoked between four and six packs a day for his entire adult life. He had decided to seek treatment after increasing pressure from his wife, children (ages 8 to 10), and physician had convinced him to get assistance in trying to stop. After several unsuccessful programs, he had decided to seek the help of a therapist. In addition to his smoking problem, he had a variety of other severe difficulties, particularly in dealing with a narcissistic and controlling boss. It was decided that the smoking issue would be the first addressed (and completed), and that the other problems would be dealt with later.

Hector was given 16 biweekly hypnotic sessions. Audiotapes were also made. The suggestions made in trance to Hector included his being able to breathe easily, getting rid of his chronic hacking cough, realizing that his health was improving, and being reinforced by his wife and children for his smoking cessation. In later sessions, suggestions included feeling disgusted with the taste of tobacco, being turned off by the smell of smoke, being nauseated, and so on. It was also suggested that the smoking being "out of control" was a metaphor for his lack of control regarding his job situation. By the 3rd session Hector had greatly reduced his smoking, and by the 12th session he had stopped completely.

Melissa, in her mid-30s, had smoked two packs a day since the age of 14. She was hoping to become pregnant with her third child and wanted very much to be able to stop smoking. During her first two pregnancies Melissa had been unable to quit, even though she had made numerous efforts with and without structured programs. Although her children had been healthy, she felt great fear that her smoking would hurt her next baby or that "passive smoking" would be harmful to her two little girls.

Initially Melissa was seen for 15 twice-per-week 20-minute visits. In these sessions, she was taught relaxation procedures to use at those times that she became tense because she was not smoking. She was also asked to do rapid smoking within the session, which led to nausea, headache, and throat discomfort. This aversive reponse was then reinforced in a hypnotic trance. She was asked to remember how uncomfortable smoking could be, as well as its other negative aspects.

Over the first several weeks, Melissa was able to cut down to three to five cigarettes per day. The next week, however, she had a severe relapse and began to smoke a pack a day again. She felt frustrated and almost ready to give up. At that point, the therapist asked her to come in with her husband, Gordon. Gordon, a nonsmoker had been hoping for years that Melissa would quit. The therapist requested that Gordon act as "cotherapist" for Melissa. He was taught some relaxation and hypnotic techniques that he could use to help Melissa if she so requested. She made the decision that with Gordon's help she would try to go "cold turkey" over the next week. The therapist asked both Gordon and Melissa to sign a contract that stipulated just what Melissa would do and how Gordon would attempt to help her in her smoking cessation efforts.

Having the couple work on the problem together and having her husband administer the hypnosis as needed proved to be the turning point in the treatment. Melissa was able to quit smoking for the very first time in her adult life. She was seen periodically thereafter to work on relapse prevention.

Obesity

Another habit disorder frequently treated by hypnosis is obesity (Mott & Roberts, 1979). A recent study by Cochrane and Freisen (1986) supported the efficacy of hypnotherapy in the treatment of obesity. Data indicate that depending upon the criteria used, between 19% and 35% of males and between 28% and 40% of females may be classified as obese (Stunkard, 1985). Although old beliefs that psychopathology is the cause of obesity are no longer accepted, it does appear that obesity may lead to a variety of emotional difficulties. For example, the obese person may have an extremely negative body image (Stunkard & Mendelson, 1967), which may lead to great self-consciousness and impairment of social function.

Any hypnotherapy program for obesity should be part of a larger program that includes diet management and behavior modification. The behavior management component of the program (Stuart, 1978) should involve self-monitoring, nutrition education, increased physical activity, and cognitive restructuring. Often such elements can be brought together in a lay-led program, such as Overeaters Anonymous or Weight Watchers. It is with the individual for whom enrollment in such lay-led programs or work with a nutritionist has proven insufficient that hypnotherapy may be useful.

The hypnotherapy aspect of a weight control program for an obese individual emphasizes helping the patient maintain better control over his or her eating and increasing motivation by having the patient imagine himself or herself thinner and pleased with his or her body image.

Miriam was an obese 24-year-old woman who sought therapy for her weight problem shortly after her boyfriend of 3 years ended their relationship. She had dieted periodically and usually with minimal success since she was 16 years old. At various points Miriam had seen diet counselors, attended Weight Watchers and Take Off Pounds Sensibly (TOPS), or used diet books. Generally, after losing 10 or 15 pounds she would "go off the wagon," begin bingeing again, and gain back all the lost weight (plus several more pounds).

Miriam felt that it would be impossible for her to be attractive to men in her current state (more than 65 pounds overweight). She also felt ashamed of her body and unhealthy. The therapist urged Miriam to join Overeaters Anonymous, he felt that it would be useful and important for her to have a good deal of continual and ongoing support in her weight loss efforts. He also began a 10-session series of hypnotherapy visits that spanned a total of 6 months. During these visits, two somewhat different suggestions were given to Miriam in trance. The first set of suggestions related to her visualizing herself at her desired weight trying on attractive clothing; walking by store windows and seeing how good she looked in her reflection against the glass; being reinforced by coworkers, friends, and family members; and so on. Of the second set of suggestions, one involved her being in a supermarket about to buy the types of fattening foods she loved (such as ice cream), and, as she was about to put them into her shopping cart, feeling a surge of motivation to lose weight. At that point in her imagined scene, she would return the fattening food and leave without it. A similar imagined suggestion was that as she went to her refrigerator or cupboard to get fattening food to eat, she would think about how useful it would be for her to be able to lose weight, be more attractive and feel healthier. She would think these thoughts while imagining the tempting food in her trance. At that point she would imagine herself putting the food back, feeling pleased that she was really accomplishing a great deal in her weight loss efforts. Over the 6-month period in which she was treated, Miriam lost about 40 pounds. When seen again a year after the completion of the hypnotherapy, she had maintained her initial weight loss.

Underlying Severe Pathology: A Caution

It should be emphasized that hypnotherapy should not be viewed as a "cureall" for habit disorders, particularly if they are part of a very severe underlying pathology. In a case of trichotillomania (hair pulling) treated by one of us using hypnotherapy, gains could not be sustained because of the patient's severe interpersonal difficulties. In addition, this patient had such great problems regarding intimacy that the hypnotic work did not function to establish a strong therapeutic alliance—one that could then have been the basis for examining other issues.

Lorraine was a computer programmer in her early 30s who had been pulling hair out of her scalp since she was 12 years old. Her problem was so severe that she always had to wear a wig in public. The patient's entry into therapy was clearly related to a sense of developmental dysynchrony and a desire to be able to form a successful relationship with a man. Her trichotillomania kept the patient worried and preoccupied, with fears of "being discovered" arising whenever she began to go out with someone new. Subsequently, she would break off any relationships that appeared to have potential for success. Lorraine also came from a very disturbed family situation, with a father who had been alcoholic and psychotic throughout her growing-up years. The patient made it clear that she did not want to open up "a Pandora's box" either about her family or about her current problems with relationships. She insisted that the therapy focus only on the hair pulling.

Lorraine was initially seen for 3 months. During this period, treatment involved a combination of cognitive–behavioral (counting hairs pulled, keeping logs of her cognitions during the pulling, etc.) and hypnotherapeutic (imaging herself with a full head of hair, combing it, seeing it grow) approaches. The treatment moved in what was an apparently successful direction: Hair on her scalp began to grow again, and some areas filled in completely. However, presumably because she was asked out by a man at work, Lorraine became very anxious and pulled out most of her new growth over a weekend. Shortly after this, she began missing appointments with the therapist and dropped out of treatment. Because so many other intimacy issues that she would not or could not address related to her trichotillomania, the hypnotherapy was unsuccessful. Furthermore, for Lorraine the developing relationship with the therapist also appeared to be cause for anxiety. Her fears of closeness seemed to be very intertwined with her habit disorder, and it proved to be impossible to treat one without treating the other.

Anxiety Disorders

Since relaxation has often been viewed as a major component of hypnotic treatments (Barber, 1984b), hypnotherapy approaches may fit well into the symptomatic therapy of anxiety-related problems. Although hypnosis, for the most part, has not been shown to be superior to other therapies in the treatment of anxiety, it does appear to have an effect equivalent to those of biofeedback and progressive relaxation (Lehrer & Woolfolk, 1984).

The symptomatic treatment of anxiety disorders is quite similar to the treatment of insomnia. The patient is first asked to track his or her anxiety over the course of a week: When does it occur? What seem to be the precipitants? What is the patient thinking about before and during the event (i.e., the "anxiety attack," if this is part of the problem)? Following this period of tracking, the therapist elicits from the patient information about places or events with which feelings of comfort, well-being, and relaxation are associated. The patient is then taught to imagine the comforting scene vividly in trance. An audiotape is made eliciting the relaxing scene. The patient is then urged to try to quickly visualize the relaxing scene whenever he or she is beginning to feel anxious, perhaps with the aid of a signal (e.g., unobtrusively touching two fingers together).

An alternative strategy for a specific fear-provoking situation, such as public speaking anxiety, is to have the patient view himself or herself during trance in that specific situation. The patient should be assisted in viewing the scene as clearly as possible; therefore, the therapist, before beginning the trance, should clarify in minute detail just what that situation is like. To use the example of public speaking fears, the therapist might ask, "What do you think the room you will be using looks like? How many people will you be speaking to? What will the smells be like?" and so on. During the trance the patient is guided through a detailed visualization of the feared situation, but with feelings of calmness, enjoyment, and self-efficacy.

At times (as will be seen in one of the examples below), we have used hypnotic approaches not only to treat anxiety symptoms directly, but to help clarify for ourselves and our patients the problems underlying their anxiety.

Marie was a 25-year-old salesperson. For more than 2 years, she had suffered from severe and at times almost incapacitating bouts of anxiety. These would affect her at what seemed to be unpredictable moments. She had gone to a variety of physicians for treatment, believing or being told at different points that her symptoms were attributable to inner ear problems, sinus difficulties, thyroid imbalance, or hypoglycemia. Finally, after exhausting a variety of medical routes, and with increased responsibility and public exposure on her job, the patient was encouraged by a close friend to seek therapy. This she failed to do until 3 weeks prior to an 8-week business trip. The patient feared that unless she received help quickly for her anxiety, she would be too incapacitated to travel (which was essential for her work) and would risk losing her job.

Marie was seen for six visits prior to her trip, mainly focused upon hypnotherapy for her anxiety. She kept a log on her anxiety attacks for a week; from this, it appeared that many of them were associated with public situations during which she was with several people and perceived herself as being judged or evaluated. She was then taught to evoke pleasant imagery whenever she was in a circumstance that had been clarified (by her log) to evoke her anxiety attacks. In addition, the therapist made a relaxation–hypnosis tape, which Marie played for herself in the morning and at night. By the time she left on her business trip, her fearfulness had been greatly reduced. She continued to use the relaxation tape while away, and when she returned she reported having had only about one relatively mild anxiety attack per week while away, as compared to 15 or 20 *a day* previously.

Marie was seen on a biweekly basis for several months following her return. During this time, a number of issues related to her job were addressed. At the end of that period, she reported infrequent and very mild periodic episodes of anxiety in times of severe stress. She felt that the hypnosis had provided her with a very useful tool for dealing with her problem.

Hypnosis can also be used to elucidate the underlying basis for a given symptom, which can then be addressed nonhypnotically. This was the case with Randy, a 39-year-old divorced man who complained of the recent onset of panic attacks in tunnels, theaters, and other large public places. Since his separation from his wife 10 years earlier, Randy had had a variety of relationships with women, most of which had proved frustrating, painful, and unsatisfying. Many of these relationships had ended in the woman's leaving Randy for reasons unclear to him. Three months prior to seeking treatment, Randy had met Kim, a 34-year-old divorcée, and his relationship with her was becoming very serious.

A hypnotic trance was used to clarify the underlying nature of Randy's panics; once hypnotized, he was asked to imagine himself in a feared situation. Specifically, he was asked to visualize himself in a theater with Kim having a panic attack (an event that had occurred several weeks prior to the therapy session). In the hypnotic scene, he was asked to imagine himself *not* running out of the theater (as he had actually done), but staying and "allowing your worst fears to be realized; see what actually happens if you stay [in your imagination]." When the fantasy was later discussed with the therapist, a great deal of valuable data emerged. Randy pictured himself screaming and crying in his seat at the theater. Suddenly, two men in white uniforms arrived and placed him in a stretcher and then into an ambulance. In the ambulance he realized that he was being brought to a cemetery because he was dead; neither Kim nor anyone else was with him. This imagined scene, when discussed with Randy in later sessions, proved quite useful in his therapy. He realized that he felt panicky about being left by Kim (as he had been by so many other women) and worried about growing older and dying without achieving some of his goals, such as having a home and family.

Pain

Of all the clinical application of hypnosis described in this chapter, the clearest and most unambiguous support exists for its use in pain control (E. R. Hilgard & Hilgard, 1983; Wadden & Anderton, 1982). Over the years, a number of excellent studies have compared hypnosis to other treatment modalities, both in the laboratory and in clinical settings. For the most part, hypnosis has been shown to have significant utility in the relief of pain, above and beyond nonspecific and placebo effects (Wadden & Anderton, 1982). Stern, Brown, Ulett, and Sletten (1977), for example, in a laboratory study of pain control (i.e., the pain was developed in the subjects by having them immerse their arms in very cold water or by tightening an arm tourniquet), compared hypnosis, acupuncture, morphine, aspirin, diazepam (Valium), and placebo. They found that hypnosis provided the greatest pain relief, followed by morphine, acupuncture, aspirin, diazepam, and placebo (in that order).

In a clinical context, J. A. D. Anderson, Basker, and Dalton (1975) compared hypnosis and medication for migraine headache pain. It was found that during the first 6 months, patients in the two treatments did not differ significantly in the frequency or intensity of attacks (although during this period, results did tend to favor the hypnosis condition). In the second 6 months, however, hypnotic treatment was clearly superior to medication. Furthermore, a much larger number of patients in hypnosis had a complete remission in the final 3-month period of the trial.

There are three frequently used methods for pain control described by E. R. Hilgard and Hilgard (1983): direct suggestion of pain reduction; altering the experience of pain, even though the pain may persist; and directing attention away from the pain and its source.

Direct Suggestion of Pain Reduction

Since most patients have experienced the pain-reducing properties of local anesthesia during dental work, this image is frequently evoked as a method of hypnotic pain control. For example, in treating back pain, the therapist may induce a trance and then ask the patient to imagine that he or she has had his or her hand injected with Novocaine. As the numbness spreads, the patient is urged to experience the coolness and/or tingling associated with local anesthesia. The hypnotherapist then has the patient touch the affected pain area with his or her numbed hand and tells the patient to "allow the anesthetized feeling to spread to your back." Melzack and Wall (1982) reported great success with this method for the management of back pain.

A patient treated by one of us for severe and chronic discogenic back pain frequently used a heating pad while lying in bed to reduce her discomfort. The therapist helped the patient, while hypnotized, develop the imagery of experiencing a "warm, healing blood flow" in the painful areas of her back and buttocks. An audiotape of these suggestions was made and used by the patient several times a day. This technique proved extremely helpful in allowing the patient to function more effectively on her job, and to begin to walk and exercise on a regular basis.

Altering the Experience of Pain

The therapist may use hypnosis to modify the pain by localizing it, moving it to another area of the body, or changing its intensity of duration. For example, Erickson (1967/1980) described the displacement of pain in a terminally ill patient. Dying of prostatic metastatic carcinomatosis, the patient suffered from intractable abdominal pain. Erickson taught him to displace the pain to his left hand. In this location, the patient found the pain far more tolerable and lived with less distraction from his pain during the last months of his life. In another case described by Cooper and Erickson (1959), a patient with 5- to 10-minute episodes of intractable stabbing pain from cancer was taught to experience these as if they were lasting 10–20 seconds.

Directing Attention Away from the Pain and Its Source

In the third method of pain control, the therapist refocuses the patient's attention away from the pain and onto pleasant comfortable and relaxing imagery. E. R. Hilgard and Hilgard (1983) reported the hypnotic treatment of a 14-year-old boy with leukemia. The patient had lesions in his brain, liver, and chest, and suffered from terrible pain in his chest. The Hilgards used hypnosis to have the boy imagine himself prior to his cancer playing Little League baseball. This method of pain reduction was usually effective and helpful for him.

In general, it has been estimated that in approximately 50% of the cases to which hypnotic pain control is applied, there is a beneficial impact (E. R. Hilgard & Hilgard, 1983; Kroger, 1963; Morphis, 1961). Thus, hypnosis is clearly worth a trial in circumstances where the patient's central symptom is in the area of pain management.

CONCLUSIONS

As we have indicated, we believe that hypnotic techniques do have a place in the therapist's battery of treatment methods, particularly in circumstances where the patient is presenting with a major focus upon symptomatic concerns. In our view, and that of others (Cautela, 1975; Dengrove, 1976; Kroger & Fezler, 1976; Spanos & Barber, 1976; Weitzenhoffer, 1972), hypnotic approaches have remarkable similarities to cognitive–behavioral practices and can easily be applied by the experienced clinician. It is important to remember, however, that the therapist must always maintain a clear sense of the broader dynamics of a given situation, and should not merely apply a set of techniques in an unthinking way or in a manner that dehumanizes the patient.

9

Treating Personality Disorders

There are persons who always find a hair in their plate of soup for the simple reason that, when they sit down before it they shake their heads until one falls in.
—Christian Friedrich Hebbel, *Herodes and Mariamne* (1850/1939)

Of all the varied problem areas presented by patients, none challenges the brief therapist's skills and capacities as much as the area of personality (or character) disorders. Because patients with these disorders were so difficult to treat in short-term therapies (or perhaps therapies of any length), many brief models implicitly or explicitly establish criteria that exclude such patients (e.g., Mann, 1973; Sifneos, 1972). Other methods posited by prominent brief therapists for dealing with patients who display personality pathology are as follows: (1) ignoring character issues in favor of maintaining a clear, manageable, and circumscribed focus (e.g., Klerman *et al.*, 1984); (2) appealing to the patient's healthy side, in an attempt to sustain a cooperative effort to address the difficulty in question without excessive characterological interference (e.g., "You are far likelier to improve if you do your therapy homework assignments than if you don't"; Beck *et al.*, 1979). Both of these approaches attempt to circumvent characterological difficulties and avoid addressing such problems "head-on" (at times a most desirable strategy). Some recent brief therapies, however, do make character pathology the central focus of treatment (e.g., Luborsky, 1984; Strupp & Binder, 1984).

Most patients neither need nor want to address characterological problems. However, for one subgroup of patients, personality difficulties present such pervasive impediments in various aspects of their lives (including the ability to profit from therapy) that if any treatment intervention is to have even a chance of success, it must in part deal with personality issues. In this chapter, we address the brief therapy of patients with personality problems. A focus on personality disorders should be undertaken only if it is clear that the patient's characterological trends so intrude upon the work of therapy and/or upon the patient's abilities to interact with others that any improvement must be predicated upon such a focus. The brief therapist, in choosing this focus, acknowledges that the course of treatment will probably be longer than the usual course for the other foci described in this book. As with other foci we have presented, however, it is important that the clinician remember that all the work of treatment need not be done at the same time, and that, almost by definition, the characterologically impaired patient will be seen for many courses of treatment over many years.

It is also important that the brief therapist take a perspective that goes against the more standard analytic therapeutic approach to the detection and treatment of personality disorders. That is, rather than seeing character problems as the area that *must* be treated before any other difficulties can be addressed, the brief therapist should assume (until convinced otherwise) that even those with severe characterological impairment can profit from treatment aimed at one of the foci discussed elsewhere in this book. Only after attempts at addressing one or more of these foci have been hampered by the patient's characterological impediments should the therapist turn to a personality focus.

THE NATURE OF PERSONALITY DISORDERS

Initially, psychoanalysts were interested in character pathology only insofar as it intruded upon the target symptoms addressed in treatment. Rapidly, however, character resistances and their analyses began to take center stage and became a distinguishing feature of most psychodynamic therapy approaches (Frances & Widiger, 1986).

Characters disorders are generally viewed as consisting of behaviors and traits that are found in "normal" as well as disturbed populations. For those with personality disturbances, however, "personality traits are inflexible and maladaptive and cause either significant impairment in social or occupational functioning or subjective distress" (American Psychiatric Association, 1980, p. 305). Thus, personality disorders are a matter of degree and may be difficult for even skilled clinicians to distinguish with accuracy and reliability (American Psychiatric Association, 1980, p. 24). Furthermore, even though personality disorders are supposedly characterized by inflexibility and consistency over time, research in personality psychology indicates that most people show great variability in social behavior from situation to situation (Mischel, 1983).

Studies of the epidemiology of character disorders indicate that they occur at a relatively high rate in unscreened general population samples (Bremer, 1951; Essen-Moller, 1956; Lagner & Michael, 1963; Leighton, 1959). Merikangas and Weissman (1986), reviewing a large number of studies, write: "The best estimate of the prevalence of personality disorders considering all of the studies was approximately seven percent" (p. 265). When one takes into account the fact that personality disorders are probably six or seven times more common in a patient population than in an unscreened community sample, it is clear that a number of patients seeking mental health treatment suffer from character pathology.

Research on the natural course of personality pathology is still at a very early stage. The studies that have been done, however, appear to indicate a relatively high level of stability over time for those disorders examined, such as schizoid and schizotypal personality disorders (McGlashen, 1986; Plakun, Burkhardt, & Muller, 1984; Wolff & Chick, 1980) and borderline personality disorder (Pope, 1983). Such stability is not apparently as true for antisocial personality disorders, which appear to evidence a great deal of spontaneous improvement in middle age (Robins, in press).

Merikangas and Weissman (1986) conclude their review of the epidemiology of personality disorders with the following sobering assessment:

> There is a general agreement that the personality disorders have a chronic course characterized by persistent impairment in social functioning and increased risk of psychiatric symptomatology and diagnoses. . . . [P]ersonality disorders constitute one of the most important sources of long-term impairment in both treated and untreated populations. Nearly one in every 10 adults in the general population, and over one-half of those in treated populations, may be expected to suffer from one of the personality disorders. (p. 274)

CLASSIFICATION OF PERSONALITY DISORDERS

There are 11 major character disorders listed within the *Diagnostic and Statistical Manual of Mental Disorders*, third edition (DSM-III; American Psychiatric Association, 1980). Rather than describing each individually, we have chosen to present the character disorders in "clusters" as a prelude to discussing their treatments. This "Cluster" concept has been described by Siever and Klar (1986), with supporting validity data offered by Kass, Skodol, Charles, Spitzer, and Williams (1985) and Stangl, Pfohl, Zimmerman, Bowers, and Corenthal (1985). The disorders are grouped into clusters according to their major unifying characteristics. Thus, for example, the "odd cluster" is typified by strange, eccentric behaviors; the "dramatic cluster" by histrionic and dramatically exaggerated behaviors; and the "anxious cluster" by tension, anxious distress, and behaviors (such as compulsions) aimed at alleviating anxiety.

The "Odd Cluster": Schizoid, Schizotypal, and Paranoid Personality Disorders

Patients in the "odd cluster" are often characterized by an aloofness and detachment from others. For those with more paranoid trends, this is often accompanied by suspiciousness, anger, and fear of being used or exploited. The schizotypal patient may have an odd or peculiar manner, dress, or set of cognitions about the world.

At times, patients in this cluster may be somewhat difficult to differentiate from patients who might be diagnosed more accurately as having borderline personality disorder, because of the psychotic-like thinking sometimes found in both (Gunderson, Siever, & Spaulding, 1983).

The "Dramatic Cluster": Borderline, Antisocial, Histrionic, and Narcissistic Personality Disorders

Patients in the "dramatic cluster" tend to behave in exaggerated, dramatic, and overly reactive ways. They frequently display extreme anger, depression, and impulsivity, particularly in interpersonal relationships. At times one may find extensive sexual seductiveness and "acting out," and/or excessive use of drugs and alcohol. In antisocial personality disorder, there is also frequently a history of criminal behaviors. Patients with narcissistic character disturbances often display grandiosity, exhibitionism, entitlement, and a marked lack of empathy or ability to "stand in another person's shoes." Overall, these patients show enormous instability in their interpersonal relationships and great lability of affect (Clarkin, Widiger, Frances, Hurt, & Gilmore, 1983). Their relationships with therapists are frequently typified by idealizing the clinicians at one moment and despising them the next.

The "Anxious Cluster": Avoidant, Compulsive, Dependent, and Passive–Aggressive Personality Disorders

Patients in the "anxious cluster" are characteristically anxious and preoccupied. Although their impairments may be quite extensive, they frequently lack the frank deficits found in patients in the first two clusters. They feel fearful, worried, and tense much of the time, and participate in behaviors that they hope will lessen their anixety. For example, the person with passive–aggressive personality disorder may continually put off or "forget" tasks he or she would prefer to avoid. The obsessive–compulsive's perfectionism and controlled emotionality about finding the "right" partner may allow him or her to avoid the anxiety associated with commitment to a relationship. Siever and Klar (1986) suggest that avoidant patients in this cluster may be differentiated from patients in the "odd cluster" in an interview situation. The "odd" patient cannot overcome his or her peculiarities even after being helped to feel more comfortable with the interviewer, whereas the avoidant patient who has had a chance to become more comfortable does not display extensive deficits in rapport or engagement.

The three cluster categories described, we believe, "make sense" clinically; we frame our specific treatment approaches using them as a context.

PSYCHOTHERAPY WITH
PERSONALITY-DISORDERED PATIENTS

Addressing Previously Described Foci

For many patients, even those with severe personality disorders, addressing the psychotherapeutic foci already described in previous chapters may provide helpful and sufficient therapy. The clinician should never jump to the conclusion that because a patient's character structure clearly fits within Axis II of DSM-III, he or she cannot be helped by a course of brief therapy addressing loss, interpersonal conflict, or the other foci we have recommended. Even the most experienced psychotherapist may on occasion be surprised by the enormous strides possible for patients with major character pathology when they find themselves in a relationship with a therapist whom (for whatever reason) they can trust, feel an affinity for, and perceive as being understanding and empathic. It may be very difficult at times to predict in advance how a given patient will respond to psychotherapy. If the therapist is fortunate enough to treat a patient at a developmentally "fluid " time (e.g., the midlife crisis for a patient with an antisocial personality disorder, when he or she has decided that there is more to life than sex, drugs, and rock and roll), a minimal intervention may be sufficient to begin "channeling" the patient into a less dysfunctional life style.

In discussing the issue of predictability of change, Carl Whitaker (personal communication, 1984) has said:

> Who knows why people change. You never can tell. I heard a story once about a cop who was trying to get a guy down off a bridge. The guy was trying to commit suicide. The cop kept trying to talk him down with no luck. Finally, the cop got so frustrated that he pulled out his revolver and said, "If you don't come down I'll shoot you." The guy came right down.

The "ripple effect" may also be extremely important as it applies to the personality-disordered patient. That is, for a patient in the "odd cluster" to feel a sense of contact with even one person about the death of his or her mother, or for a patient in the "dramatic cluster" to feel a sense of control regarding his or her sleep disturbance, or for a passive–aggressive patient in the "anxious cluster" to tell his wife he is angry at her may go a long way in helping such a patient make other relevant modifications in other aspects of life.

In an interesting finding with relevance in this regard, K. Holroyd (personal communication, June 1982) studied a number of patients who had been treated with biofeedback for tension and migraine headaches. He found that those whose headaches improved often spontaneously reported other life changes, such as being more assertive at work, clarifying needs with a spouse, and so on. Improvement and control in one aspect of these patient's lives seemed to have an impact upon other areas that had never been discussed or addressed. Such may often be the case for patients with characterological disturbances, as well as others seeking psychotherapy. That is, mastery over one set of issues may have important impact for other difficulties and even for one's overall personality structure.

As an example of a patient with severe character pathology who was treated with a limited focus, we briefly describe a woman named Norma.

Norma came from a severely disturbed family of eight children, four of whom had been hospitalized for psychosis, alcoholism, or drug abuse. Aged 32 when she sought therapy, Norma was seen intermittently over a 5-year period. She came to treatment because of severe depression that appeared to be related to pressures from her family to "do more" to take care of one of her adult sisters, who had become psychotic and suicidal and who had recently been hospitalized. Norma had also had many extremely disrupted relationships with men in a romantic context, and with her employers of either gender (she worked as a commercial artist). The patient's characteristic interactions with people would place her in the "dramatic cluster" of personality disorders. She was often impulsive and at times explosive. In her 20s, Norma had used alcohol and drugs to excess, although this behavior had ended by the point at which she entered treatment. Throughout therapy Norma's tendency was to idealize the male clinician who was treating her, and her characterological issues did not impede the treatment but appeared in some ways to facilitate it. The initial focus was on the issue of developmental dysynchrony. Norma's family had always made her the "parentified child" and had placed inordinate pressures upon her to take care of them all (including her mother and father). The therapist helped her to examine the fact that, being in her 30s, she was too young to be the mother and father to her parents and siblings, and she was also too old to be just "a good kid" in the family.

The initial focus in treatment was upon helping Norma take the necessary steps to separate from her family in a developmentally appropriate way. Since one of the precipitating events that had brought Norma in for treatment was the psychotic break and subsequent hospitalization of her sister, and her parents' pressure for her to "manage" this sister's hospital care, the opportunity to address the problem directly existed *in vivo*. Over eight weekly visits (one with Janet, Norma's "healthiest" sister), the patient addressed the issue of dealing with her parents in a more developmentally appropriate way. Norma took a very useful step when she, with the therapist's help, refused to attend several meetings at the psychiatric hospital in her parents' stead. She was also able to begin to explore the ways in which her familial interactions made her afraid of being "smothered and controlled" in intimate relationships.

After the initial eight visits, Norma was not seen again for about a year. When she returned, she was seen again for four visits focusing upon a developing relationship with a man. She had been handling things with her family far better, and without getting "sucked in" as she had so many times in the past. Over the subsequent 3 years, Norma was seen for a total of 10 visits focusing, for the most part, upon issues of work and relationships. Norma also wrote to the therapist every 6–8 months describing her current situation. She appeared able to incorporate much of what went on in treatment, and carried it with her during the extended periods between her visits. Over the 5 years during which Norma was treated, she established a friendly but separated relationship with her parents and family. (She did not, for example, agree to have her brother's severely disturbed, alcoholic 16-year-old daughter move in with her, withstanding great pressure to do so.) She also started a free-lance business, which allowed her to be her "own boss." Her subsequent business relationships were much improved. Finally, although Norma did not have any interest in getting married, she had extended and positive relationships with several men during the period in question.

Norma's basic character structure was not extensively addressed; however, she appeared to make some useful and substantial changes in her overall style of relating. This was achieved in fewer than 25 visits over a 5-year period.

When Other Foci "Don't Work"

Although there are many patients with personality disorders who, like Norma, can respond to the more standard foci described, some cannot or do not. How is the therapist to know when the emphasis in treatment should be upon character issues and his or her major focus should be shifted? We believe that two major factors contribute to the decision to emphasize a characterological focus:

1. The patient's personality style intrudes so severely upon the work of therapy and/or upon the establishment of a therapeutic alliance that little is achieved. For the clinician, the experience of working with a patient under such circumstances may be one of frustration and/or despair about being unable to provide anything useful or beneficial.

2. Although the patient appears to be at least moderately receptive to treatment while in the office, there is an apparent lack of "follow-through" outside. Homework assignments are rarely done; activities are seldom un-

dertaken that might change typical forms of interaction; and "nothing ever changes" in the patient's real life.

We describe below a patient for whom a focus upon the issue of loss proved ineffective because of her severe personality maladjustment.

Natalie was aged 31 and single when she sought treatment. Although she had achieved a good deal academically, she wandered through a variety of insubstantial part-time jobs during much of her adult life. Her professional difficulties reflected the fact that she was usually at odds with her employers and would get fired or quit after brief periods of time. Natalie, who had been in psychotherapy a number of times in the past, sought treatment 3 years after the tragic and prolonged death of her father, who had been injured in an industrial accident. He had lingered on for months after this accident, receiving medical treatment and surgery that proved fruitless. The patient viewed herself as suffering from "an unresolved grief reaction." She stated that she never felt rested after a night's sleep, and was always depressed and upset. She had poor, hostile relationships with men and women and almost always felt abused by others. Natalie also was obsessed with the thought that she would be in some type of accident, like her father, which would eventually lead to her death. She "hated the medical establishment" for their "abuse" of her father.

In first beginning to treat the patient, the therapist began with a focus upon the loss of her father. Because of Natalie's pervasive personality pathology (falling at times in the "anxious cluster" and at other times in the "dramatic cluster"), it was necessary to abort this focus in favor of a characterological orientation. Some transcript excerpts may give the reader some sense of how difficult the loss focus was to maintain with Natalie.

The following excerpt is from the first session. The therapist and patient had agreed upon a focus of loss, examining the nature of Natalie's relationship with her father. The father had been a "weak but abusive" man, who had been addicted to prescription narcotics for many years prior to his accident and death. The patient had frequently been beaten and verbally attacked by her father, but her two younger brothers had not been abused. Her mother had been unhelpful, and also quite critical of the patient during her childhood. Natalie's typical behavior with men was to be somewhat seductive, passive, and advice-seeking, and then quickly to feel controlled, betrayed, and angered—a set of behaviors that clearly intruded during the therapy.

Patient: I don't know if you can offer me the type of in-depth therapy that I need. It's not clear to me whether to talk about my father and his illness, or my mother and what's gone on with her, or my brothers, or what. It would really be easier if you could direct me and tell me just what to address and what to say.

Therapist: I'll try to give you some sense of structure, but I sure can't tell you what to say.

P: I hate it when therapists are just silent. I went to a therapist once who didn't speak to me for weeks—what a jerk. I really need help in knowing just what to talk about.

This constant pushing for structure and control continued through the first two visits. After the second session, the patient had felt upset regarding her memories of her father. She called the therapist, who discussed the situation briefly with her and then asked her to bring it up at their next visit, which she agreed to do. Below is an excerpt from that session.

P: Did you feel like I was asking too much of you the other day [when she called]? You sure did rush me off the telephone.

T: I felt like you wanted to talk about the session.

P: No (*angrily*), not the session—my feelings about my father.

T: The session and your reaction to it. I thought we could talk about it briefly and then go into more detail when we met today. I also felt that if you continued to feel distressed, you could call me back.

P: Even after you were so quick and rude to me? You acted like, "Everyone deals with it, why can't you? Don't bother me."

T: That's not what I felt. I felt like you could handle it, and if you felt badly you would call. I also felt that not much could be done to change the situation at the time. We are talking about pretty painful stuff here.

P: I have two things to say about that: I'd rather call an anonymous hotline than get rebuffed by you again and be humiliated by you again. You acted like, "She's being a cry baby."

T: (Continuing to try to explain his behavior on the telephone:) I see you as a basically strong person who can handle your life pretty well.

P: Thank you, but no thanks. Now you're putting me in a corner so I have to be strong, just like outside.

The session continued with Natalie thwarting almost any attempts by the therapist to work with her or to maintain a focus. She repeatedly turned their interaction into a struggle: Any efforts to structure the session were seen as "too controlling," while allowing her to discuss any area of her choosing was viewed as *laissez-faire* and ineffective.

Patients with this type of personality impairment are like the characters at the beginning of Woody Allen's film *Manhattan* who say, "The food here is terrible." "Yeah, and the portions are too small!" One simply cannot avoid the personality focus under such circumstances. Regardless of how the therapist chooses to intevene, the patient's character pathology looms constantly as an intrusive, inhibitory factor, detracting from or preventing therapeutic work.

We believe that a focus on personality impairment requires a particular shift in intervention, which we describe below. We first present the theoretical basis for such intervention, and then present a clinical structure and case examples.

A THEORETICAL MODEL FOR INTERVENTION WITH PERSONALITY-DISORDERED PATIENTS

For the patient with severe characterological impairment, it is often the case that all or most significant relationships (including therapeutic relationships) carry with them so much negative valence from past interactions that the patient repeatedly plays out his or her anachronistic, self-defeating patterns almost regardless of the circumstances. In treating patients for personality disorders, the therapist's goals become these:

1. To help the patient experience and realize his or her self-defeating patterns of interaction.
2. To allow the patient to feel that other modes of interaction are possible.
3. To enable the patient to "test out" new, more functional patterns of relating.

These goals can be achieved by focusing upon current transactions between the therapist and patient as an *in vivo* laboratory for exploring those issues. Similar goals may be accomplished by examining the patient's interaction within the context of a therapy group or a conjoint marital treatment.

It should be noted that, as Strupp and Binder (1984) state, "the patient will unconsciously seek to draw from the therapist behaviors that reenact the role assigned to the object in the patient's enduring scenario" (p. 35). That is, the patient behaves in ways that are provocative and pull from the therapist the reactions that the patient expects others to have. Natalie, for example, described above, believed that most people were harsh, controlling, and punitive (like her father). Her interactions with the therapist were often efforts to have him "show his true colors" by attempting to control her, or not giving to her, or ultimately rejecting her out of frustration.

The characterologically impaired patient tends to have a distorted world view that is self-perpetuating; the term "self-fulfilling prophecy" has been applied to this phenomenon (Carson, 1982). When the male obsessive–compulsive reports that "all women in my life are so explosive and hysterical," he may be correct. What he does not see, however, is the impact that his endless nitpicking rumination and preoccupation with detail has upon others.

In part, the patient's characterological impairments are an attempt to cope with a frightening and disturbing world view. This world view usually develops in childhood and is maintained by the patient's eliciting reciprocal behaviors in others (as described above) and/or by choosing as significant people in his or her life individuals with marked capacities to fulfill the reciprocal roles in the patient's life drama (e.g., the sadistic lover, the ever needy but selfish friend, etc.).

The Corrective Emotional Experience

In 1946, Alexander and French initially described the concept of the corrective emotional experience. They believed that the central goal of therapy is "to reexpose the patient, under more favorable circumstances, to emotional situations which he/she could not handle in the past" (Alexander & French, 1946/1974, p. 66). They felt that insight alone is often insufficient to help patients make substantial behavioral modifications. Rather, it is the opportunity to experience the interaction with another person *without* the feared consequences, or with outcomes contradictory to those anticipated, that leads to change. G. T. Wilson (1981) has commented upon how strikingly similar this perspective is to the behavioral desensitization paradigm.

As we have mentioned in Chapter 1, Alexander and French described as a vivid example of the corrective emotional experience the case of Jean Valjean from Victor Hugo's novel *Les Miserables* (1862/1938). Valjean, a lifelong criminal, is taken in and cared for by a Catholic bishop. Although the bishop catches Valjean trying to steal from him, he continues to be warm and forgiving. This experience has a tremendous impact upon Valjean, and is the cause of his transformation into an honest man. Thus, Valjean's transformation takes place because the bishop does not get "pulled" into relating to him in a "typical" retaliatory manner. That is, although he observes criminal behavior on Valjean's part, he refuses to treat Valjean as a frightening or detestable person. Rather, he continues to treat him with kindness and compassion. It is this disconfirmation that produces the corrective emotional experience and thereby leads to behavioral changes in Valjean.

Strupp (1980a, 1980b, 1980c, 1980d) has indicated that it appears often quite easy for a therapist to be drawn into the reciprocal (i.e., counter-therapeutic) role with a character-disordered patient. The patient, after all, has been able to elicit particular responses from his or her environment over a lifetime, and without great care the therapist may not be immune to the evocative power of this interaction. Under such circumstances, therapy may be ineffective at best or may lead to destructive consequences and even greater impairment at worst (Mays & Franks, 1985).

For Alexander and French (1946/1974), helping to provide the patient with a corrective emotional experience involves, in part, "manipulating the transference." That is, rather than acting as a "blank screen" for the patient's attitudes, fantasies, and projections (an impossible task, since doing nothing has as many meanings and implications as doing anything), the therapist's behaviors need to contradict the reactions expected by the patient. Thus, for example, for a patient who expects cold, controlling relationships with parental authority figures, the therapist needs to be warm and noninterfering. The corrective emotional experience occurs when, as Kiesler (1982) says, "the therapist breaks the transactional cycle by not continuing to be hooked or trapped by the client's engagements or pulls" (p. 19).

The Intervention Sequence

Fromm-Reichmann has indicated that patients need experiences, not explanations (Strupp & Binder, 1984). This is particularly true for character-disordered patients. Whereas others may be able to use understanding and clarification alone to modify their behaviors, the patient with a severe personality disorder has a very fixed set of perceptions about the world and an "automatic" response style. Therefore, emphasizing the therapeutic interaction *in vivo* and experiencing a corrective emotional interaction may prove most beneficial in helping the patient to change. This emphasis in no way precludes the examination of other issues described earlier (e.g., losses or dysynchronies). It is the area, however, that we believe should be foremost when working with characterologically disturbed patients.

It is interesting to note that Lane (1986), in a review of differential change factors in psychotherapy, indicates that more disturbed patients appear to respond best to empathy and support, while less disordered patients seem to respond better to interpretation and cognitive input. In this regard, he writes: "Some patients, those with more serious developmental deficits, may need to draw more on the relationship so as to benefit from therapy; others may need to draw on the therapist's skill to provide meaningful explanations in order to make therapeutic gains" (p. 3). In our view, a key factor in treatment of the patient with severe personality impairments is the development of a "safe" environment in which the patient can risk modifying his or her rigidly maintained interactional approach. In individual therapy, this means being highly empathic and supportive, *along with* any confrontation of the patient's defenses that occurs. In group therapy with such patients, the leader must keep an even greater vigilance regarding the group cohesion than with less impaired patients.

Whereas a healthier patient may be able to overcome or overlook less favorable therapeutic circumstances, the patient with severe character impairment readily falls back upon his or her common modes of interaction under adverse conditions. Furthermore, these patients often elicit less favorable environments from those around them, making change even less likely. In this regard, Wachtel (1982) has written: "Thus . . . the early pattern persists, not in spite of changing conditions but because the person's pattern of experiencing and interacting with others tends to continually recreate the old conditions again and again" (p. 48).

A beneficial intervention sequence with characterologically impaired patients includes many of the following elements:

1. Display of the pathological behaviors and interactions in the treatment
2. Examination of the in-therapy interactions
3. Strong affective involvement
4. Therapist's (and/or therapy group members') descriptions of the patient's dysfunctional pattern
5. Disconfirmation of the response the patient anticipates

Display of the Pathological Behaviors and Interactions in the Treatment

The behaviors that impair some patients' interactive abilities are readily and clearly apparent. Others' dysfunctional patterns are more subtle and far less perceptible. With the characterologically impaired patient, it is the task of the therapist to observe and experience the self-defeating patterns in question.

As an example, June, a 40-year-old divorced lawyer, sought therapy after Joe, the man whom she had been dating for 3 months, suddenly broke off their relationship and refused to see her any longer. This type of situation had occurred on numerous occasions in the past with many other lovers. The focus in the therapy was upon dealing with the loss of Joe, but also related to trying to examine the patterns that repeatedly led to June's rejection in intimate relationships.

A telling incident occurred several months into the therapy. June, who was a superb amateur musician, was soon to be performing at a recital. When she mentioned this to the psychologist, he asked June to inform him when the recital was scheduled. A week later June brought a flyer about the recital to the session. As she handed it to the clinician, June went into a lengthy explanation about how it would not be worthwhile for him to attend: It was too long; she had not had enough time to really rehearse; she had selected the music poorly; and so forth.

The session after the therapist had attended the concert (and found it to be excellent), June began by again discussing all of the shortcomings of the recital. The therapist realized at that point that *he* was beginning to wonder whether he had not misperceived the concert. Perhaps the music had been poorer and less well performed than he initially thought; maybe there were too many selections played; and so on. Once he realized his reactions, he said to June, "You almost have me believing that the concert, which I enjoyed, was awful. Perhaps you're eventually able to convince most of the men in your life about all of your inadequacies." It began to be clarified to June at that point that what she perceived of as being "humble" and "not tooting my own horn" could be perceived very differently by others.

Examination of In-Therapy Interactions; Stong Affective Involvement; Descriptions of the Dysfunctional Pattern

Because the next three elements of the treatment sequence are very closely related, we discuss them together. It is an important part of the therapist's work to try to clarify and elucidate for himself or herself as well as for the patient what types of self-defeating behaviors are repeatedly evidenced. The examination of immediate in-therapy behaviors is usually a more intensely emotional process than abstractly describing behaviors or events outside of the treatment. Yalom (1985) believes that such affective intensity is a very significant element in an interpersonal approach to psychotherapy.

Exploring *in vivo* interpersonal issues in psychotherapy frequently involves the therapist's talking with the patient about how he or she is feeling right now (in the therapy), as well as the therapist's exploring his or her own responses within the treatment. It also may include "stopping the action" and looking at "what just went on."

Tina, a young woman with chronic job and relationship problems, complained that people never gave her any clear feedback, and therefore jobs never worked out and men would leave her precipitously. Her style in therapy was to come into a session talking about her concerns and difficulties over a given week, occasionally asking rhetorical questions, and hardly giving the therapist the opportunity to respond to what she was saying. It proved to be useful to her when the therapist indicated that he felt "blocked out" and that she really did not appear to want feedback from him, because she rarely left him with the opportunity to provide any.

Andy, a 36-year-old divorced man who complained that he "could never really get close to anyone," was describing his marital breakup to the therapist. He went through an extended presentation, talking about his ex-wife, Ramona, and her numerous infidelities during their marriage. She had "suddenly" told him that she no longer loved him, had not cared for him for many years, and wanted a divorce. For 3 years afterwards he had not dated or gone out, and had spent most of his nonwork time alone in his apartment or going to movies. After hearing his story, the therapist commented:

"You've spoken about a series of terrible events—your wife's affairs, her sudden breakup with you, being forced out of your home—but you're describing it all like it happened to someone else. There are no real feelings or emotions expressed. It's as if you need to distance yourself from these things as much as possible." (In fact, Andy's presentation of almost every topic was monotone and uninvolved.) This input proved helpful in allowing the patient to begin to try to express his emotions more than he had previously. Patients who are disconnected from others are often disconnected from themselves and their own emotions as well.

Disconfirmation of the Response the Patient Expects

As we have described, people expect others to respond to them in a particular manner. Shy, timid people expect that others will be uninterested or critical; hostile, suspicious people expect that others will be attacking and belligerent; and so on. Since their own behaviors have frequently drawn such responses from others in the past, their expectations are often realized. It is one of the (sometimes difficult) tasks of the therapy to help the patient disconfirm his or her expected transactional outcomes.

This was the case with Herbert, a 34-year-old man with a severe avoidant personality disorder ("anxious cluster"). (The patient was a preschool teacher at the same nursery school that he himself had attended as a child!) He rarely went to social functions except when he was virtually dragged out of the house by one of his few "interested acquaintances." Herbert spent nearly all of his non-job-related time working on his collection of stamps. Although he was not an unattractive or unintelligent man, he had not gone out on a date in more than *14 years*! A significant turning point came for Herbert about 6 months into the 18-month time-limited group of which he was a member. Veronica, another group member, had been having a great deal of difficulty regarding her living situation. Over the course of several meetings Herbert had asked her on a regular basis about her problems, had been receptive and concerned, and had tried to provide whatever support he could. When in one meeting Veronica turned to Herbert and said that she felt that he was "wonderful" for being so concerned and that she found him to be an "interesting person," Herbert turned beet-red and started to stammer a reply. Several other group members asked him what was wrong, and what had happened. A few moments later when Herbert was able to begin speaking again, he said, "No woman has ever called me an 'interesting person.' I don't know what to say." Herbert's participation in the group had allowed him a corrective emotional experience to counter the limited, safe experiences he allowed himself in his own life. This brief encounter proved quite significant for him later in his therapy.

Wendy, a stunningly attractive 30-year-old, had "always had hopeless, horrible relationships with men." She would find herself involved either with inappropriate men with whom a relationship could not develop (because they were married, gay, alcoholic, etc.) or with men for whom she felt little and whom she quickly rejected. Wendy's father had been physically, emotionally, and sexually abusive, and although she recognized the importance of her relationship with him, "that doesn't help make my life any different."

Her therapeutic interactions had also been highly destructive. She had had a sexual relationship with a clergyman she had gone to for pastoral counseling, as well as with one of the psychiatrists who had treated her. "Everybody is out to get what they can from you," was Wendy's (not surprising) belief.

At one point in her treatment, the patient began to come to therapy sessions (during the summer) wearing increasingly revealing and provocative clothing, and to describe in breathless detail to the male psychologist the sexual relationship with her latest inappropriate lover. During this same visit she developed a painful back problem, which required her to "lie down on the couch, because it hurts too much sitting." As she lay down, the therapist, who had repeatedly explained to Wendy that part of the focus in therapy would be examining in-therapy interaction, asked her how she understood what was transpiring:

Patient: (*Smiling broadly*) You're not going to interpret some of that "You're trying to be seductive" bullshit, are you? My back and neck just hurt, and that's why I'm lying down here.

Therapist: I don't think it's so much seductiveness as testing me out to see how I'll react.

P: What do you mean? What am I testing?

T: I think in moving onto the couch like that, you basically trust me not to get angry at you and not to attack you.

P: Sexually?

T: Yes, but I think even though you trust our relationship and trust me not to be attacking, you need to make sure.

P: (*Begins to cry*) I don't know why you've been nice to me so far. I wonder what you're waiting to get. Most men are trying to get something. It's hard for me to feel comfortable if a man isn't getting something from me. I wait for the next shoe to drop.

This session was beneficial to Wendy, who eventually developed a very positive therapeutic relationship with the clinician. She was also gradually able to stop needing to test the therapist's intentions and acceptance of her, which transferred to other significant relationships.

The Therapist's Role in the Treatment of Character Disorders

For the patient with a significant character disorder, as we have indicated, there is often an (unconscious) attempt to place others in the reciprocal role in his or her unhappy life script. "I'm always victimized," "No one is ever interested in me," and so on all represent central themes in such impaired characterological life scripts. The expected reciprocal role for the "victim" could be the "abusive lover"; for the "shy, withdrawn individuals," it might be the "bored listener"; and for the person who "always gives but never gets," the "selfish, narcissistic friend" will often fill the bill. A important aspect of the therapist's role with a character-disordered patient is to attempt to get a sense of what the patient is trying to "draw out" of him or her, and also of how the patient experiences the therapeutic encounter.

When the therapist is focusing upon characterological issues in a patient with a severe personality disorder, he or she should always keep the following questions in mind:

1. *How am I reacting to this patient*? Does he or she act in such a way that I feel unusually unsympathetic, bored, angry, helpless?

2. *What is the patient's general way of reacting to me*? Does he or she appear detached, hostile, idealizing, aloof, disappointed?

3. *Is there an interactional theme developing across sessions*? For example, does the patient deal with me as a frightening authority figure? Is he or she becoming *more* anxious as our sessions go on? Or, as the patient gets to know me better and reveals more of himself or herself, is he or she at the same time becoming increasingly hostile and suspicious?

4. *How do my reactions to the patient and his or her reactions to me "fit" with his or her usual problematic scenario with people*? (and/or *How do these reactions "fit" with life history issues?*)

These same questions are relevant when treating character-disordered patients in group or in conjoint couples therapy, except that the perspectives are widened. That is, one also considers the patient's reactions to his or her spouse or lover, or to other group members. Indeed, in marital and family therapy, these sorts of characterological transference reactions to the therapist are significantly reduced or muted, since the focus of such characterological conflicts almost always involves family members.

When the therapist is thus able to clarify how the patient is displaying his or her enduring scenario in the treatment, it is easier to stay out of the "trap" of playing the reciprocal role (or helping others to stay out of this trap in a group or conjoint therapy). In addition, the therapist can help the patient examine his or her self-defeating processes, and can thereby make him or her more cognizant of how they occur.

The therapist emphasizing character issues will often ask the patient, "How are you feeling at this moment?", or will ask of an interactional sequence, "What just went on between us?", or will offer his or her own reaction to a sequence of events in the therapy (e.g., "I felt as though you asked me what I thought, but didn't really want to hear my response"). This examination of the in-therapy processes may be done in different ways, depending upon the type of patient being dealt with. In general, it should be remembered that focusing on immediate, in-therapy processes can often be powerfully evocative and effective for the patient. For some patients who either are "too emotional" or are easily confused or overwhelmed by their emotions, such material must be greatly titrated by a focus on various other, less intense, more cognitive matters.

TREATMENT OF SPECIFIC CHARACTER CLUSTERS

We focus our discussion of the treatments of specific character disorders upon the three character clusters described earlier: the "odd cluster," the "dramatic cluster," and the "anxious cluster." Although particular DSM-III Axis II diagnoses within a given cluster may require some technical modifications, the overall thrust of our approach is similar within a given cluster.

We are in general agreement with the principle posited by Liebowitz, Stone, and Turkat (1986):

> [The treatment of character disorders] is in line with guidelines once given a medical school class about the treatment of a dermatologic disorder: "if it's wet, dry it; if it's dry, wet it." We encourage the histrionic patient, who tends to have a poor sense of chronology and indifferent punctuality, to become more attentive to matters of schedule, and to "cool it," with respect to emotional display. We become more "orderly" and "logical" in our demeanor with this type than with other types of patients. With the compulsive, we adapt in an opposite way, often expressing in a rather dramatic way ("You mean to say your father died last Saturday, and you didn't even mention it till now!") what the patient may characteristically report in a perfunctory and affectless manner. (p. 358)

This "principle of opposites" must be applied in a nonattacking and nonjudgmental way, along with the elucidation and elaboration of the patient's interpersonal style described earlier. At the same time that one is attempting to introduce to the patient an approach contrary to his or her usual mode of interacting with the world (e.g., being more affective or more cognitive), one must remain aware that this cannot be done too quickly. The patient has acted in particular ways for a lifetime; to attempt to force such a change is doomed to failure. Before beginning to present the patient with the "opposite" position, it is often useful in early visits to present material that helps the patient shift his or her position *slightly*, but is still related to his or her own usual perspective. Often, with such patients, posing out-of-session tasks as "experiments that might help both of us understand your situation better" rather than as directives is useful toward this end.

A considerable body of data indicates that therapist–patient similarity is a fair predictor of treatment outcome (Beutler, Crago, & Arizmendi, 1986). In addition, people probably do not take kindly to being confronted with pressure to make large and rapid changes in their styles of relating to others. Thus, the therapist to a paranoid patient in the "odd cluster" might say, "You can never be too careful about who you trust, but Frank acts as though he might like to spend a bit more time with you." Or, to a narcissistic patient in the "dramatic cluster," the following might be appropriate: "The group therapy I am considering for you is *very* special and *very* unusual. Only a small percentage of my patients with problems like yours enter such a group." Finally, one might say to the compulsive patient in the "anxious cluster": "Take plenty of time in making that job decision. Don't rush yourself and don't feel compelled to come to a conclusion until you feel a bit more comfortable with what you want to do."

None of these statements should be made insincerely or with a paradoxical intent; they all maintain a recognition of the patient's personality style, and accept it prior to moving toward change.

Treatment of "Odd Cluster" Patients

As described earlier, patients in the "odd cluster" are usually characterized by aloofness and detachment from others. Often these individuals present with a history of great isolation, loneliness, and an inability to connect with others. Those who tend to be more in the paranoid personality range also present a history of suspiciousness and strong beliefs about the general malevolence of others ("They'll screw you if they can").

With such patients, it is central to try to develop a supportive, trusting relationship. These patients are easily injured by even minimal slights (which often go unnoticed by others). It is important to try to keep a constant gauge on the quality of the relationship with questions such as these: "How are you feeling about our meetings?", "What was the last visit like for you?", "Is it getting any easier to talk about things here?", and so on. At the same time, with a patient in this category it may be most appropriate to "titrate" sessions by meeting for 30-minute visits and/or meeting every 2–3 weeks. Coming on too strong or too fast with patients in the "odd cluster" leads to premature termination and the patients' flight from therapy. Many novice clinicians, intuitively sensing the "principle of opposites" cited earlier, will attempt to be too warm too quickly with such patients, and will be viewed with suspicious scorn, or fear regarding their "true" motivations.

The major foci mentioned in other chapters in this book may apply to individuals in this cluster, just as they may apply to all patients with severe character pathology. Problems such as loss, developmental dysynchrony, interpersonal conflict, and various specific symptoms are universal. When working with those who have severe and impairing personality disorders, however, the therapist often maintains a "blended" focus, which includes examining and addressing the characterological difficulties as well as other foci.

A major goal for the therapist treating a patient in the "odd cluster" is to help the patient to trust him or her, and thereby to trust others more; the ultimate aim is for the patient to become less isolated and alone in the world.

When he sought mental health care, Darrell was 39 years old. He was referred to therapy by his internist after his physician had failed to find any medical basis for a persistent and atypical pain problem. As Darrell's current difficulties and related history were revealed in the first several visits, it became clear that he had since childhood been isolated from, suspicious of, and uncomfortable with most people.

Growing up in a small, rural town, Darrell had always been viewed by others as brilliant but peculiar. He "could not stand" most of his peers and spent much of his time when out of school functioning as an "altar boy and general helper" to the local priest. When he was in his early teens, he decided to join a religious order and to go to a monastery. Shortly after he arrived there, he became frankly delusional, believing that all the monks were plotting against him. Following a brief hospitalization, he returned home; a short while after this he began college. Although he was again tremendously isolated and had little contact with others outside of class, Darrell achieved excellent grades. He was able to get a full scholarship to go to graduate school in an obscure area of music history. Once he left home to attend college, he completely cut himself off from his family, and never saw or communicated with them again. Also while a graduate student, Darrell admitted to himself that he was "homosexual." (He would never initially describe himself as "gay": "I'm not gay, in the true sense of the word. That is, I'm never happy. Therefore I won't use the word.") He would periodically visit gay bath houses and find anonymous sex there. At no point in his adult life had he ever been with the same lover on more than two or three occasions.

His work history had been mixed. Although he had lost several good positions in the past because "I didn't play politics," he had been able to get a stable position recently, but did not enjoy the work that he was doing.

As an initial answer to the question of "Why now?", it appeared that Darrell was dealing with a problem of developmental dysynchrony. He was nearly 40 years old but was totally isolated in the world, feeling little career satisfaction or connection with anyone or anything around him. Although in treatment he would talk about his loneliness and increased desire to "make some type of connection with people," he clearly had great fears about the therapist's motivations. Along with focusing initially upon the developmental opportunity that the patient now had to make some of the changes he had been unable to achieve earlier, the therapist also examined with Darrell their relationship. Talking about "what you are afraid I [the therapist] might do to hurt you" proved to be quite beneficial, and allowed the patient to put on the table some of his terror of being humiliated and taken advantage of.

Over the course of 3 years of treatment (usually about once or twice a month), a number of significant issues were addressed with Darrell. An important change in the therapy occurred when, after being seen for approximately a year, he began finding it somewhat easier to socialize with people during nonwork times. The patient was encouraged to try joining a local chess club, which he did. (Prior to this he had only played chess through the mail, never meeting his opponents face to face.) This club membership proved to be a significant turning point for Darrell. He began to attend meetings and tournaments on a regular basis, and even on some rare occasions went to dinner with other club members.

Darrell remained a peculiar and unusual person throughout the therapy, but he did make useful changes. He did not continue to deteriorate and did not become more depressed and isolated—a direction in which he seemed to be moving when first seen. He also began to socialize on a limited but structured basis through his chess club. At the end of treatment he was regularly attending these meetings, and felt "almost friendships" with some people who were isolated, regular attendees like himself. He also felt a sense of trust in the therapist and was seen periodically on an as-needed basis (usually during the Christmas holidays) over the next several years.

For some patients, even meeting goals that many people might consider insignificant must be viewed as an important accomplishment. With such patients it is essential that the therapist try to maintain *realistic* and *reachable* goals, rather than striving to accomplish the impossible, which can lead to frustrating, protracted, and expensive therapy.

Treatment of "Dramatic Cluster" Patients

In general, patients in the "dramatic cluster" display behavior that is provocative, exaggerated, and excessive. Those in the antisocial category may have histories of criminal behavior or difficulties with the law, while patients with more severe narcissistic difficulties may have a sense of grandiosity, exhibitionism, and entitlement. In general, patients in this cluster may demonstrate great lability of affect, often with "storms" of anger directed toward and/or idealizations of significant people in their lives. There is often a history of instability in relationships with many friends and lovers, who are first held in very high regard but are later despised, rejected, devalued, and vilified (Adler, 1986). There also may be excessive use of drugs and/or alcohol. Finally, patients with borderline personality disorder appear to have a very high rate of occurrence of major depression (Docherty, Fiester, Shea, 1986).

Because substance abuse is so prevalent in this population, the therapist must be sure to clarify this issue early. Also, some agreement from the patient to work on substance abuse when it appears to be a problem is critical. Patients in this cluster almost always look far worse when they are using drugs and/or alcohol extensively. It may be extremely difficult to get such a patient to begin to address substance abuse problems; however, if this is not done prior to or concomitant with psychotherapy, we believe that the benefits of treatment will be minimal at best. The man with a borderline personality organization who gets drunk and then has explosive fights with his girlfriend, or the woman with an antisocial personality disorder who uses drugs ("recreationally") but then goes on a shoplifting spree, is unlikely to gain much control over these behaviors as long as the substance abuse continues.

For patients in this cluster, the "Why now?" question is of major importance. A significant aspect of all character problems is that they are often seen as ego-syntonic (i.e., accepted by the individual as part of himself or herself, and thus having low susceptibility to change). This ego-syntonic quality tends to be present more often for the antisocial and narcissistic patients in this cluster and to a lesser degree for the borderline and histrionic patients. Therefore, ascertaining why the patient has chosen to seek therapy now allows some opening for the establishment of a relationship with the patient. Understanding where it hurts, why it hurts, and how it hurts now may allow the therapist to begin to establish an empathetic connection with an antisocial or narcissistic patient, who might under most circumstances not allow such contact with another person.

For example, Walt, a 38-year-old computer programmer, sought therapy with his wife, Mary, 3 months after their young son suddenly died. Walt had used alcohol excessively and had "chipped" heroin on weekends for 15 years. As an adolescent and young man, he had spent time in reformatories and in prison. It was only the tragic and sudden death of his son that allowed him to begin to address some of his issues.

Frederick a 29-year-old writer for a science publication, began therapy after a "crazy" 3-year relationship with a woman broke up. He had been with Barbara in a "mutually destructive and symbiotic relationship," during which both spent much of their nonwork time together drunk or stoned on marijuana (behaviors in which Frederick had participated since he had been

15). The two had also been drug dealers for much of their first year together. Frederick had decided after the relationship with Barbara ended that he would really like to get close to a woman, "settle down," and eventually have a family. Once out of the relationship, however, it rapidly became clear to him that he lacked the skills and abilities to relate socially and that he had severe problems with impotence and premature ejaculation.

Both of these men had completed college and were extremely intelligent, but under an adequate social veneer they were highly disorganized, depressed, and dependent upon drugs and alcohol. Each entered therapy because of problems other than their addictions or character difficulties. It was only after their substance abuse was confronted that they were able to make any real progress. With patients in the "dramatic cluster," the therapist hopes to help the patients make "better," more reasonable judgments; to relate to others in a less self-centered and in a more genuine manner; and to modify their pervasive view of the world as an unstable, constantly changing, and unsafe place.

Willie, when first seen, was 33 years old. He had been "kicked out" of the apartment he shared with Vivian, his girlfriend of 3 years. Willie's patterns with Vivian were similar to his behaviors with other women in intimate relationships. After several months of being "infatuated," he would begin to feel increasingly hostile and sexually cold. He would surreptitiously see other women "just for the sex." All the while, his principal relationship would deteriorate, until there was constant sniping and anger and no sex at all. Although he claimed to love Vivian, Willie's hostility and sexual indifference had infuriated her and finally led her to leave the relationship. At that point, Willie was surprised and could not understand why Vivian was unwilling to "work on things."

Willie, who had been a designer for 10 years, had had nine different jobs during that period. He would invariably get into terrible struggles with his employers, leading to his angry dismissal. In one job, the patient had been given a special set of keys so that he could work in his office at his own convenience, late in the evening or on weekends. By giving him extra responsibilities and privileges, his employer had felt as though he could "transform" Willie from a gifted artist who had a reputation for being impossible to work with to a valued employee. After working late one weekend evening, Willie had "forgotten" to lock the office doors or to reset the alarm. Consequently, when the office was opened the next day, the first person in found all of the typewriters, computers, and radios gone. Willie was dismissed the following week. Again, he could not comprehend his boss's anger or unwillingness to give him a second chance.

Willie had a history of several previous courses of psychotherapy.

When he entered treatment with one of us and was questioned about these therapies, his discussion of these interactions was shallow and superficial. He could recall almost nothing about the clinicians he had seen, how long the treatment had lasted, what had been discussed, and so on. He also (not surprisingly) indicated that little had come out of these interactions.

Although Willie would periodically drink too much or use cocaine, he complied when it was recommended that he reduce his alcohol consumption and cease his cocaine use. Therefore, this never became a major issue in the treatment.

Willie was initially seen for several sessions with Vivian. She was a bright but very constricted woman who had great difficulties in expressing her emotions. She could not really articulate to Willie how pained and angry she felt by his treatment of her. It was clear to the therapist, however, that she experienced herself as beaten down, ignored, and finally enraged by Willie's self-centered, ungiving, and hostile demeanor.

After four individual sessions, focused in part upon Willie's reactions to the loss of this relationship (which was closely followed by the loss of yet another job), the major focus turned to characterological issues. Part of the clinician's efforts were directed toward helping Willie see how his behaviors affected other people—in particular, how they were affecting the therapist and the course of treatment. An illustrative interaction occurred in the fifth visit when, for the fourth time, Willie arrived 15 minutes late for a 50-minute session.

Therapist: It makes it much more difficult for us to use the time effectively when you arrive so late.
Patient: I really wanted to be on time today, you know, but I'm never really on time, anywhere. It's gotten so bad that my friends call me "Speedo." If you think that this is bad, you should see when I'm invited to dinner or something like that. Thirty minutes is, you know, early. Usually they say, "Invite him but give him the wrong time, or else he'll never show."
T: Don't they get angry or annoyed with you?
P: (*Laughs*) Why should they? I'm basically a very nice guy. Everybody puts up with it.
T: Is it the same thing here [in therapy]? Are you wanting me to "put up with it" in the same way because you're such a nice guy?
P: Well, it's really hard for me to catch the train at the right time. There are so often delays at [his train stop].
T: What do you think that the lateness *means* between us?
P: I don't really understand.
T: What's the *meaning* of it? What are you trying to say or tell me through the behavior?
P: Tell you? It's still not . . .

T: I guess what I'm wondering about is maybe you're saying that you're angry at me about something. Sometimes I think that the kind of behavior that you describe toward people, the lateness and lack of consideration, is perhaps your way of being angry.

P: I don't know.

T: Some of these things you've done make me wonder if maybe you play out your being angry indirectly.

P: It's hard to know. I don't really get angry much. [A discussion ensued regarding the patient's almost total inability over the years to get angry at his parents. In an attempt to deal with some of Willie's passive-aggressive behaviors by paradoxical means, the therapist said to the patient later in the session:]

T: I would predict that gradually you'll find yourself more and more angry toward me. You'll probably start coming to sessions later and later, and there may even be some where you fail to show altogether.

Because of the patient's strong passive–aggressive trends, he "refused" to do as the therapist predicted and began to attend most sessions for the complete period allotted. After a relatively short course of 10 individual visits, Willie was referred to a time-limited 18-month group for those with character impairments.

The patient's course in this group was very beneficial. He was initially a "nice guy" in the group, but his narcissistic self-involvement began to become increasingly obvious. He also became more and more flirtatious with several of the women in the group. Finally, about 8 months into the group, a number of the members began to confront Willie with his unwillingness to give anything of himself in the sessions, or even to listen to what others had to say. With sufficient repetition (and a willingness to stick with the therapy rather than flee), the patient began, at first tentatively and then more definitively, to express concern for and involvement with other members. He came to be a well-liked and respected part of the group.

During the course of the treatment, Willie met a woman with whom he had had a casual sexual "fling" several years before. Upon meeting her again, Willie realized that she was "a terrific person." Six months later they were living together, and in another 6 months they were married. Willie was followed for 3 years after the end of treatment as part of a study of psychotherapy outcome. When last contacted, he and Becky (his wife) were still doing well. He had a young child of whom he was very proud. In addition, Willie had decided that he simply did not enjoy working for a boss. Therefore, he had started his own free-lance design business, which was doing quite well. In his follow-up discussion with the therapist 3 years after the end of treatment, Willie said, "I was able to change because of the love, warmth, and support in the group and because of your [the therapist's] great caring and support."

Treatment of "Anxious Cluster" Patients

Patients in the "anxious cluster" are frequently anxious, ruminative, and preoccupied. Their lives are often plagued by intense apprehension and worry. When patterns such as compulsions or passive–aggressive behaviors are present, these should be seen as ways of binding anxiety. Often, these patients may be viewed as stiff, overintellectual, or constricted.

For several of the disorders in this cluster (particularly the compulsive and dependent disorders), there is a good deal of overlap with Axis I anxiety and affective disorders. Furthermore, as has been mentioned, patients with avoidant personality disorder may look more like those in the "odd cluster." For patients in the "anxious cluster," it is most important to help them "loosen up"—be less tight, inflexible, and/or self-critical and frightened.

These goals may be achieved in a variety of different ways, depending upon the situation in question. However, whereas patients in the "odd cluster" need to be able to trust more, and patients in the "dramatic cluster" need to learn to exert more control and better judgment in regard to their behaviors, those in the anxious cluster often need to be less controlled and more open to their experiences and interactions.

Because of the somewhat varied presentations of patients in this cluster, we provide several different case examples to illustrate treatment.

Aged 30 when she was first seen by one of us for treatment, Liz presented with a severe depression. She was confused and uncertain about remaining in her career as a veterinarian or leaving this field completely and going into a totally unrelated area. She also felt lonely and worried about the possibilities of ever establishing an intimate relationship with a man. Throughout her adult life, Liz had suffered from extended periods of depression and anxiety, with chronic feelings of low self-esteem. She also had a severe eating disorder, which had developed in her late teens; her bouts of bingeing and purging would last for weeks at a time. During these periods, Liz would call in to work ill until "I finally see how crazy I'm being."

She had lived and worked in many parts of the United States and Canada, never feeling comfortable or safe, and inevitably moving on. Liz had had numerous courses of brief and extended psychotherapy, and although the outcomes of these treatments appeared vague and rather nonspecific, the patient spoke warmly of her previous clinicians.

Liz's family of origin was rigid and controlling. She had two older sisters, both of whom were anxious and perfectionistic people, and both of whom had severe eating disorders. Her parents were ungiving people who emphasized money and appearances. Her mother also seemed to have an eating disorder; she took great pride in her own emaciated appearance and the fact that all of her daughters were so skinny.

In answering the question of "Why now?" with Liz, it appeared to the therapist that she felt as though she stood at a crossroads in her life. Should she continue in her career? How could she establish an intimate relationship? And could she finally get her bulimia under control after being dominated by the guilt, shame, and anxiety associated with this symptom for so many years?

It was decided with the patient that the first focal area should be helping her deal with the symptomatic problem of her bulimia. Although a number of other foci were possible, such as developmental dysynchrony or character issues, the symptomatic difficulties were undertaken because they were so influential in Liz's life. As noted, she frequently missed work, and she also had difficulties with dating and friendships because of her bulimia.

A variety of strategies were undertaken. For example, since the bingeing–vomiting cycle often began at times of anxiety and tension for Liz, she was taught self-hypnosis relaxation and given an audiotape to use on a regular basis. It was also planned that whenever she began to feel as though she were about to begin the cycle, Liz would immediately write an extensive letter to the therapist describing her feelings at the time. Over a 5-month period, during which she was seen approximately once every 2–3 weeks, Liz wrote the therapist three such letters. They proved to be very valuable in helping her to stop herself *before* the bulimia "took over." During the initial course of therapy, Liz's mastery over her eating problem increased until she rarely began the bingeing–vomiting cycle.

At that point, the focus shifted toward Liz's character, relationship, and career issues. It became clear that the patient's overwhelming fears and pervasive sense of uncertainty and anxiety about herself and her abilities influenced both her work and her interpersonal relationships. Although she was a caring and supportive person to others, she always "put on a good face" and rarely disclosed her own fears, problems, or needs. (Her bulimia obviously fit well with this overall style.)

Liz was a "good" patient with the therapist and was able to act appropriately open with him. However, they decided that in order for her to make more substantive changes, it would be useful for Liz to participate in a short-term group for young adults. This she did with a different clinician.

In her 15-session short-term group experience, Liz initially played her familiar role of helper to others while hiding her own feelings of uncertainty, fear, and depression. When she did talk about her issues, it was in a stiff and abstract manner with little real feeling or expression. A significant turning point in the group occurred for Liz in the ninth session. At that point, with the therapist's support, Liz began to talk about her eating disorder and her familial pressure to stay thin. She also described her fears that people would get to know her too well and her chronic insecurity in jobs and relationships. This was a very moving session for Liz and the rest of the group. Many of the members responded to Liz's openness and strong affect by being open, emotional, and supportive themselves. They also told Liz how difficult it had previously been to give her support in the group. Her coolness and distance in talking about her own problems had made it very hard for group members to become involved with her and what she was saying. They also noted that her behavior in this session was very different and presented a great contrast to what had come previously.

In subsequent group sessions, Liz was able to consolidate some of the changes that had occurred in this session. As part of a study of process and outcome in short-term group psychotherapy, Liz was interviewed 1 year following the completion of her short-term group. At that time, she had become involved in what appeared to be a very positive relationship with a man. In addition, she had made a decision to stay with veterinary medicine and had found a much better position than those she had held previously. Her eating disorder remained in good control, and she could not remember her last bout of bingeing and vomiting.

Liz remembered her individual and group treatments very clearly and felt that the therapeutic work which she had done had been enormously beneficial. "My therapists were both terrific."

Reggie was a 33-year-old bank auditor. When first seen, he said (quite seriously), "Although both of my parents are mental health professionals, I never feel anything about anything." He initially sought therapy because of "a dilemma": He had been dating Harriet for about 3 months but "couldn't react" to the relationship. "She's right for me—everyone says so. She's pretty, she's smart, she's the right religion, she comes from a good family, and she loves me. I think I'm supposed to feel something for her, but I don't feel anything."

Reggie's relationships with people tended to be superficial and distant. He could never be clear in regard to his feelings for women about whom he was "supposed to" care. Almost invariably, women would become angry at his ambivalent and often passive–aggressive approach to relationships. In his work situation he was tense and unhappy, never feeling as though he was doing enough, and at the same time being in a constant state of uncertainty and ambivalence about continuing in his career.

When he first began therapy, Reggie was tight, constricted, and withholding during sessions. He would complain about his work and romantic situation, bemoan his ambivalence, and endlessly describe the impossibility of taking any beneficial course of action. In an early visit the therapist requested that Reggie come in with Harriet, which he did. She was an expressive woman who described her great frustration in communicating with Reggie. Most of her attempts to get closer to him were met with hostile or noncommittal responses. Since she appeared to be considering the possibility of quitting the relationship unless things changed, and was herself rather uncertain about whether or not she could continue to tolerate Reggie's mistreatment of her, Harriet was seen with him only once.

Shortly after the visit with Harriet, Reggie began an 18-month time-limited therapy group. It had quickly become clear to the therapist that Reggie's withholding, passive–aggressive style made it difficult for him to respond quickly in a beneficial way to the individual treatment. Even when his distant and ungiving approach was interpreted to him in the treatment, Reggie seemed to have great difficulty making use of this data.

In the time-limited group Reggie quickly became a regular and committed member, albeit a generally quiet one. A significant turning point in the group occurred for Reggie in the fourth month of treatment. Reggie started a session by saying that he wished to talk. He then launched into a litany of issues that made him feel that he was "probably unhappy"—"I don't smile enough. I don't laugh enough. If I am with friends and we hear a joke everyone laughs; I just grimace." Beverly, a very explosive and dramatic group member, began to laugh. "You won't give anybody anything, will you? You go somewhere where everyone thinks things are funny and you just give out a grimace." Beverly continued to express anger and frustration toward Reggie intermittently during the session. Finally, at one point, Reggie turned on Beverly and quietly and calmly began to point out the fact that she had never had a long-term loving relationship with a man, and that since her mother and father were alcoholics she might never be able to do so. When the therapist asked Reggie what he was feeling as he criticized Beverly, he denied any hostile intent: "No, I am *not* angry. She can say what she likes—no matter how dumb!" When he was asked to again examine his feelings, he admitted to "maybe a very little anger."

This session proved to be very helpful to Reggie in beginning to be more relaxed and less controlling regarding his emotions. It also opened up to him the enormous power of his controlling and passive–aggressive behavior to frustrate and enrage others.

INTERMINABLE BRIEF THERAPY FOR SEVERE BORDERLINE CHARACTER DISORDERS

For some people with severe characterological problems (usually borderline personality disorders), there is the possibility of major deterioration if they do not have a therapist in their lives for some type of ongoing maintenance. The following case history describes such an individual who, while in ongoing and at times intermittent treatment, did relatively well. After this was discontinued, the patient lost ground and regressed.

Shelley was a very attractive woman, aged 26 when first seen in therapy. She had a history dating back to high school of severe alcohol and narcotics abuse. (She did not admit to these addictions until many months into treatment.) Shelley, although she had completed all of the course work for her doctorate in biology, had quit graduate school and for the past 2 years had worked as a receptionist/secretary at various small companies. She would almost invariably become sexually involved with much older, married men in positions of authority at these companies. When she became increasingly demanding, wanting to spend more and more time with the man or pushing him to leave his wife, she would find herself fired. Shelley was married to a passive, alcoholic man named Jed. He, too, had done all of his graduate work toward a PhD, except for his dissertation. Although she flaunted her indiscretions, Jed was unable or unwilling to challenge her about them.

Shelley sought medical care when, after being fired in what for her was a typical scenario, she began developing debilitating phobias and pain problems. Shelley found herself amost unable to leave the house, and several times each day was wracked by excruciating abdominal pain. She was first seen by a mental health therapist after she had fought with her primary care doctor over his reluctance to give her any more narcotic pain relievers or Valium.

Shelley was a person for whom it quickly became clear that a personality focus was necessary. She would deal with the mental health clinician in a whining, child-like manner, complaining about her pain and/or about how badly everyone (including the therapist) was dealing with her. Shelley was treated intermittently by the same therapist over a period of 10 years. She was first seen weekly for a 3-month period, then on a biweekly basis for 6 months. After a 4-month break, she was seen in an 18-month time-limited group. Following this group, she was not seen for about a year; then she was seen on a weekly basis for 6 months. After another year-long break, she was seen monthly and then about four times a year until she moved to another area.

A major focus in the treatment was upon the ways in which Shelley related to the therapist. Particularly in the beginning of therapy, her imma-ture attempts to get the psychologist to "do something" for her were fol-lowed by bursts of anger and threats to terminate treatment, as well as by direct and indirect threats of suicide. Aside from the character focus, a variety of other areas were also examined. Quite early in the treatment, Shelley was seen with Jed. Having him in allowed the clinician to clarify the state of her marriage, to understand Jed's perceptions of Shelley, and to try to do some work on the interpersonal conflicts in their marriage. It was in these sessions that it became obvious to the psychologist that both Shelley and Jed were addicted to alcohol and drugs. After several months of joint work, the therapist pushed for the couple to begin attending AA and to get some drug and alcohol counseling. Jed never followed through; Shelley attended AA herself only sporadically, but she began to reduce her alcohol intake and stopped taking drugs.

The couple separated during the conjoint therapy, and Shelley con-tinued to be seen alone. During this part of the therapy she was treated mostly by herself, but was also seen for several visits with her mother, father, and two adult sisters. It appeared that both of her parents were severely disturbed people who had not provided her with any type of caring or support in growing up. Her father, an alcoholic physician, was a "pill pusher" who treated every one of Shelley's problems or difficulties with one medicine or another; her mother, an immature and whining person (in some ways not unlike the patient), had been a terrible somatizer who took to her bed at the slightest provocation.

In the time-limited therapy group, Shelley was confronted by group members about her unwillingness to listen to them and her inability to express even minimal caring for others. Slowly, she began to modify her behavior and took a far more mature and interested approach in her interactions. A key point in the group therapy for Shelley was when Walter, another alcoholic member who had been attending AA for many years, insisted that she go with him on a regular basis for one month. Shelley agreed to do so, became committed to staying sober, and began to go to three meetings a week.

Once she was no longer taking drugs or drinking, Shelley began to profit much more from therapy. She was able to get better jobs and to keep them, and got a divorce from Jed. Toward the end of the group and periodically afterwards, Shelley had lapses regarding both her substance abuse and her relationships with men; in general, however, her improvement was substantial. For the first time in her life, she was able to maintain friendships with other women; she developed some reasonably healthy relationships with men; and she found a high-level administrative position with a large medical center. She continued to be seen infrequently through the years, "just to touch base" and to let the therapist know how things were going.

During the 10th year of her treatment, Shelley's therapist became very ill and was unable to see her for a number of months. At this point, she precipitously left her job and moved to another city. Her therapist later learned that in that city Shelley had taken another responsible position, but had quickly become romantically involved with her married boss. This man, who was also an alcoholic, "encouraged" her to begin drinking and taking drugs again. When she was last heard from, Shelley was very depressed, drinking heavily, and in the process of being fired from her current position.

It appears to us that for some patients brief therapy is interminable (Bennett, 1983). Even minimal contact may be valuable and significant in assisting the patient to maintain his or her equilibrium, sobriety, overall adjustment, and so on. As always, this does not mean that a patient must be treated weekly or twice a week for many years. It does mean that, for some more disturbed patients, having a therapist in their lives may be extremely important and is to be encouraged.

CONCLUDING COMMENTS

Overall, patients with personality disorders present a major challenge to the brief therapist. It must, however, again be stressed that if one does not emphasize the concept of "cure," the goals and approaches to treatment become far more manageable and "do-able" with a time-effective model. Even with those who have severe characterological impairments, it is possible to do "pieces" of work spread out over many years. As the reader will have observed, within our model for most patients with characterological difficulties, we believe that a time-limited therapy group along the lines described in the next chapter is beneficial. This is particularly true for patients in the "dramatic cluster" and the "anxious cluster." Our experience of treating "odd cluster" patients in time-limited groups has been less favorable. Such patients generally have been too frightened, suspicious, and distrustful to profit from their group experience; therefore, they tend to be fringe members of the group, just as they are often at the fringes of life. Even 18 months of group participation is often too short a time to allow them to begin trusting and interacting more openly with others.

There is also the category of patients who, like Shelley, must always have a therapist in their lives. Without some type of even minimal support and contact, the patient's own resources for coping and using good judgment are quickly depleted and become ineffective. Therefore, if the therapist perceives substantial deterioration in a patient's coping abilities during treatment-free periods, he or she must reassess the situation and make a decision about possibly continuing support without any breaks in treatment.

The therapist who is working from a model similar to ours has numerous options and possibilities when it comes to treating those with severe character pathology. These options are not available to those who view therapy as long-term *or* short-term, complete *or* incomplete, cure *or* failure.

10

Time-Limited Group Psychotherapy

Effective group treatment has been viewed as being, by necessity, very long-term, typically lasting from 2 to about 5 or more years. There is, however, little research evidence to support this stance. Furthermore, a theoretical rationale that could adequately explain why group therapy should take many years to be effective, while brief individual treatments may have their impact in a fraction of this time, also appears to be lacking. It is our belief, backed by a growing body of research evidence and many years of clinical experience, that group therapy structured along appropriate lines need not be of indefinite and open-ended duration in order to be highly beneficial.

For a variety of reasons, it is becoming increasingly important that clinicians doing group therapy must consider ways in which to make this treatment clearer, more efficient, and better-defined. Just as individual treatments have come under increased scrutiny to insure their efficacy, as well as the quality of their administration, group therapy will surely soon be subjected to such scrutiny as well.

As is also true of psychotherapies in general, patients use group treatments in the ways in which *they* (not their therapists) find most appropriate. For example, Stone and Rutan (1984), two traditionally oriented long-term group therapists, examined the duration of group treatment in private practice groups that they each ran. Much to their surprise, they found that nearly 40% of the patients in their groups left before the end of the first year. They also discovered that 75% of the patients who entered their groups had left by the end of 2 years, and fully 90% before the end of 4 years. Thus, two highly experienced therapists, working with a relatively select population of private outpatients, rarely kept these patients in their groups for the full length of time implied by their model (Rutan & Stone, 1984)—that is, several years. Other figures, which we have cited in earlier chapters, also indicate that many patients come for relatively short periods when they do arrive for therapy (Garfield, 1980). Similarly, Klein and Carroll (1986) found that in their community mental health setting, over half of the patients (52%) who actually began group therapy were seen for 12 or fewer sessions. For those who began group treatment, the mean number of group sessions was 18.8, the median was 11.7, and the mode was a single visit.

In this chapter we describe, in detail, a generic model for short-term experiential group psychotherapy. We use the term "experiential" because the model to be described is more than simply an economical way to treat several unrelated individual patients or couples simultaneously. Rather, the emphasis is upon those interpersonal factors (e.g., cohesion, group development, feedback, self-disclosure, etc.) that are believed to be pivotal elements of any experiential group treatment. Merely to have a number of patients with similar problems sit together for a brief series of "classes" or do sequential individual treatments in a group does not make the best use of the unique elements available in such a potentially rich interpersonal environment.

LENGTH OF TREATMENT IN SHORT-TERM GROUP PSYCHOTHERAPY

Before describing the important therapeutic elements in short-term groups, we address the issue of treatment duration. Although it would be easiest to define short-term group psychotherapy as always being fewer than a given number of sessions in length, or as always running for under x number of months or weeks, our view of brief treatments in general does not permit such an overly rigid and simplistic approach. In line with the definition of brief treatment that we have provided earlier, it is not only that a particular short-term group runs for fewer than a given number of sessions that defines it as such. The treatment also is parsimonious, uses the time allotted in the most efficient and effective manner possible, and rations the time allocated to the therapy.

Whereas in individual therapy it is possible to ration time by having a given patient come for visits in any of a variety of flexible ways (e.g., weekly, biweekly, monthly, semiannually, or any of the possible combinations of these), such varied scheduling is usually impractical or impossible for a whole group of patients. Therefore, almost all of our short-term groups have been weekly and time-limited. The approximate length of the time limit is determined by the *shortest* period in which the particular focal goals of a given group are likely to be achieved. In general, the time limits of the short-term groups we have run have varied between 8 and 60 sessions.

In a group focused upon a relatively clear, circumscribed issue, such as dealing with a life crisis (e.g., loss of a job or relationship, a recent move, illness, etc.), we have used a time limit of 8 sessions (Donovan, Bennett, & McElroy, 1981). For groups focused upon developmental life transitions, such as dealing with the problems associated with young adulthood, midlife, or later midlife, we have found a 15- to 20-session limit to be preferable (Budman, Bennett, & Wisneski, 1981). In groups that have as their purpose the treatment of patients with very rigid and enduring characterological problems, we have applied a time limit of 60–70 visits. These time limits may apply to the group as a whole, with the entire membership beginning and ending the group together; or there may be a rotating membership, with each member continuing the group for only the allotted number of visits before rotating out. In a group with a closed membership, group developmental themes are clearer and more prominent than they are when time limits apply to individuals, and membership rotates.

Some may take issue with our description of up to 60–70 visits as still being short-term; however, we are most interested in the *effective and efficient* use of time in treatment. It appears to us that for some individuals with severely impaired modes of interpersonal interaction, such as those with borderline conditions, beneficial and effective treatment in slightly over 1 year of weekly group therapy must certainly be viewed as "brief." In order to be considered planned short-term group psychotherapy, we believe that a group must have a predetermined time limit (either for the group as a whole or for each member); that this time limit must be circumscribed and well defined; and that the group's focal issue or issues must be treated in the shortest feasible, most efficient, and parsimonious time frame.

In this consideration of the issue of time in short-term group therapy, it is also important to place this treatment mode within the primary practice model of therapy that we have described earlier in this book. That is, a patient's group therapy experience probably will not be his or her first or last course of psychotherapy. Patients return to therapy at various points in their lives. Assuming that as a therapist one can (or should) provide a patient with a "definitive" treatment is like assuming that a teacher should provide the definitive class, that a physician should provide the definitive antibiotic, or that a travel agent should provide the definitive vacation. What one hopes is that the group therapy provided has had sufficient impact to alleviate some of the problems with which the patient presented upon entry into therapy, and that the patient takes with himself or herself some useful tools for dealing with similar problems in the future. To attempt to rid the patient now and forever of emotional problems and difficulties leads to continuous, open-ended therapy. Such therapy often gains a life and momentum of its own.

CENTRAL ASPECTS OF SHORT-TERM GROUP THERAPY

A number of elements are uniquely relevant to short-term, time-limited groups. The four that we view as most important are these:

1. Establishing and maintaining focus in the group
2. Pregroup preparation and screening
3. Group cohesion
4. Existential factors and the time limit

It should be obvious to anyone examining this list that these elements blend into one another, and that the demarcation line between them is quite arbitrary. However, for the sake of clarity, we treat these elements here as if they were to a great degree independent.

Establishing an Early Focus

The most important aspect of any brief therapy is a clear and well-defined focus. Such a focus is a central aspect of time-limited, short-term group treatment as well. However, in such therapy a focus may be harder to obtain and maintain than is the case in short-term individual or conjoint marital therapy.

Obviously, in a group, the task for the therapist is to help establish a focus or foci that are relevant not only to each individual, but to the group as a whole. The short-term group psychotherapist walks a very fine line between establishing a focus that is so general and applies so loosely to everyone that it has no real vividness or relevancy for anyone, and establishing a focus that is so specific to individual members that it does not allow a group theme to emerge.

Clarifying the Working Focus

There are a variety of possible approaches to establishing the "working focus" of a short-term group. We call this primary focus a "working focus" because the leader works with it in finding appropriate patients for his or her group, in planning time limits and group structure, in "advertising" the group to other therapists and patients, and so on. The "working focus" is differentiated from the "emergent focus," which develops over the course of a group when one has had the opportunity to meet with patients together in the actual therapy situation. Development of the emergent focus in the group is due to the fact that people are not theories. All depressed patients, all midlife patients, all patients in crisis, and so on are unique. One may choose patients who share a given set of characteristics or similarities, but one must always realize that the unique aspects of these patients and their particular styles of dealing with issues will emerge over the course of a group. Furthermore, it is never clear until a particular group of patients begins to meet what these specific personalities will draw from one another.

The working focus is initially addressed by choosing a particular issue, problem, or set of concerns, and by opening group membership to a *relatively homogeneous* population of patients who share these. This emphasis upon homogeneity is one of the first ways in which short-term and long-term groups differ. Indeed, it is often seen as most desirable in a long-term group situation that through heterogeneity a true microcosm of the interpersonal world will develop (e.g., the elderly woman who is depressed will be forced to deal with people who are like her hostile and uncaring middle-aged son; the young woman who has never been able to deal with older authority figures like her father will have the opportunity to do so). In general the objects for transference will be more numerous and varied under conditions of heterogeneity than under conditions of homogeneity. We have been struck, however, by just how long a heterogeneous group may take to break through individual differences and begin to unify as a group. It is our impression, on the other hand, that in a short-term group situation, homogeneity along one or more important dimensions will allow the group to "come together" more quickly and to circumvent some of the issues that may arise when such similarities are not present.

To give an example, a group of mildly to moderately disturbed young adults will often share a sense of concern about their abilities to be close to others and/or worries regarding career issues. Shared issues such as these, whatever the specific diagnoses of the patients in question, offer an initial unifying element in the group. To give another example, a therapist who decides to run a short-term group may choose as the initial working focus the issue of recent life crises. This would mean that when he or she is planning or organizing the group, it is labeled as a group for people dealing with a variety of life crises (e.g., a recent death, loss of a relationship, job changes, etc.). The group should be relatively homogeneous in regard to this issue. Also, the structure of the group should be related to a knowledge of the normative phenomena of such crises. For example, since most crises resolve within 6–12 weeks (H. J. Parad, 1971) and often tend to be most acute at the beginning, the patients might be seen for no more than 6–8 weeks and more than once each week. Such a group is described in detail by Donovan *et al.* (1981).

The initial step of clarifying and presenting the working focus is essential. When one fails to elucidate such a focus to oneself, to potential group members, and to one's colleagues who will be referring patients, the best that one can expect is to do truncated long-term therapy. Piper, Debbane, Garant, and Bienvenu (1979) have found such "short-term-by-default" group therapy to have minimal efficacy.

The first two questions that the short-term group therapist must ask himself or herself are these:

1. What will the focus or foci of this group be?
2. What are my goals for this group?

One can, for example, decide to run a short-term group for posthospitalization schizophrenic outpatients. If one's focus is upon helping patients deal more effectively with this transitional period, and the length of the group is six sessions, one's goals should be relatively modest and realistic. The therapist should not plan to modify profoundly the patients' home situation, employability, or the like. If goals are limited and realistic, this will also help the therapist and patients feel positive about even small steps, rather than feeling inadequate because more dramatic results have not occurred.

Let us assume for the moment that the therapist has adequately developed a working focus and goals for his or her short-term group. Furthermore, let us assume that because of organizational exigencies, the therapist's interests, and patients' needs, this group will be a short-term young adult group. What are the concrete steps to be taken in using this focus for the construction and initiation of such a group? First, the therapist should clarify what aspects of the young adult experience he or she wishes to emphasize. One of us (Simon Budman) and his colleagues at the Harvard Community Health Plan in Boston believe that from an adult developmental perspective, a major issue for many young adults concerns their willingness and capacity to form close, intimate relationships. If dealing with and working on such developmental issues is the stated purpose of the group, the therapist should make it clear and explicit that this is the case. He or she can and should set age range criteria, criteria regarding severity of pathology, and criteria regarding other factors that would necessarily exclude certain patients from participation.

A series of actual examples of working foci for different time-limited groups and their related criteria follows. These are obviously not exhaustive of the relevent possibilities, nor are their entry criteria suitable for the needs of every setting. They are presented as illustrative examples of types of foci possible, and their related exclusionary or inclusionary criteria.

1. *Young adult group.* This group will focus on issues common to those in their 20s to 30s. Of particular interest are issues of intimacy and closeness in interpersonal relationships. The members of this group have often been able to form reasonably workable and satisfying friendships, but have frequently had difficulty in beginning or maintaining longer-term, sexually intimate relationships. Potential members should not be psychotic, suicidal, or homicidal. While the intimacy issue need not be their only concern, it should be a major and sustained concern. Patients who view their problems solely or primarily in somatic terms generally do not do well in such a group. In our experience, a successful group of this sort might run for 20 weekly 1½-hour sessions with no members being added after the group's first meeting.

2. *Crisis group.* This group will have as its central focus recent life crises. Members may be dealing with a variety of recent life events, such as the death of a spouse or a child, a marital separation, job loss, a move or impending move, and so on. This group will be open to adults of all ages. Potential members should not be actively psychotic, alcoholic, homicidal, or suicidal. Members will enter the group, which meets twice a week for 1½ hours, for a total of eight sessions. There will be a rotating membership.

3. *Marital therapy group.* This group is for couples dealing with problems of poor communication and/or frequent conflict. Those participating should agree to participate as a couple; should not be actively abusing alcohol; and should not be psychotic, homicidal, or suicidal. The group will meet for a total of 15 weekly 1½-hour sessions. All couples will begin and end the group together.

4. *Time-limited group for those with chronic and severe difficulties in intimate relationships.* This group will focus upon interpersonal problems of a persistent and chronic nature. The group can be particularly useful for those who have had repetitive problems of withdrawal, explosive anger, isolation, severe depression, and/or anxiety when they are attempting to become engaged or disengaged from an intimate relationship. Potential members for this group have frequently experienced numerous failed attempts at such relationships. They may have had experience with a number of group or individual therapies, sometimes with little reported benefit. Members will begin and end the group together. The group will meet weekly for 1½ hours for a total of 65 sessions.

The reader will observe that each of these four foci is interpersonally oriented rather than symptom-oriented. This means that rather than emphasizing, for example, the depression or anxiety experienced by those dealing with strained relationships, it is the nature of these relationships *themselves* that is examined. The interpersonal environment of the group is uniquely suited to the examination of such issues.

It should be noted that each of the focus descriptions above (1) defines the problem in interpersonal terms; (2) explicitly states exclusionary and inclusionary criteria; and (3) sets a time limit.

Development of the Emergent Focus

The emergent focus may gradually become the secondary focus in a short-term group. If and when such a focus develops, it is most useful for the therapist to attend to this issue and support the group's examination of this topic along with the exploration of the working focus. As an example, in a couples therapy group, it (coincidentally) turned out that three of the four couples had at least one spouse with an alcoholic parent. In addition to discussing their interpersonal conflicts, the couples spent much of their time talking about how their early parental deprivation had affected their current marital relationships. As another example, in a group of young adults that had as its working focus the exploration of relationship issues, it developed that a number of the participants, although not clearly gay, had had questions about their sexual orientations. These questions were examined as the emergent focus, and were beneficial to all members in regard to overall questions of intimacy.

Pregroup Preparation and Screening

It is far more difficult for most patients to "know" just how to use group therapy than is the case for individual therapy. Furthermore, for most people, group treatment is (at least initially) more anxiety-provoking and unpredictable than individual therapy.

Although good preparation and screening approaches may be important in many modes of group therapy, it is nowhere more essential than in a short-term group. A long-term group with a number of dropouts or inappropriate members has sufficient longevity to recover from such problems by the addition of new members or the time-consuming working through of these difficulties. A short-term group must "hit the ground running." A time-limited, closed-membership group that sustains numerous dropouts, or one that must deal with a monopolistic member or a member who is far more disturbed than the others, may be well on its way to termination before these issues can be addressed adequately. Worse still is the short-term group that never really "gels" because so many members are inappropriate to the working focus of the group, or are inadequately motivated to engage fully in the group experience.

We have tested a variety of pregroup preparation and screening approaches, and have chosen to use one that is experiential in nature. It is based upon the fact that when using interviews alone, clinicians are relatively poor predictors of ingroup behavior (Piper *et al.*, 1979). Furthermore, it is simply not possible to predict the dynamic interactions between members without actually seeing what they are like together. Being experiential means that members are given a live, structured small-group experience before the actual group. In this way, they experience what it is actually like to be a member of such a group in a way that cannot be achieved by a therapist's description.

Individual Sessions with Potential Group Members

We describe below a method of experiential pregroup preparation and screening developed over a number of years at the Harvard Community Health Plan in Boston. Before proceeding with this description, however, we would like to discuss the issue of individual orientation with potential group members. Although this issue was not as clear to us earlier (Budman, Bennett, & Wisneski, 1981), it now appears essential that the short-term group therapist have at least some minimal contact on an individual basis with possible group members. This contact is not mainly for the purpose of screening or providing the patient with information about how the group operates; all of this will occur in the experiential pregroup workshop session. Rather, this individual session is an opportunity to help the patient reframe his or her presenting problems in a way that is coherent with the focal theme of the group. To some degree, this reframing may have begun with individual sessions that the patient may have had prior to the group referral. However, if one is taking referrals from other therapists and not just drawing from one's own practice, it is difficult to be assured that the patients being sent to the group have a shared understanding of the basic aim of the group and the way in which their own concerns fit with the working focus.

Some illustrative examples follow here to suggest some of the ways in which such sessions might be used.

Darleen was a 21-year-old woman originally referred for mental health treatment because of a chronic feeling of depression and low self-esteem. She had been repeatedly sexually abused by her father between the ages of 11 and 14. Once the sexual abuse was discovered by local authorities (Darleen had revealed her secret to a warm and concerned teacher), she and her three younger siblings had been moved together to a foster home. During and before the years of living in foster care, Darleen had been forced to fill a maternal role for her younger siblings, as her mother was a weak and inadequate woman. Darleen had little opportunity to become involved in after-school activities, and had virtually no ongoing contact with peers. The therapist referring her for a short-term young adult group felt that in such a situation, she would have the opportunity to interact closely with other people her own age and begin to learn how to develop peer supports. The referring therapist also believed that her reason for seeking care at that particular point in time ("Why now?") was her recent move to the Boston area. She had lived most of her life in a very isolated and rural farming community. Although she was quite lonely there, she had had a fairly structured environment and was close to her pastor and his family.

The group leader, upon meeting Darleen for her individual orientation session, emphasized the nature of the young adult group for which she was being interviewed. It was stated that most young people in their 20s deal with intimacy problems. Because of her background, Darleen was probably having more problems being able to establish herself in Boston than others might. The group was described as an opportunity for Darleen to learn more about relating closely to others and about developing intimate and supportive relationships. Her depression and low self-esteem were described as being a function of her isolation and inadequate opportunities to learn about peer involvement.

Carl was a 32-year-old man with numerous somatic, pain, and anxiety problems. He had come for therapy after a failed relationship with a woman caused him to begin questioning his sexual identity. Although he had always felt a strong sexual attraction toward men, these impulses frightened him so much that he would constantly run away from them by beginning unsuccessful, unsatisfying relationships with women. Carl had many friends; however, he felt such intense shame that this issue of sexual orientation was never discussed. Carl was offered a young adult group. In the initial session with his group therapist, it was explained that joining the group might give him the opportunity to talk openly with a group of people, many of who were struggling with similar fears and concerns about identity and intimacy. Also, if Carl chose to "come out" regarding his sexual feelings, the group could be a safe environment in which to do so. Since the group members did not work with him at his job and were unlikely to be in ongoing social contact with him, the group could be the chance to try out the open expression of some of his inner concerns about sexual identity.

The important issue for the therapist in the individual pregroup session is to help the patient clarify whether and in what way his or her issues tie in with the overall focal theme of the group. The group focus is only real to the patient to the extent that he or she can see its personal relevance.

The Pregroup Workshop

Following the individual pregroup session, the patient is invited to a pregroup workshop. This workshop, usually consisting of between 8 and 15 individuals, is held several weeks after the individual meeting.

Purposes of the Workshop.   The workshop serves a variety of useful purposes.

1. *Reduction of dropout rate.* In studies by Piper *et al.* (1979), a similar pregroup approach reduced dropouts significantly. Budman, Clifford, Bader, and Bader (1981) also reported substantial reductions in dropout rate using the method to be described. It is probably more accurate to state that some patients drop out *prior* to the official start of the group after their workshop experience. However, such dropouts are clearly preferable to having patients leave during the group when their leaving could have a demoralizing effect on other members. In addition, some patients who might well have become dropouts during the difficult early period of the group "bond" to another member or members in the more comfortable structure of the workshop exercises, and continue to discuss these experiences periodically throughout the group itself.

We believe that another aspect of the lowered dropout rate after the workshop may be the anxiety reduction that comes with the structure and support of this type of pregroup preparation. The format of the workshop is such that members go from smaller- to larger-group exercises and from more to less structure. Participating in the workshop can lead to a greater sense of mastery and readiness for the group. After a workshop, one member stated, "It's like we're all in a ship that has been cut loose and set out to sea."

Clearly, the expectation that members will stay with the group is strong. Studies by the Harvard Community Health Plan mental health research group (Budman, Demby, & Randall, 1980) indicate that those who drop out of short-term groups tend to have poorer social interactions and fewer close friends than those who do well and remain in the groups. The potential dropouts may begin the group with considerably more anxiety and discomfort than most other patients. Thus, the structure of the workshop may also allow some patients to stick with and perhaps benefit from the group who might under other circumstances not have continued.

2. *Skills training in desirable group behaviors.* It is a more difficult process for the client to understand and be aware of desirable patient behaviors in group therapy than in individual psychotherapy. Though most people in our society have had exposure to individual therapy through books, movies, television, or personal contact, this is not the case for group treatments. Furthermore, individual therapy "fits" with the Western model of going to an expert for help. In primitive cultures, much healing occurs in groups (Frank, 1973), and in public and community settings (Ellenberger, 1970); this is not the case in our society.

In order for the patient to learn how to use the group most appropriately, some explicit skills (e.g., giving and getting feedback, interacting in a small-group situation, appropriate self-disclosure, etc.) should be identified and taught. As will be explained, the pregroup workshop is an attempt to address these needs.

3. *Improved patient selection.* It is clear that pregroup workshop behavior is a far better predictor of in-group behavior than is a one-to-one interview with a therapist (Budman, Clifford, Bader, & Bader, 1981) prior to the group. Furthermore, research also indicates that after observing patients interacting in a workshop situation, therapists are able to make some fairly accurate predictions of the relative degree to which the patients will benefit from a therapy group (Piper *et al.*, 1979). The pregroup workshop can be an opportunity to screen out problematic and disruptive patients; those who simply cannot fit in well with the other members of that particular group; or patients who are too anxious, acutely disturbed, or disorganized to profit from a particular type of group, at least prior to more individual treatment.

4. *Informed decision by the patient.* It is of great importance that the potential group member make an informed decision regarding the joining of the group. Without such a decision, the patient may never really take full responsibility for this choice. We have often heard patients entering short-term groups (begun without a workshop) explain that they were in this group "because Dr. Jones sent me." Many short-term groups are sufficiently brief that a patient can cling to such an explanation without ever feeling that he or she has taken an active, willful role in being a member of the group. Patients prepared with the workshop are encouraged to use

the pregroup session to make their own decision about becoming group members.

Components of the Workshop. The workshop is a single 1½-hour session. Generally, between 8 and 12 patients are asked to the workshop, with the assumption being that several will choose not to join the group itself after this initial meeting. The workshop has three components: introductions, "the task," and a whole-group exercise.

To begin the workshop, the leader or leaders inform the group that the workshop will give each of them some sense of what group therapy is like. Furthermore, they will be able to decide whether or not they wish to join the group. It is also explained that the group itself will be considerably less structured than the workshop.

1. *Introductions.* In the first part of the workshop, members pair up and introduce themselves to one another. Once introductions have been made in these dyads, members are asked to return to the larger group. At that point, each member is asked to introduce the other member with whom he or she has been speaking (not himself or herself). Variations of this introduction have also been done with couples (in marital groups), where two couples pair up and then introduce each other to the rest of the group.

2. *"The task."* In the second structured exercise, participants get together in three- or four-person groups. The task of these small groups is dependent upon the central focus of the group. For example, in couples groups, we ask two couples to work together in this part of the workshop. One couple at a time is asked to role-play their "most frequent argument." In young adult groups, one participant at a time describes "a problem with another person that you wish you had handled differently." The members of the small group are then asked to role-play this problem situation with one another. The significant aspect of this "task" is that it closely relates to the major theme of the group. In addition, members have the opportunity to present their difficulties, to offer potentially helpful input to one another, and to suggest alternatives to problematic interactions. After a member has described and role-played a situation that he or she wishes had been handled differently, or after a couple role-plays their most frequent argument, other members are asked to role-play alternatives to this problematic interaction. For example, in a workshop for a young adult group, a woman described a situation in which her roommate had called her from the airport at 1:00 A.M. to request a ride back to their apartment. The woman, Linda, who had been sleeping, had felt angry and used, but had gone out and gotten her roommate anyway. The situation was role-played first as it had happened. Then it was role-played again with Joan, one of the members of Linda's small group, playing an "alter ego" for Linda. That is, Joan would state aloud the feelings that she assumed Linda was having but was unable to express. Finally, the situation was again role-played, with another member of the

small group playing Linda's part and politely but assertively stating that she would not come to the airport for the roommate.

3. *Large-group exercise.* In the third and final exercise of the workshop, all participants work together in a group task. Again, in this part of the workshop, we are attempting simultaneously to teach, to screen, and to give participants sufficient experience in the group situation to make an informed decision about participation in the treatment.

The large-group exercise is often related to the type of group being planned. For young adult groups, members are asked to imagine that they are part of a club or are living in a communal house, and are all organizing a party together. They are asked to discuss how the party will occur, when, who will be invited, who will bring what, what the entertainment will be, and so on. Similarly, couples are asked to organize a block party with the same type of tasks. The leader does not participate in this large-group exercise. Rather, after giving the group its instructions, the leader observes how the group goes about achieving its task.

After all three exercises have taken place, the leader summarizes what has gone on, asks for questions, and requests that members consider carefully whether or not they wish to join the group. Generally, the group itself begins 1 or 2 weeks after the workshop. Workshop participants are asked to contact the leader within several days of the workshop to state whether they are planning to join the group.

What to Look For in the Workshop.   The leader should be carefully observing what goes on throughout the workshop. In particular, the following should be noted:

1. Are some members unable to take part? That is, are some people so withdrawn, frightened, or constricted that they cannot give or get from other members? If this appears to be the case, the leader should try in the second exercise ("the task") to see whether it is possible to draw such patients into the proceedings by supportive questioning.

2. Are some members so monopolistic that they severely limit others' participation? If one or more members seem to talk insensitively and without apparent regard for other participants, the leader should also use the second exercise to test the members' responsiveness to input about "giving other members a chance to talk," "listening to what others have to say," and so on.

3. Do some members appear to be too severely disturbed for a given group, or to be very different from other members in a way that will make the group focus irrelevant? For example, in some young adult group workshops, it becomes clear that one or two of the participants are clearly dealing with issues far more closely related to separation from their parents than to intimacy with other adults.

4. Is the number of members in the group sufficient? Are there enough

men? Enough women? There have been occasions when, after we have drawn from our group waiting list, only 4 out of a possible 15 members have shown up for the workshop. Again, it is useful to know that a sufficient number of members is not yet available, and that the start of the group should be delayed.

The leader can and should use the workshop for screening purposes. If the leader has specific questions about one or more members, these people can be brought in for an additional interview, can be referred to another group, or can be referred for further individual therapy prior to re-referral for group treatment.

Group Cohesion

Before discussing the process of short-term group therapy, we would like to examine the concept of group cohesion. We believe that it is an often-discussed but little-understood dimension of group therapy, and one that is of central importance in any short-term group approach.

Most group therapists carry with them an internal model of cohesion. They "know" whether it is or is not present, and can describe to others (such as supervisors, colleagues, trainees, etc.) group events that affect it. However, what is actually meant by "cohesion"? The research literature has generally defined "cohesion" as "the total field of forces which act on members to remain in the group" (Festinger, Schacter, & Back, 1963, p. 164). As will be seen, our view of cohesion is much broader and, we believe, closer to the concept maintained by practicing clinicians.

A Model for Cohesion

Over the past several years, a team of clinicians and researchers at the Harvard Community Health Plan has been studying this very important dimension in group treatment. We have developed scales for its measurement, and tracked its change and progress over the course of both short- and long-term psychotherapy groups. Our Group Cohesiveness Scales (GCS) are reproduced in Table 10-1. Before readers turn to these, however, it might be useful for them to describe to themselves a definition of "cohesion" to see just how closely their own concepts parallel ours.

We view group cohesion as a multidimensional concept with the following parts (scales on the GCS):

1. Withdrawal/Self-Absorption versus Interest/Involvement
2. Mistrust versus Trust
3. Disruption versus Cooperation

Table 10-1. Harvard Community Health Plan Group Cohesiveness Scales
(HCHP-GCS)

Evidence of Global Fragmentation				
−5 Very strong	−4 Strong	−3 Moderate	−2 Slight	−1 Very slight
Pushing away from self-examination or examination of process; individual differences only further the separation; factionalism and/ or individualistic behavior of group members; extreme lack of unity; hostility or active distancing.		Predominantly separate individualistic interactions without active hostility and distancing; lack of identification with other members; no attempt to identify common group themes or issues.		Individualized presentations around common themes, but without any attempt to connect to other members; lack of empathy or shared dilemma; narcissistic quality to disclosures.

☐ NO EVIDENCE; CAN'T BE RATED ON THIS DIMENSION

Evidence of Withdrawal/ Self-Absorption				
−5 Very strong	−4 Strong	−3 Moderate	−2 Slight	−1 Very slight
Autism; sleeping; strong passive–aggressive quality to silence.		Slumped, apathetic posture; no eye contact; looking bored and disengaged; looking around aimlessly.		Limited verbal activity; quiet and expressing only sporadic nonverbal interest and/ or attention; depressed quality. Sporadic evidence of interest and/ or attention (verbal or nonverbal).

☐ NO EVIDENCE; CAN'T BE RATED ON THIS DIMENSION

Evidence of Global Cohesiveness				
+1 Very slight	+2 Slight	+3 Moderate	+4 Strong	+5 Very strong
Tentative, superficial, and/ or inconsistent attempts to connect with others around common themes and/or issues. Lacking in depth. Inconsistent responsiveness to others.		Consistent, empathic responses to common themes; some acceptance of individual differences; some depth and trust.		United, purposeful; feeling of "we-ness"; acceptance of individual differences. Marked depth.

Evidence of Interest/Involvement[a]				
+1 Very slight	+2 Slight	+3 Moderate	+4 Strong	+5 Very strong
Quiet but obviously attentive/ interested. Body language indicators: leaning forward; eye contact; facial expression showing attention.		Sustained eye contact; sustained attention; verbally and nonverbally responsive to discussion/issues/ feelings.		Enthusiastic quality to responses; deeply felt and affectively significant responsiveness (questions, feedback, etc.).

Table 10-1. (*Continued*)

Evidence of Mistrust				
−5 Very strong	−4 Strong	−3 Moderate	−2 Slight	−1 Very slight
Total inability to share due to overwhelming fear and/or discomfort; a definite paranoid quality, where destructive motives are inappropriately assigned to therapist or other members.		Unwillingness to discuss an issue; clear inability to share personal material due to strong discomfort or fear.		Slight suspiciousness; slightly guarded discussion of issues; some evidence of struggling with clear discomfort/ fear of sharing personal material.

☐ NO EVIDENCE; CAN'T BE RATED ON THIS DIMENSION

Evidence of Disruption of Therapeutic Work				
−5 Very strong	−4 Strong	−3 Moderate	−2 Slight	−1 Very slight
Leaving group; attacking; interrupting; subplays (e.g., counterconversations, subgrouping); extreme acting-out or bizarre behavior; collusion around resistance to working therapeutically.		Nonverbal or verbal redirection of attention from therapeutic work; active resistance (e.g. eye rolling, sighing, looking away, changing subject); active blocking or avoidance of affective exploration (e.g. false reassurance, intellectualizing).		Superficial advice giving; passive avoidance or blocking of affective exploration; social interactions not contributing to therapeutic work.

☐ NO EVIDENCE; CAN'T BE RATED ON THIS DIMENSION

Evidence of Trust				
+1 Very slight	+2 Slight	+3 Moderate	+4 Strong	+5 Very strong
Peripheral, tentative attempts to disclose feelings and issues.		The ability to share personal issues with clear comfort, and with some depth and affect.		Truly genuine, meaningful openness, sharing observable in all group members.

Evidence of Cooperation toward Therapeutic Goal				
+1 Very slight	+2 Slight	+3 Moderate	+4 Strong	+5 Very strong
Some verbal and/or nonverbal evidence of helpfulness; meager, early-stage or precursor quality to attempts to support, help, confront, engage others in therapeutic task.		Significant amount of active verbal and/or nonverbal supporting, helping, confronting, clarifying responses.		Explicit, strong sense of unified effort toward common therapeutic goal ("We are all working together to change things").

Table 10-1. (*Continued*)

Evidence of Being Unfocused				
−5 Very strong	−4 Strong	−3 Moderate	−2 Slight	−1 Very slight
Each member brings up a separate and dissimilar topic; each member as a different agenda and direction that he or she attempts to pursue.		Aimlessness; rambling; tangential discussion; unintegrated material; unidentified process themes. Increased superficiality and disorganization would merit a higher (negative) rating.		Some disconnectedness, unresponsiveness, and/or indifference to topics addressed by others.

☐ NO EVIDENCE; CAN'T BE RATED ON THIS DIMENSION

Evidence of Abusiveness				
−5 Very strong	−4 Strong	−3 Moderate	−2 Slight	−1 Very slight
Verbal hostile attack; blatant lack of respect; condescension, hostility, critism, fault-finding, blaming; abrupt leave-taking behavior. Hurting others intentionally; exploitation of others' feelings.		Clear disregard/ ignoring of others' feelings; unconstructive fault-finding; unsympathetic ridiculing.		Passive nonattending to others' feelings and issues; unresponsiveness to others' feelings or issues.

☐ NO EVIDENCE; CAN'T BE RATED ON THIS DIMENSION

[a]For Interest/Involvement scale, verbal activity doesn't necessarily denote positive interest and involvement. Rate the *quality* of the verbal *or* nonverbal activity

Evidence of Being Focused				
+1 Very slight	+2 Slight	+3 Moderate	+4 Strong	+5 Very strong
Superficial associations to topics presented; limited attempts to concentrate on a particular issue or theme (either individual or group).		Some identified themes and patterns, somewhat developed, with various perspectives attended to. A higher (positive) rating would reflect a maintained/sustained, common, identified theme or deeply felt issue.		There is a willingness to focus on a common theme or agenda; members put aside their own topics or relate these to the issue(s) being addressed in the group.

Evidence of Expressed Caring				
+1 Very slight	+2 Slight	+3 Moderate	+4 Strong	+5 Very strong
Showing limited responsiveness and some concern; tentative attention to others' feelings.		Openly recognizing and/or pursuing exploration of others' feelings; verbalized support and concern or nonverbal expressions of clear interest and concern.		Clearly empathic responses; emotions brought up, engaged and stayed with; sustained ability to move beyond intellectual discussion toward emotional involvement; observable affect, caring, and concern. Evidence of members' feeling understood (e.g., "Yes, that's *just* how I feel").

    4. Being Unfocused versus Being Focused
    5. Abusiveness versus Expressed Caring

We also have a global scale:

    6. Global Fragmentation versus Global Cohesiveness

How Is Cohesion Important for Short-Term Groups?

Many authors consider cohesion to be the group counterpart to the therapeutic alliance in individual therapy (Budman *et al.*, 1987). As such, it presents the members of a group with an environment in which to get feedback, support, information, and advice, as well as an opportunity to try out new behaviors and ways of being.

    For those in short-term groups, some of the most important therapeutic events may relate to cohesiveness. Most studies of therapeutic factors in brief groups find cohesion to be consistently among the most important elements described by members (Butler & Fuhriman, 1983; Fuhriman, Drescher, Hanson, Henrie, & Rybicki, 1986; Marcovitz & Smith, 1983). In an intriguing study, Rahe and his colleagues (Rahe, O'Neil, Hagan, & Arthur, 1975; Rahe, Tuffli, Suchor, & Arthur, 1973; Rahe, Ward, & Hayes, 1979), found that in a randomized clinical trial of short-term (six-session) groups for patients recovering from myocardial infarction, group members had significantly lower morbidity and mortality at the end of 3 years than did controls. The patients in the group condition tended not to remember the specific information they had received during the treatment about heart disease; rather, they recalled the supportive atmosphere present.

    A cohesive group allows a unique experience. Many groups in our individualistic society tend to function at fairly low levels of cohesion. The most problematic aspect of cohesion, however, for the short-term group therapist is how to achieve it quickly and maintain it once it is present. In our view, the brief group therapist must be an outstanding "manager" of cohesion. Without such skills, it is not possible to help 5 to 10 people who may have experienced relatively little cohesion over the course of their lives to feel interested in, trusting of, cooperative with, caring about, and involved with one another.

    Lacking at least moderate levels of cohesion, a short-term group is likely to be minimally beneficial to its members. Over the course of a time-limited group, the leader needs to gauge and work continually with the level of cohesion in the group, along with the actual content focus of the group and the time limit itself. This level will often vary and fluctuate; however, if it drops into the negative range of cohesion (see Table 10-1) and remains there for more than one session, it may spell the premature ending of the group.

Time Limits and the Existential Focus

Since short-term groups are characterized by a clear and definite time limit, there is always an underlying awareness for therapist and patients alike that the group, as it is constituted, will end. Of course, patients may return for further treatment, and on some occasions such groups have continued on their own for brief periods as leaderless peer groups. Nonetheless, the current constellation of the group, with all members and the leader under the auspices of a given health plan, mental health center, and so on, will end at a time specified at the outset. For this reason, time-limited groups for individuals draw out powerful time-related existential issues. (This is not usually as salient an issue for married couples who leave a couples group together, since the major "transference" object in each spouse's life is his or her partner.) Members begin to think about where they are in their lives and the time still remaining to accomplish various goals or aims.

Most of us give little thought or consideration in our daily lives to issues of our own finitude and mortality. Unless we are affected by a serious illness, an accident, the loss of a loved one, or a morbid preoccupation with death and dying, most of us manage to live our lives as if our time is limitless. After a nearly fatal automobile accident, a friend said to one of us, "Obviously, I always knew that everyone dies sometime. I just felt like I might be the exception. I don't feel that way any more."

James Mann (1973), in his book on time-limited therapy, quotes the psychoanalyst Marie Bonaparte as writing: "In all human hearts there is a horror of time." Mann goes on to state:

All short forms of psychotherapy, whether their practitioners know it or not, revive the horror of time. Whatever differences there may exist among the various kinds of short forms of psychotherapy, or among their proponents, the factor common to all is the obvious and distinct limitation of *time*. (p. 9; italics in the original)

In a time-limited group, the time barriers are nearly undeniable. The group members confronted with such a barrier often respond initially by denying to themselves that the end of the 15 sessions will ever come. (We have, however, seen such denial continue into the last session of a time-limited group. In one such instance, a member, whose leader had been clear and precise about "counting down" each of the 15 sessions, "totally forgot" that the group was approaching its final meeting. She expressed shock and anger about the termination of the group when it finally came, and was surprised that the other members knew that the group was about to end.)

In general, as members realize that the group will indeed terminate, distinct issues related to life stage, prior losses, and the need to "act before it is too late" begin to surface. Under some circumstances these issues are so frightening or disruptive to members that they focus all of their energies in the final sessions toward being angry at the leader or institution for not allowing them "more time." Unfortunately, this preoccupation may preclude the useful exploration of existential issues that have been brought to the fore.

When group members are able to explore the issues raised by the time limit, the fact that is often brought into focus is that the time available in one's life is also limited. Often, this realization helps to "get members moving" who have previously been too fearful or too stuck to attempt even minimal changes with their subsequent risks.

PHASES OF SHORT-TERM GROUP PSYCHOTHERAPY

Several authors have described the different phases of therapy groups (MacKenzie & Livesley, 1983; Tuckman, 1965). In our view, the general course of most time-limited groups falls into five phases: (1) starting the group; (2) early therapy; (3) middle of the group; (4) late therapy; and (5) termination. A 6- to 12-month follow-up constitutes a sixth "phase." The model is set forth in brief in Table 10-2.

In a typical 15-session time-limited group, the five phases will frequently occur in approximately equal 3-session blocks. Of course, our distinctions between phases are arbitrary, and the phases may occur idiosyncratically under special or unusual circumstances. However, the therapist carefully observing the course of a short-term group will probably find an evolving process at least somewhat similar to the one described here.

The processes to be described have been extensively researched in a study of such processes in young adult groups (Budman *et al.*, 1987). However, because of their similarity to the descriptions offered in the literature for small-group processes in general, and because of our own experiences in a variety of time-limited groups, we would estimate that they are applicable to most briefer groups regardless of the working focus.

Starting the Group

After the workshop and individual screening, members should have at least a relatively clear understanding about the overall aim and focus of the group. Nonetheless, the group generally begins slowly, with some attempt on the part of the members to understand why others are "really" there. Questions often raised either directly or indirectly are "How were we chosen for this group?", "How do we share time here?", and "Who will be the first to risk in the group?" There is a considerable degree of tentativeness and uncertainty about how the group will operate to meet its goals, who the other members are, and what the relative safety versus danger of the group situation is.

Often during this period, after some initial searching for a starting point, one or two members emerge as the "patients." These "patients" generally display in their presentations the typical focal problems for others in the group. These problems are presented at a relatively superficial and informational level, while other group members respond with advice and suggestions about trying possible alternative solutions.

Focus in Starting the Group

In this phase, the therapist should reiterate the focus of the group frequently. He or she should open and close the group sessions with a brief discussion of how the group is addressing or not addressing the focal target areas dealt with in the group. The very first meeting should begin with a brief statement by the therapist about the goals and ground rules of the group. Here is an example:

> As I've mentioned to all of you previously, this is a young adult group that will have as its central theme problems of intimacy. Members of this group have all, in one way or another, been struggling with these issues recently. Experience indicates that a short-term group like this one can be a very useful vehicle for helping people with such difficulties. Obviously, you all have other concerns as well as those related to intimacy. To the degree that it is possible, we will talk about some of these too. However, because of our limited time working together, we will need to remain focused for the most part on intimacy concerns.
>
> The group will continue for 15 sessions on a weekly basis, 1½ hours per session. If you cannot come to a session, please call ahead and let me know.
>
> You've all been to the workshop, so you know something about what these groups are like. But, remember, the group itself will not be as structured as the workshop. If you are uncertain about staying in the group, I would ask that you give the group at least eight sessions before you decide to leave. It takes about that long for the group to really "gel" and become a smoothly functioning unit. No one will force you to stay with the group if you decide to leave sooner, but it may not be in your best interest to do so.
>
> Since we are under time constraints, it is important that we all be here promptly so that we have the opportunity to do the maximum amount of work in each and every session.
>
> Frequently in these types of groups, members may get to know one another outside of the group as well. This is OK, as long as you talk about this inside the group. Also, if one of you calls me or has any contact with me outside the group, the group should be informed about this.
>
> Finally, there is the issue of confidentiality. I would ask that you all agree to maintain the confidentiality of the group. Without such confidentiality, people never can really feel as though they can be open, honest, and safe.

Table 10-2. Phases and Treatment Tasks in Time-Limited Group Therapy

	Start	Early	Middle	Late	Termination	Follow-up
General characteristics	Group members try to clarify who else is in or out of the group. Membership and safety issues are central. How does the group work? Who else will stay?	Groups begin to show signs of improvement or of deterioration. Most group members show some signs of hopefulness that therapy will help them. There are attempts to be helpful, usually by advice or suggestions.	There is generally a period of disappointment and frustration with the group at this point. Members realize that although the group is half over, much work remains. Questions about the therapist's effectiveness are frequent.	This is a period of intensive work in the group. Members feel close and involved. They are motivated by the time limit to use the group.	This is a period of intense emotion. Members experience a sense of losing the group. Often old losses are reactivated and remembered.	This occurs 6 months to 1 year after termination. It is used to help members "mark" gains and help leader assesses their work.
Focus	Leader restates and frequently clarifies focal themes of the group; tries to illustrate intermember similarities.	Leader helps members to clarify how the focal issue is present for them in their lives, how it affects them, and how they have dealt with it.	Therapist must be willing (if need be) to set aside focal theme briefly and deal with group crisis. This is only done temporarily.	Focal issues are addressed at greater depth than ever before in group. New perspectives emerge.	Leader should help members to recall what they have learned about focal issue. How will members take gains with them?	Leader should ask members about their progress in focal area.

270

Cohesion	Leader uses focus as central building block of cohesion. Members need to be taught aspects of cohesive behavior.	Cohesion will precipitously fall, and, if the crisis is well managed, will begin to rise steeply again. Therapist must deal with crisis.	Cohesion may be quite high at this point. Leader helps members to see how supportive these interactions are.	This may well be the period of greatest group cohesion. Leader's task is to help members continue cohesion even as group ends.	Leader should ask members how group support and caring affected them.
Existential and time issues	Time limits are discussed. Brevity is described. Members usually attend minimally to time issue at this point.	Members feel the time pressure begin to mount. They will realize that unless they quickly address their problems in the group, the opportunity will pass.	Members think about the group ending soon. Some may disengage from group emotionally; most think about their life stage.	Members will feel much sadness and will recall deaths and losses. They also consider their own lives going by and their eventual deaths. Therapist should use this.	How were time limits important?
Comments	Good pregroup preparation and screening make this phase easier.	Leader may become overly optimistic or overly pessimistic. In fact, ultimate outcome is not yet set.	Group may be highly productive during this phase. Leader must use high cohesion to enhance learning.	Therapist should avoid changing or modifying time limits, even though there may be some pulls to do so.	This is a very useful aspect of the intervention.

"Maintaining confidentiality" means that if other people are mentioned, they are never identified or described in such a way that would make them identifiable. Any questions? If not, we can get started.

Cohesion in Starting the Group

Our research indicates that most time-limited, short-term young adult groups begin life at about the same level of cohesion. That is, a low but positive level of cohesion is usually found for early sessions. This is not surprising, and probably is true of other short-term groups that have been carefully formed. Most groups members probably start with some hopeful anticipation, but not with much skill in working together as a group or in being helpful and interactive with one another. It is only after several meetings that some groups begin heading toward success and some toward failure.

The cohesion task for the leader during the initial phase of the group is to help members see how they are similar and to help them tolerate the ambiguity and uncertainty pervasive during this phase. This may be achieved in a variety of different ways. The leader might frequently ask members how they are reacting to one another's statements in the group. It is also useful to point out similarities that arise as people are talking in these early sessions: for example, "Bill, you had a very similar experience to Mary's when your marriage broke up. How are you reacting to her story?" or "Everyone in the group, at one time or another, has probably felt some of the loneliness that Chuck is describing."

During this early period of group development, the cohesion task is of utmost importance. Without the therapist's emphasis on cohesion, the group may never really move toward a close, supportive environment, which we believe to be essential to good outcome. During this stage, the cohesion task for the therapist is to help members realize that they do share mutual concerns and interests, and that these concerns and interests are greater than those forces mitigating against members' trusting, caring for, and supporting one another. That is, there is more to be gained from coming together as a group than from mistrust and disintegration.

Existential and Time Issues in Starting the Group

Of course, the time limit is described and emphasized in the first few meetings of the group. However, with a few minor exceptions, most members in early sessions react overtly as if the time limit were nonexistent. This can occur to such a degree that the therapist may come to believe that the limited nature of the time is not important. This is clearly not the case, but only becomes more apparent as the group goes on and as the group's ending approaches. It is essential that the therapist continue to emphasize the limit (in spite of the members' best efforts to de-emphasize the issue).

Every single session should begin with something like this: "This is session 3; after today, there are 12 sessions remaining."

Additional Comments

The first few group sessions are often somewhat stressful for group leaders as well as group patients. Group therapists can, however, increase their chances of running a successful short-term group if they have put sufficient time and effort into the pregroup preparation and screening process. Members who are well prepared know more about how to interact appropriately in a group, as well as how to use a group for their own benefit and that of others. Leaders who have prepared a group well know the members better than they would have otherwise, have taken steps to screen out those who do not belong in a group with a given working focus, and have some sense of how the focal concern is relevant to each member.

Early Group Development

After beginning the group, the therapist finds that the early period of group development is characterized by strong indications that the group is "working" or "not working." A group's "working" means that members begin (at first perhaps tentatively) to address the concerns regarding which they first entered the group, and to attempt to pull together as a functioning unit. Failure to do so leaves members with frustration and other negative feelings about the group situation; as a result, they are more likely to drop out or withdraw, and the group may go into a generally negative spiral. It may be possible to remedy this negative situation at this point or in the next phase of group development. The therapist must, however, act quickly if the group is to achieve its specific and focused aims. In the well-functioning group, members feel hopeful and excited about their prospects.

Focus in Early Group Development

During this phase, the leader helps members clarify how the central theme of the group applies to each of them as an individual. The members generally move from broad descriptions of their issues in the area of intimacy, for example, to deeper and more personal accounts of how their difficulties with intimacy have had major and/or pervasive repercussions in their dealings with people. Without therapist assistance, this may become a period of extensive "storytelling" without much therapeutic value in some groups. In short-term groups with the poorest outcomes, we have observed that one or two members go on with such storytelling almost endlessly, much to the consternation of other members. It is the rare short-term group, however, that is so safe and cohesive that members can put an abrupt stop to such behavior. Rather, members politely (appear to) listen, with fewer people coming to sessions on time and participating actively in the proceedings. If the therapist cannot help members focus on the group task in an active and emotive manner, such a focus is unlikely to occur. Monopolistic patients, after all, do not go on in an endless manner except in the interactional context of others' not jumping into the breach. Especially in the early phase of the group's life, setting limits on the monopolist is primarily and essentially the task of the therapist.

Cohesion in Early Group Development

During this stage the leader must actively continue to teach group members cohesion-related skills. It may be possible for the group to apply such skills themselves later in the group process. In the late or termination phases of a group, we frequently see members asking one another the types of cohesion-related questions that the leader has asked earlier.

What we mean by "cohesion-related skills" are those methods of interacting that will serve to bring a group together in a supportive and mutually helpful manner. For example, the leader may frequently inquire, "How did you react to what Joan just said?" or "Why don't we go around the room and describe our feelings and thoughts about today's session?" There is a good opportunity for all members to give something to one another, to participate, to be involved, and to feel a sense of connection with the group.

Existential and Time Issues in Early Group Development

The general tendency of both members and leaders to ignore or deny the time limit continues during this stage of the group. There continues a feeling that the end of the group is far off in the future; if the issue is addressed at all, members feel that enough time still remains, and that the therapist is playing an alarmist role by regularly reminding the group of its dwindling time together.

Additional Comments

It is during this early period of the group's evolution that the leader may become aware of the fact that a screening error has been made. That is, it may become clear that one or another of the members simply does not belong in the group. We have often encountered highly monopolistic members who have not been perceived to be problematic for a given group during the workshop. This is usually due to the fact that such an individual may look as though he or she is doing just fine in the workshop, where there is a greater degree of therapist structure and control. In the more open environment of the group itself, such a member's own controls may be inadequate. Furthermore, attempts by the leader to assist the member in better participation are frequently seen as angry confrontations by that member. We have seen instances when such a member has literally demolished a group by never allowing others to speak. In one such instance, the monopolistic member later stated: "I had to keep talking. If I hadn't spoken, no one else would have. Whenever I paused, no one else spoke." Again, in the infrequent instances when this type of behavior occurs, it should be obvious that the therapist has committed not only a screening error, but also a fundamental technical error by failing to assert appropriate authority and control.

In other instances, a member may appear to become disturbed as the group continues, even though such behavior has not been displayed as clearly at any time in the patient's life previously. In one such case, a young physician in one of our groups became convinced that the therapist "had it in for" him. He would constantly describe the therapist's interventions as "fighting with me." It was learned only later that the therapist reminded the patient of a boy in his high school who had accidentally shot and killed the patient's best friend during a hunting trip.

Whatever the reason for any problems that arise, the therapist must deal with them quickly. In general, monopolistic or disruptive patients must be taken out of the group at this point. Although over the course of a long-term group such patients can be worked with (usually by the group), there is simply insufficient time in a short-term group to do so. The leader of the group has a responsibility to all members. It is easy to lose sight of this responsibility and to devote all of one's efforts to one member (the "squeaky wheel" approach). If a member is not appropriate for a given short-term group, this does not mean that he or she cannot be appropriate for another group. In all likelihood, after some additional (usually individual) work, the member may be able to function in a group in a way that is helpful both to him or her and to others in that group. Although some leaders may fear that "kicking out" the disruptive member may lead to fear on the part of the remaining members that they will meet the same fate, we have not found this to be the case. Rather, members are usually able to see themselves as different from that person. There is also a sense of appreciating that the therapist "took charge and did the best thing for the group." It may also be helpful for group members to learn that some situations are unworkable and that a separation from the group may be in the best interest of all concerned. For example, after the fourth session in a midlife group, the therapist decided to ask a woman who had been enormously disruptive and controlling to leave the group. In the following session, after the therapist explained his actions, Trish, another member of that group, began to cry and described how she had several years before been forced to send her teenage children to live with their father. She stated that her tears were in appreciation of learning that sometimes some situations were even too difficult for the therapist to handle without having to "ask someone to leave."

Members' feelings about the disruptive member's leaving must, of course, be addressed as a group issue. The therapist should be willing to recognize the ambivalence and guilt that this event may engender in the group. However, failure to act under such circumstances does a disservice to all members, including the member who is disruptive.

Middle Group Development

The middle period of short-term group development is often characterized by a growing sense of uncertainty and frustration on the part of most group members. Sometimes described as the "group crisis" (Yalom, 1985), this phase is critical to the ultimate outcome of the short-term group. Members may begin to feel that although the group is nearly half over (or, in longer-term groups, although they have been meeting for quite a number of weeks), there still remains a great deal to be done. There often is a feeling that had the group been run differently, "more would have happened by now." The form members' complaints take is direct and confrontative at some times or with some groups, and more circuitous at other times or with different memberships (e.g., "I once had this teacher who never taught me much. He always wasted his time on the trivial issues"). The leader who fails to address such dissatisfaction runs the risk of a continued process of dissatisfaction, failure to achieve the group's goals, and low cohesion. Examining this frustration head-on appears to be the most effective way to allow a group to make continued progress.

Focus in Middle Group Development

As is true in every stage of short-term group development, the focal theme should be adhered to and maintained as central. However, in this stage only, the focal theme may need to be set aside in order to provide an adequate opportunity for the "crisis" to be addressed. We have viewed dozens of videotapes of periods that we consider to be "crises" in short-term therapy groups. If the therapist is able to recognize, acknowledge, and address the crisis, there is a rapid alteration of mood in the group and attitudes, and (in our view) an almost quantum leap into a higher level of group functioning. Failure to deal with the crisis usually leads to a downward spiral with little forward movement, and a growing sense of being at a stalemate.

There are three essential steps in handling the group crisis: (1) recognizing; (2) acknowledging; and (3) addressing. Examples of statements a leader can make to accomplish these steps are as follows:

- *Recognizing*: "I have the sense that a number of people in the group are sharing Bill's frustration that more hasn't already happened here, and we're into the eighth meeting already."
- *Acknowledging*: "I certainly can understand how you might feel that way. Mary feels worried much of the time; Jim still doesn't know how he turns women off; and Bill and Russ feel like I haven't told either of them anything they didn't already know."
- *Addressing*: "The truth is, however, that I really don't have the 'answers' to your problems for any of you. I do have information I can give (which I have tried to give all along), but probably the way in which I can be most helpful to you is by helping you all interact more directly and in a straightforward manner with one another. High levels of skill, knowledge, support, and information exist in this group. If each of you uses those assets to your benefit and for the benefit of one another, the group can be a very helpful experience to all of you."

Such statements may be made in rapid succession, or may evolve over several meetings. Regardless of how this crisis is handled, it is essential that it be dealt with. This may preclude dealing with the focal concern for a short period; however, as often as not, the focal issue may be tied in with addressing the crisis. For example, in a group of young adults where intimacy is the central theme, people's reactions to the group crisis may be very closely tied in with their intimacy problems. A young man with relationship issues who tends to be shrill and hostile in his confrontation of the therapist during the crisis may realize how hard it is for anyone to deal with his magnified aggressiveness. A woman who cannot ask for her own needs to be met in relationships may realize that she, too, has unfulfilled longings during this period of the group.

Our research indicates that the therapist must actively address the crisis. Failing to take an active approach is counterproductive, since this common problem will not simply evaporate, much as the therapist may hope it will.

Cohesion in Middle Group Development

As the therapist addresses the focal task relating to the crisis, he or she is simultaneously dealing with cohesion. Dealing well with the crisis is probably the best strategy that the therapist can take in terms of enhancing and maintaining cohesion; this is because the best outcome of the crisis can be for members to feel a sense of working together. They may come to believe that "A major source of help will be our helping one another," "The therapist won't (can't?) do it for us," and "There's only a short time left for all of us to use this group in the best way we know how." As mentioned previously, if the crisis is successfully negotiated, cohesion rises precipitously and often remains extremely positive through the rest of the group's time together. If this is not the case, the group seems to move into a rather stuck, depressed, and moribund state.

Existential and Time Issues in Middle Group Development

The time pressures on both the patients and the therapist begin to mount during this stage. Half of the group's life has passed, and there is a strong sense that anything that is to be done must be done quickly. Even the therapist may begin to wonder whether, in fact, much can be accomplished in such a short period. It is crucial that the therapist remain aware of the fact that he or she must maintain a focus on limited goals, but that at the same time small changes may set the occasion for greater improvement later.

Additional Comments

The middle period is a stage of enormous importance to the beneficial outcome of the short-term group. In a long-term group, the crisis repeatedly arises in different forms; thus there are numerous opportunities to address it. This will not be the case in the short-term group. It is, however, easier for the novice to recognize the crisis in a short-term group, because it often occurs near the middle session and is frequently more of a simultaneously shared sentiment than might be true in a long-term group. It should always be kept in mind that the group will *not* rid itself of the leader (other than symbolically), and that at the same time members feel dissatisfied, they also continue to feel hopeful and involved in the group.

Late Group Development

In the late stage of the group, if the middle stage is negotiated properly, cohesion often continues to rise; group members come together in a more positive and hard-working way than in prior meetings. Problems and concerns are addressed in new ways and with greater depth. The focal issue remains central, but at a deeper level of discussion, sharing, and self-disclosure. Members feel that time is running out for them to achieve their goals in the group, and most put extra effort into addressing these goals "before it is too late."

Focus in Late Group Development

Often it will be necessary for the leader to keep pulling members back to the focal theme during this stage. Usually, members themselves are prepared to return to the focus and examine it in great detail. Members by this point have often learned from the therapist's example how to raise questions or refocus as people wander too far away from the mark. However, if the group is not doing this, the leader must remain fixed on the working focus of the group.

Cohesion in Late Group Development

The members have also often learned by this point how to share with and support one another in a manner that is cohesion-enhancing. The leader should continue to support cohesion and try to intervene in ways that increase the level of cohesion. However, if the previous phases have been successful, the leader may be able to apply himself or herself more to making interpretations, suggesting alternative strategies for patients to consider experimenting with in regard to given issues, and so on.

Existential and Time Issues in Late Group Development

Existential issues become highly prominent during this stage. As the group's ending nears, patients begin to realize (at some level) that life does not last forever. Patients often have the sense that if they are planning to go to college, change jobs, leave a spouse, or get married, the deed should probably be done "before it is too late." There is often a momentum in the group for members to try to make some useful changes in their lives before the group ends, and to call upon the group for support during this transitional period. At this point, a patient may have to be advised against the apparent wisdom of change for its own sake. During this and the next stage of the group (termination), patients who have experienced numerous painful losses may begin to recall these and bring them up in group discussion, trying to work them through.

Additional Comments

The late stage is a phase of extensive work and investment in the group. For some groups it is a "golden era." The therapist may have the idea in this or in the next stage that if he or she could only extend the group meetings, then even more of value would happen. In most circumstances, this should not be done. Lengthening the group beyond its initially set time limit is confusing, disruptive, and counterproductive. Our advice here is quite similar to Mann's approach to the same issue in individual treatment that is time-limited (Mann, 1973). In some ways, however, it may be even more difficult to stick to a time limit in a group than in an individual therapy situation, because of group pressure. Although we have rarely advocated the maintenance of a rigid therapeutic stance in this volume, we believe that the time limit is a point that generally should be steadfastly maintained. When we ourselves have succumbed to the temptation to continue a time-limited group for an additional series of sessions, the results have often been poor. Frequently, the group will "go flat," attendance begins to drop off, and members often feel the continuation to be a Pyrrhic victory.

As with all rules in therapy (or anything else), there are exceptions. For instance, toward the end (after the 40th session) of a time-limited 60-session group for those with characterological problems, the leader (Simon Budman) became severely ill. He was out of the group for 4 months. The group, remarkably, stayed together and continued to meet (with occasional input from one of the leader's colleagues); it was extended for an additional 40 sessions once the leader was healthy enough to return. The members, when interviewed (as part of a research study) after the end of the group, said that the added time had helped them enormously in accomplishing their therapeutic goals. These were most unusual circumstances; however, it probably should be kept in mind that although the leader should usually adhere to the time limit with great tenacity, flexibility is sometimes still the best policy.

Termination

Termination is often a period of intense emotion in the group. Members and leaders may experience great sadness regarding their mutual loss. Members will have shared much powerfully evocative material, will have come to feel close to one another, and will then have to give up the group. Some members may try to avoid experiencing this loss by downgrading the group or its leader. For others, there is a tendency to "forget" the termination date. Yet another reaction may be a resurgence of problems that have previously been improving. The most central aspect of this phase for the leader is helping the members review the changes they have achieved in the group, say goodbye, and plan for the future. Again, there are some strong similarities to Mann's (1973) approach.

Focus in Termination

During this phase, the focus is upon what each member has learned that can be helpful in dealing with the focal issue of the group. The focal issue may also be addressed by discussing (1) what changes have occurred for each member in regard to this issue that may be apparent to the other group members, and (2) how the participants have taken steps toward changing behaviors in their everyday lives related to their focal concerns. The therapist may usually be more structuring and directive during this stage than has been the case at earlier stages of the group's life. It is also important to focus on what the member feels things will be like *without* the group.

Cohesion in Termination

For many successful groups, this period appears to be the one of greatest cohesion. Members have usually learned how to relate to one another and support one another. They feel a strong sense of loss as the group concludes. It is the leader's task to help the group separate while at the same time supporting this feeling of cohesion. It is essential to remain alert to the fact that for some members, the most familiar way to leave people who have come to mean a great deal to them is to become angry and devalue those from whom they are separating. It is always valuable for people to learn that they can separate and still retain the feeling of closeness to and caring for others.

Existential and Time Issues in Termination

It is truly in this period that existential and time issues are most clearly available for examination; indeed, they may well dominate the awareness of group members. The sense that the group will soon end makes it apparent once again that, like life, therapy does not continue forever. Patients who have been stuck or unable to take risks in the group may use this time as an opportunity to finally take advantage of the group.

Additional Comments

It is not uncommon for members to push for added sessions at this point, or for patients who have made little progress to claim that 5 or 10 more sessions would surely allow them time to improve. Like Ulysses tied to the mast, the leader must (usually) adhere steadfastly to his or her (and the group's) original commitment to stop at the predetermined time. It is generally unlikely that such added sessions will be of major benefit. It is far better to allow the group to end—for members to take what they have gotten from the group and reflect on their experience for a month or two— and then for anyone desiring additional treatment to recontact the therapist. The leader should advise members that it does take time for most people to consolidate gains, and that they should see how things go for a while before jumping back into treatment. The door, however, is always open if they should wish to return.

For some groups, termination is so painful that the group may continue on its own without the leader for a period. To the best of our knowledge, such groups almost always end within several months of the formal group termination.

Follow-Up

Just as the pregroup preparation is essential to group functioning, planning a group follow-up is important to the benefit of the group and the maintenance of changes that have occurred. During the termination phase, the members are advised that the leader will contact them for a reunion meeting in 6 to 12 months. The purpose of this meeting is to allow members to hear what has transpired in the lives of the members since the group ended, and to help the leader increase his or her knowledge about the outcomes of his or her groups. We have found that members appreciate such follow-up meetings and experience them as illustrating the therapist's general interest in their welfare. For leaders, it is truly a way to improve their abilities to predict longer-range outcomes from their clinical work.

The follow-up session is a highly structured meeting, the goals of which may be described to the members in this way:

> I'm glad that you all could come today. In order to have time for all of you to inform us of how you're doing and what has occurred since the group ended, we'll have to keep it to about __ minutes apiece. Maybe we can go around, starting with Mary, and find out just how you have been. I'd especially like to hear how you've done regarding _____ [the focal problem]. I'm also interested in learning what aspects of the group stayed with you and were useful, and which were really not helpful. You can all certainly ask questions as we go around. Let's start with you, Mary. How have things been for you?

The follow-up is a very significant intervention. Being away from the group helps people see more clearly what they have been able to achieve on their own and what still needs to occur in order for them to continue to make the changes in their lives that matter to them.

CONCLUSIONS

Time-limited groups are an important therapeutic modality for the brief therapist. Such groups can, for some patients, be at least as effective as individual treatment (Budman *et al.*, in press). For the therapist who is concerned about issues of time, efficiency, and organizational or financial constraints, time-limited groups may offer a significant opportunity for treating homogeneous populations of patients. Although it still remains unclear who will profit the most from group as opposed to individual therapy, we believe that with many people this "either–or" choice does not need to be made. Since a patient's group therapy, in our model, can be perceived of as part of an overall course of treatment, it is only one element in the broad array of tools available to the brief therapist.

11

Time and Termination

Look upon that last day always. Count no mortal happy till he has passed the final limit of his life secure from pain.
—Sophocles, *Oedipus the King* (ca. 429 B.C./1949)

It ain't over till it's over.
—Yogi Berra

THE USE OF TIME IN BRIEF PSYCHOTHERAPY

Most brief and long-term psychotherapists have applied a notably low degree of creativity to the use of time in treatment. Perhaps because of convenience, insurance restraints, and habit, there is nearly universal application of the 50-minute, weekly psychotherapy session. Groups and families tend to be seen for about 90 minutes, also on a weekly basis. The major "mainstream innovation" in the last 80 years regarding the application of time in psychotherapy has been the use of clear time limits set early in the treatment. However, the most truly novel uses of therapy time about which we have heard or read are Milton Erickson's (1980) approaches to this issue, and Alexander and French's (1946/1974) time utilization.

Erickson, in some cases, would see people for very brief sessions (sometimes just several minutes), and at other times he would see a patient for many hours without a break. On occasion some patients would be seen for daily visits; on other occasions an individual might be seen very intensively and then not again for many months. As with so many other aspects of Erickson's approaches, it is not usually easily discernible from his writings how and why he made his differential decisions regarding whom he would treat in one way as opposed to another.

Alexander and French (1946/1974), in many of their case studies, described strikingly flexible and innovative uses of time. For example, in their "Case P" (pp. 293–297), a young man of 19 came for treatment because of severe and debilitating depression. He was to leave for the Army in less than 3 months, and because of scheduling difficulties he could come in for only very brief (15- to 20-minute) interviews once or twice a week. The therapist saw him for a total of 35 visits, which appeared to have been extremely helpful. He had two more brief contacts with the therapist several years after entering the Army. In addition, Alexander and French (1946/ 1974) provided many examples in their book of increasingly "spread-out" sessions as a method of weaning the patient away from therapy, (e.g., "Case K," pp. 234–244). The authors also presented a number of other cases in which the therapists seemed to use time in a variety of flexible ways.

We believe that even if a therapist does not often choose to modify his or her uses of time, it is important for him or her to be aware that there *are* infinite possibilities for its use. We also believe that some clinical and empirical principles may be applied when the therapist wishes to maintain a time-effective perspective and does have the inclination and opportunity to modify his or her time utilization more radically.

Our empirical data regarding this issue come in part from D. H. Johnson and Gelso's (1980) excellent review of the effectiveness of time limits in psychotherapy, and in part from Howard et al.'s (1986) analysis of the dose–effect relationship in psychotherapy. One of Johnson and Gelso's conclusions is as follows:

> Apparently a minimal amount of counseling may be needed to get improvement started; after this point, the actual duration of the counseling is not predictive of long-term improvement. Thus, with at least weekly treatment contact to begin the improvement process, time alone (with or without counseling) seems to be the actual variable in producing optimal improvement in our clients. In other words, it may be that it is not "the more counseling time the better" but "the more time after beginning counseling the better." (pp. 73–74)

Howard et al. (1986), on the other hand, conclude that up to a certain point (about 52 weekly sessions) there is a clear, positive dose–effect relationship in psychotherapy; that is, for the first year, the more once-a-week therapy the better. How can these seemingly different findings be reconciled? It appears to us that neither the studies reviewed in the Johnson and Gelso (1980) paper nor those cited in Howard et al. (1986) compared, in a careful, randomized experimental design, therapy that was provided intermittently over an extended period of time with therapy that was provided weekly (or more frequently) over this same extended period of time. In the absence of such research, what is apparent from a careful examination of both sets of data is that the early stages of an episode of treatment (the first six to eight visits) are extremely important in initiating the change process. (Howard and his colleagues believe that 50% of patients treated in psychotherapy will show some response to therapy with six to eight sessions.)

Thus, if the therapist wishes to use time in an innovative, time-effective manner, he or she might consider seeing a patient initially for longer visits (more than 50 minutes) and/or for a number of sessions close together. Once the treatment has been initiated (after perhaps four to eight visits), the therapist who is continuing to see a patient might move to briefer visits and/or visits that are "spread out" over longer periods. Most importantly, the therapist should remember that there is nothing sacred about seeing patients in a particular way as regards the timing of visits. We have found that even the most disturbed patients can respond to the flexible use of time in a favorable manner. Indeed, setting up twice-a-month visits with such patients may at times be viewed as a vote of confidence in their abilities to survive without the therapist. Even less disturbed patients may profit considerably from such unusual scheduling of appointments. In addition to suggesting the patients' capacity to "survive" without the commonplace weekly meeting, such scheduling—particularly when used in the context of the active, focused style of intervention described in this book—also implies the need for patients to work on their problems outside the therapist's office. That is, dependency is minimized, and self-responsibility is enhanced. The therapist should consider the fact that time and timing are just as much types of interventions as are interpretations, tasks, and so on, and need not be applied in an unquestioned, unchangeable manner. In any case, the flexible brief therapist should place particular emphasis upon making maximal use of early sessions in a given episode of care, and may consider a move to less frequent or less "time-intensive" visits later in a given episode.

THE ISSUE OF TERMINATION

Psychoanalytically oriented thinkers, in particular, have been interested in the issue of termination in psychotherapy. Since "good" treatment is viewed as having a prophylactic effect, the need for additional treatment once the therapy is "completed" is often perceived as indicating a therapeutic failure. The following excerpt from Firestein's (1978) review of psychoanalytic termination criteria will give the reader some idea of what many analytically oriented thinkers see as the ideal state for the terminating patient:

> A typical characterization would indicate approximately the following: Symptoms have been traced to their genetic conflicts, in the course of which the infantile neurosis has been identified, as the infantile amnesia was undone ("insight"). It is hoped all symptoms have been eliminated, mitigated, or made tolerable. Object relations, freed of transference distortions, have improved, along with the level of psychosexual functioning, the latter attaining "full genitality." Penis envy and castration anxiety have been mastered. The ego is strengthened by virtue of diminishing anachronistic countercathectic formations. The ability to distinguish between fantasy and reality has been sharpened. Acting out has been eliminated. The capacity to tolerate some measure of anxiety and to reduce other unpleasant affects to signal quantities has been improved. The ability to tolerate delay of gratification is increased, and along with it there is a shift from autoplastic to alloplastic conflict solutions. Subli-

mations have been strengthened, and the capacity to experience pleasure without guilt or other notable inhibiting factors has improved. Working ability,
under which so many aspects of ego function, libidinal and aggressive drive
gratification are subsumed, has improved. (pp. 226–227)

Furthermore, not only must the patient be in this extraordinary (and
unlikely) state of mental health, but there should be no looking back. That
is, "when you are done, you are done."

Ticho (1972) strongly advises against reassuring the patient that he or
she can recontact the analyst if the need arises. Indeed, such reassurances
are viewed as suspect. The therapist's need to make such a statement and the
patient's need to hear this reassurance probably mean that the treatment is
not really complete and perhaps should not be terminated.

This rigid and unrealistic view of termination in psychotherapy and
psychoanalysis has pervaded long-term dynamically oriented thinking
(Panel, 1969; Panel, 1975). In a modified form, this view has also influenced
brief dynamic therapies (Davanloo, 1978a; Mann, 1973; Sifneos, 1972,
1979). That is, little attention is paid to the possibility of the patient's
returning, because successful treatment will have been curative, and additional therapeutic input should not be required. Indeed, as Davanloo (1980)
writes regarding his approach, "[A]t the time of termination there is definite
evidence of the *total resolution* of the patient's core neurosis" (p. 70, italics
added). Moreover, this minimizing of the possibility, need, or appropriate-
ness of the patient's returning contradicts the theoretical and research
evidence we have considered in previous chapters in favor of an I-D-E
framework for brief psychotherapy. The Davanloo position would seem to
deny the likelihood of developmental changes across the life span.

Mann and Goldman (1982) warn against telling the patient, in their
form of time-limited therapy, that there will be a follow-up interview about
1 year after termination. They write:

At no time during the treatment does the therapist make any mention of a
follow-up interview. It is incumbent on the therapist to make certain that the
separation phase of treatment is *unequivocal*; anything less will suggest to the
patient that the separation is not genuine, that more time will be available.
(p. 13, italics added)

Thus, in their model, the termination is presented to the patient as absolute
because to do otherwise would intrude upon the fantasies, anxieties, and
"working-through" process evoked by the separation. In brief behavioral
treatments, termination appears to be seen as an issue of no major importance and is generally addressed only minimally (e.g., Beck, Emery, &
Greenberg, 1985), if at all. When the issue is addressed by cognitive-
behavioral therapists, return for treatment is viewed (pejoratively) as indicating a "relapse" (see Beck *et al.*, 1979, p. 327; A. A. Lazarus, 1981, p. 30).
(Should those who return to physicians or dentists for more care be viewed

as "relapsers" or "treatment failures"? We hope not. However, this terminology and the underlying mythology pervade mental health care.)

In contrast to the views expressed in such illustrations from the psychoanalytic and behavioral literature on the matter of returning patients, our experience has been that a patient's returning often indicates not only that a positive working alliance has been established, but also that the patient has derived some benefit from his or her initial therapy experience.

"Working Through" Termination in Brief Dynamic Therapy

Strupp and Binder (1984) write:

> A central purpose of psychodynamic psychotherapy is to help the patient come to terms with previous separation and object losses, whether these be emotional or actual. Accordingly, one may say that many patients enter psychotherapy because they failed to resolve reactions to earlier traumas or losses. Symptoms and complaints often embody a return to earlier lost objects with whom the patient has unfinished business. (p. 260)

In working out a "better" ending for the treatment, the therapist tries to help the patient change his or her previously unsatisfactory pattern of handling separations.

Mann's (1973) emphasis in time-limited therapy upon termination issues has as its goal the working through of separation–individuation issues:

> It is absolutely incumbent upon the therapist to deal directly with the reaction to termination in all its painful aspects and affects if he expects to help the patient come to some vividly affective understanding of the now inappropriate nature of his early unconscious conflict. More than that, active and appropriate management of the termination will allow the patient to internalize the therapist as a replacement or substitute for the earlier ambivalent object. *This time the internalization will be more positive (never totally so), less anger laden and less guilt laden, thereby making separation a genuine maturational event.* Since anger, rage, guilt, and their accompaniments of frustration and fear are the potent factors that prevent positive internalization and mature separation, it is these that must not be overlooked in this phase of the time-limited therapy. (p. 36, italics in original)

Although dealing with and "working through" terminations in psychotherapy have taken on almost mythical proportions, there are no empirical data of which we are aware that indicate any relationship between outcome and focus upon termination. Indeed, Clara Hill (personal communication, June 20, 1986) and her colleagues, in their interesting study of process and outcome in time-limited therapy, found that the highly experienced therapists in that study tended to spend extremely short periods of time discussing termination with their patients.

Furthermore, although the termination of psychotherapy is often described as a very painful event for the patient, engendering strong emotions of grief, loss, anger, and abandonment (Edelson, 1963; Firestein, 1978; Mann, 1973), the single careful study on the topic of which we are aware seems not to support this contention. Marx and Gelso (1987), in a field study of former counseling center clients, reported: "Perhaps the most surprising finding of the study was participants' pervasive positive reactions to ending counseling in sharp contrast to the literature's emphasis on termination as a painful loss. . . . it is clear that clients in the study expressed largely positive feelings about ending" (p. 8).

We do not mean to imply by what we have said that termination is an inconsequential issue which should be ignored by the brief therapist. Certainly, in our description of time-limited group psychotherapy (see Chapter 10), the ending of the group is viewed as one of the important foci in the treatment. Similarly, we believe that for those individual patients and/or couples for whom a "break" in the therapy engenders major insecurities or issues regarding previous losses, the separation should be examined and clarified. There may, however, be numerous circumstances in which excessive focus upon the so-called "termination" is unwarranted. This may be because such issues have little relevance to the particular patient in question and his or her circumstances, or because the "intermittent" and "as-needed" nature of the treatment relationship has been emphasized by the therapist and accepted by the patient. It may be unnecessary to analyze the "termination" if one is simply "interrupting" treatment for some period of time.

We also believe that the view that therapy is *totally* terminated at a given point has led to some serious ethical issues. In a national study of psychiatrists (Gartrell, Herman, Olarte, Feldstein, & Localio, 1986), it was found that 10% at one point developed a sexual relationship with a patient. The vast majority of such liaisons developed after the formal termination of therapy. This study has moved the American Psychiatric Association to consider revising its ethical standards so that a "dual relationship" with a patient is eschewed *at any time*. Once a person is a patient, he or she is always a patient.

The Reality of "Finality"

As we have mentioned earlier in this book, the data on how patients actually make use of psychotherapy appear to tell a different story from that told in the theoretical literature. Many patients return for multiple courses of mental health treatment over the span of their lives.

In a research project by V. Patterson, Levene, and Breger (1977), about 60% of the patients in brief psychodynamic or brief behavioral therapy who were studied returned within 1 year for more treatment. Furthermore, it was learned that almost 60% of the patients interviewed had had psychotherapy prior to entrance into that study. Kovacs, Rush, Beck, and Hollon (1981), in a randomized clinical trial comparing cognitive–behavioral therapy and imipramine for depression, found that about 50% of the patients studied in either condition had had additional treatment after the formal termination of the study therapy. Weissman *et al.* (1981), comparing pharmacotherapy and interpersonal therapy for depression, reported at the 12-month follow-up that "most patients received some treatment. . . . Only about one-third of the patients received no psychotherapeutic drugs and did not see a mental health professional during the year [following therapy]" (p. 52).

The phenomenon of patients' returning to treatment after the formal "termination" of a course of therapy is not limited to brief approaches. Goldensohn (1977), in a survey of graduates of the William Alanson White Psychoanalytic Institute, found that 55% had additional therapy after their analyses. Hartlaub, Martin, and Rhine (1986) surveyed analysts at the Denver Psychoanalytic Society, who reported that within 3 years of termination two-thirds of their "successfully analyzed" patients had recontacted them. Grunebaum (1983) and Henry *et al.* (1971) also found that psychotherapists themselves had received many courses of long-term treatment over their life spans, and that return for more therapy was unrelated to the perceived quality and/or outcomes of previous therapies. In fact, Grunebaum reported that in his sample the most striking determinant of returning for treatment was the patient/therapist's age: The older a therapist, the more likely it was that he or she had received more episodes of therapy.

Several years ago, one of us had an interesting experience that highlighted the (frequent) interminability of brief psychotherapy.*

I was asked to do a consultation at a local mental health center on a somewhat problematic outpatient. As the patient was described to me by the psychiatrist who was treating him, I had a *déjà vu* experience. I wondered whether I had supervised some of the patient's previous therapy. Suddenly, I recalled that this was a man I had seen presented (on videotape) at a large national mental health conference, by one of the nation's foremost practitioners of brief dynamic therapy and described as a stunningly successful case of short-term therapy—a "cure." When I later met the patient face to face for a consultation interview, I asked him if he had, in fact, seen Dr. X in therapy.

"Oh, yeah," he said. "Dr. X was a great guy. I saw him for some sessions before I left computer school. Then when I moved here I got into a therapy group to work on some of the issues that had come up later. After that, me and my wife went into about 6 months of couple therapy with Dr. Y. Following that, I felt like I needed to work more on my own issues,

*For the sake of clarity, this description is written in first person singular.

so I saw an individual therapist for awhile. After a year we began to have trouble with our kid, so we came here and started being seen."

It was my impression that Dr. X had done an excellent job. He was remembered fondly by the patient, and had helped the patient view "talking with someone about my problems" as a very beneficial endeavor. However, in contrast to the impressions conveyed in Dr. X's writings and lectures, the therapy was far from definitive.

In our view, although a therapist may "terminate" a patient's treatment by arbitrarily setting a date after which the therapist will no longer see that patient, patients can and do (with great frequency) seek out more treatment elsewhere when they want and need it. While there do exist circumstances in which it may be useful for the therapist to emphasize what it is like "to separate" from another person, we believe that this can be accomplished by the use of "treatment-free" periods. That is, we often suggest to the patient that after a course of brief therapy, he or she might wait 3–6 months before seeking more treatment. This period without therapy may be most helpful in allowing the patient to clarify and consolidate gains. Of course, if the patient needs to be seen before the end of this period, we are flexible and accommodating.

From our perspective, it is usually best to maintain a primary care perspective with patients—that is, to keep in mind a model of care like the model maintained by the family general practitioner. He or she may first see a patient for the flu, later for a back problem, and still later for family or emotional issues.

Both of us have seen patients for as many as 15 years in successive courses of brief therapy, and have treated children (now grown) of some of our early cases. As we say to psychology and psychiatry trainees, "There is nothing easier than getting a patient *not* to come back." Indeed, many therapists seem to have exceptional innate skills in getting patients never to return to them. We believe that patients can and should return as needed. This perspective does not preclude doing therapy efficiently and effectively, and it encourages a more flexible perspective of "not needing to do it all at once." Moreover, even relatively few visits may be viewed as sufficient if seen in the larger context of an overall primary care relationship. On the other hand, a rather large number of visits may be experienced as depriving if this is understood as *the* definitive course of therapy.

CASE EXAMPLES

In this section, we describe a number of case examples that illustrate the flexible use of time and a primary care model of brief treatment.

As a first example, we return to Helen, whose initial interview is presented at the end of Chapter 2. Helen, as described previously, was a 25-year-old woman who was very depressed and demoralized when she initially sought treatment. It readily became apparent to the therapist that much of what was going on for Helen related to the fact that although she wished to separate from her mother and go to graduate school, at the same time she felt tremendous guilt and responsibility toward her. This guilt and responsibility related to the fact that Helen's father had died when Helen was 5. Her mother had herself lost her father at nearly the same age, and in some ways looked to Helen to take care of her and be *her* parent.

Helen was treated initially in a total of nine sessions over a period of 20 weeks. In keeping with some of the views we have mentioned previously in this chapter regarding the use of time, Helen was first seen with a good deal of "time intensity." That is, sessions were initially held weekly, and the second one lasted 2 hours. Subsequent visits were set up on about a bi-weekly basis. As the reader may recall, after nine visits Helen entered school in a distant city. Over the next several years, the therapist received some brief notes from Helen describing her experiences in her graduate program.

Almost 4 years (to the day) after Helen had begun treatment for the first time, she returned for another course of therapy. Following graduate school, Helen had joined a volunteer organization and spent a year in Africa teaching science. Unfortunately, while abroad she contracted an unusual disease, requiring her to return to the United States for treatment. Once she was recovered and healthy, the realization set in that she was back home, living with her mother, and unemployed. She again began to feel depressed and hopeless, particularly when she contrasted her current situation with the one she had enjoyed in Africa, where she had felt effective and well liked. While abroad, she had for the first time in her life begun (tentatively) to develop a relationship with a man. Furthermore, her colleagues had often praised her for her fine work. Upon her return, her mother remained critical and demanding and to some degree began to escalate her guilt-evoking pressure for Helen to remain at home, presumably because Helen's younger brothers had moved out to live on their own.

In the second course of treatment, Helen was seen for three 1-hour visits over a 1-month period. Much of this second course of therapy was spent in helping Helen review the changes she had made following her initial treatment. The therapist attempted to help her look at all of the progress she had made since her last period of treatment. (Helen had a hard time taking credit for many of these changes and tended to attribute them to "dumb luck.") The clinician pointed out to Helen that *she* had ultimately made the decision to go to graduate school, and then had been able to achieve the grades necessary to get her degree. In addition, *she* had decided to go to Africa, and had done an outstanding job there until her illness forced her to return. Also, *she* had allowed her guard to drop sufficiently so that a man began to develop an interest in her.

It was again clarified how much pain Helen had previously experienced and continued to experience regarding her father's untimely death, but she appeared to be dealing with it more effectively. That is, she was able to discuss the death readily and to understand its impact, but it did not dominate her behaviors as totally as it had 4 years before. Furthermore, Helen felt far less responsive to her mother's demands than she had earlier. By the third visit she had decided to make "the big move" across the country. Although Helen had considered such a move many times in the past, she had never felt the "courage" to do so. The week after her third visit, she moved to a distant city (after having discussed the decision with the therapist).

Helen appeared much improved during the second course of treatment. Although she still clearly had many issues to be addressed, she had changed extensively, and in many ways her behavior seemed much more age-appropriate and less like that of a little girl. It is fascinating to note that at one point Helen spontaneously mentioned to the therapist that she now felt "20 or 21" (rather than 12, as she had previously felt), but wished that she could finally feel her chronological age of 29.

As another example, we describe Dennis, who was 25 years old when he was first treated. At the time of his initial evaluation, Dennis was having frequent anxiety attacks and was becoming increasingly agoraphobic. He could only drive in a limited area of the city without being overwhelmed by his terror. He also found himself unable to enter a subway, elevator, or airplane. Thus, his professional and recreational activities were becoming increasingly constricted.

Dennis also had extensive social deficits. He had had only one girlfriend in his life (for 3 weeks) and had never had a male friend for any extended period of time. To complete the picture, he hated his dreary and tedious job as a bank teller. His most extensive social contacts were with his eight younger siblings and his parents, all of whom lived in the area. However, even in his family, he felt lonely and depressed. His parents were initially described as "hard-working, generous, and strict people." Dennis's characterization of them changed quite dramatically over the course of the therapy.

The first area of focus for Dennis and his therapist was upon his agoraphobia and anxiety. Over a series of six individual sessions, it was clarified that his anxieties had become much more severe during a period 3 months prior to his initial visit with the therapist. That month, July, represented the second anniversary of the brutal rape and near-murder of his youngest sister, Nicole. During this crisis Dennis' parents had been completely unable to cope and to help Nicole deal with the trauma. Instead, they put great pressure on Dennis to deal with the police, lawyers, counselors, and so on. At the same time, they were harshly critical of and dissatisfied with the things he would do to be helpful. It became clear to Dennis after several individual therapy visits that although his agoraphobia was "real" and not contrived, its severity prevented him from being able to travel to his parents' home—a trip that would have required him to drive or take public transportation.

Following the individual therapy, Dennis was treated as part of a time-limited 15-session psychotherapy group for young adults. It was felt that this would be beneficial regarding some of his social (developmental dysynchrony) problems.

As it turned out, much of the focus in the group for Dennis was on his sister's rape. In talking about this trauma and his parents' reactions to it and to him, Dennis became far clearer about his feelings. Many of the group members were incredulous that his parents would be so attacking and belittling, when it was they who had abrogated their responsibilities toward their daughter. For Dennis, who had always tried to be the "perfect son" and never would be overtly critical of his parents, these reactions were eye-opening. By the end of the group Dennis was doing much better symptomatically, and was beginning to express a sense of hurt and anger regarding his parents' harsh treatment of him.

At the completion of the group, all of the members were asked to take several months to consolidate their gains before getting more treatment. Dennis did this and recontacted the therapist after about 6 months. He was now traveling freely by car and train, but still was frightened of traveling by airplane. He had begun to be more direct with his parents and had had several confrontations with them about their dealings with him. Dennis had profited a great deal from his group experience and wished to be in another short-term young adult group. This time, he wanted to "learn more about relating better to women." In his second short-term group, Dennis was able to begin to be more open and interactive with men and women. He could be a caring and supportive person and was therefore very positively regarded by the other members. Also while in this group, Dennis made plans for getting some additional training in a new line of work.

A little more than a year after this second group ended, Dennis was seen individually once again for about 4–5 months. This time the treatment focused upon the difficulties he had been having with his girlfriend, Bette. She was beginning to pressure Dennis to get engaged and to move in together. He did not wish to do so at the time. Bette was determined that the marriage would be "now or never." They therefore separated, got back together, and separated again. Dennis came in shortly after the second separation. During this course of treatment Dennis also discussed his continued problems with his parents. He wished to get closer to and perhaps marry Bette, but at the same time "could not imagine" being with someone and having a relationship "the way my parents have a relationship." Dennis's fears about getting too close to Bette were examined in light of his family of origin.

Over the next several years, Dennis was not seen. He then called at one point to say that he and Bette were back together and thinking seriously about marriage. He came in with Bette to talk about issues in their relationship. After about 3 months of couples treatment, Dennis and Bette decided to move in together.

A short while later, Bette received an offer for an outstanding job in another city. She and Dennis decided that they would get married the following spring and that he would join her at that point in that city. Dennis had done very well in his new field, and was reluctant to leave an outstanding job situation. However, his relationship with his parents had continued to deteriorate, and he was not altogether unhappy with the thought of moving. In the next course of treatment, which lasted about 6 months, Dennis tried to prepare himself to go to the new city and mourned his increasing alienation from his parents.

About 3 months after he had moved and married, Dennis called the therapist prior to coming back to town for a business trip. His fears of driving had returned, and he wished to deal with this problem "very quickly," since it had begun to impede his work (which required extensive travel). Dennis was seen in a 2½-hour visit directed toward the hypnotic/ behavioral treatment of his symptom. The stimuli for his panic were elicited. Once these were specified, a variety of posthypnotic suggestions were given to him. Also, a hypnotic relaxation tape was made for Dennis's home use. When Dennis called back later in the week, he was much calmer and was getting over his driving phobia.

Dennis has continued to visit the therapist about once a year. Altogether, he has been seen for relatively few visits over a period of 10 years. He has developed an extremely successful career and marriage. At this point he has one child. There remains a major rift between him and his parents, which may be unchangeable. His psychotherapy has been very beneficial to him; it is not possible to determine whether he would have done better or worse in long-term, open-ended treatment. As it is, however, his outcome to date has been most favorable, and has been achieved in a highly cost- and time-effective manner.

As a third example of the flexible use of time in a primary care model, we describe Arnold and Rhonda J. Arnold and Rhonda were both in their mid-20s when seen for the first time; they had one young son and had been married for 4 years. Their relationship had always been a "rocky" one. The two had met in high school and had been together ever since. They sought treatment when Rhonda began to question whether or not she wished to have another child with Arnold and remain married to him. Arnold was a very depressed, dissatisfied man who was chronically worried about other people's reactions to him. Rhonda was an isolated and unhappy woman, who described herself and her husband in their first therapy interview as both being "damaged goods": "We both come from horrendous backgrounds and never really learned how to be together with another person."

Both Arnold and Rhonda were very needy people who came from ungiving and abusive families. Rhonda's father was an alcoholic who was "thrown out" of the family home repeatedly by the patient's wealthy but manic–depressive mother. When Rhonda was 12, her father took an overdose of pills and died after one of these angry brawls with his wife. After this, Rhonda's mother forced her into the role of the "parentified" child with her younger siblings and was constantly demeaning and critical.

Both of Arnold's parents were alcoholic, but at the same time they were "pillars" of their small, rural Southern community. Although they were at times very critical of him, they tended in general to ignore Arnold and his younger brothers. Being deeply committed to community activities, they "gave at church, gave at the town council, gave at the school committee, but never gave at home."

Arnold had developed a pattern of whining and chronic complaining to get support from Rhonda. She, on the other hand, "gave till it hurt." At that point she would become furious with Arnold; he in turn would martyr himself ("Yes, you're right. I am a shit. I'm just a horrible person"). Rhonda would feel guilty and responsible for his suffering, and so it went. At the time of their entry into treatment Rhonda was beginning to question whether it might not be better to be alone than to continue in this terribly painful pattern.

During the initial course of therapy, the clinician attempted to help them look at and begin to modify their dysfunctional patterns of interaction. There was also a goal of clarifying how their relationships in their families of origin affected their marriage. The therapist had the couple together examine photo albums of their families of origin. Since Arnold's parents lived in the local area, the therapist had them and his brothers come in for a joint session with Arnold. Gradually, it became clearer to the couple that part of their current difficulties related to how hard it was for them to separate their family-of-origin relationships from their current marital relationship. They both became increasingly able to "stand back" from their characteristic patterns of interacting. Arnold began to try to ask Rhonda for help and support more directly than before, rather than acting childish and whining. Rhonda, too, began to try to get more for herself rather than subjugating her needs to the needs of those around her. The blowups between the couple were reduced, and Rhonda gradually began to feel increasing interest in continuing the marriage.

After about 5 months of biweekly conjoint sessions, Arnold and Rhonda were referred to a time-limited couples group that lasted 4 months.

The group allowed a great deal of input and feedback between the members. Rhonda was supported in her striving to do more for herself; at the same time, she was urged to be more direct with Arnold. As soon as she felt that he was being childishly demanding, she would tell him, so that things would not develop to the point of an explosion. Arnold was pushed by members to be more attentive to Rhonda's needs and to be less self-preoccupied. Following the couples group, Rhonda and Arnold were seen for two more conjoint visits to help them consolidate their gains. After this they were not seen for nearly 10 years.

Rhonda recontacted the therapist 1 year after she had been found to have and had been treated for cancer. Since the cancer was found at an early stage, treatment appeared to have been successful. Rhonda's immediate reason for seeking therapy at this point was that "My mother is destroying my life." After Rhonda's diagnosis of cancer, her mother had been singularly unsupportive and unhelpful, and had been most preoccupied with the impact upon herself. Nine months following Rhonda's surgery, her mother had become psychotically depressed and hospitalized. Upon discharge she had moved into an apartment in Rhonda's city and tried to spend as much of every day at Rhonda's home as possible. When her mother again began to become severely depressed, Rhonda called the therapist. In the second course of treatment Rhonda was seen initially weekly and then every third week over an 8-month period. Every third or fourth visit, she was seen with Arnold.

A great deal had transpired for Rhonda and Arnold over the 10 years since they had previously been in therapy. They had had another child who was now 8 (their older child was now a teenager). Arnold had found a satisfying and lucrative line of work. He appeared far more self-confident and open in the couples sessions, and appeared to have increased the directness of his communication with Rhonda. She in turn seemed, although clearer about her needs, still somewhat tentative in stating what she wanted. The major issue for the couple at this point appeared to be Arnold's lack of time away from his work, and the fact that both were beginning to drink too much.

A number of issues were dealt with simultaneously in this course of treatment. Rhonda was helped to set limits with her mother and not to allow herself to be ruled by her mother's needs. In addition, Rhonda discussed her reactions to her illness and the terror she felt at being diagnosed as having cancer. There was also some examination of how Arnold could be more involved with his wife and children, in spite of a long and arduous schedule. Rhonda was referred for vocational counseling and began to train for a career. Finally, the couple were later urged to reduce their drinking (which they successfully did). This second course of therapy again proved to be very useful to Arnold and Rhonda. Their vivid recollections of their previous treatment with the therapist were striking. They saw that period of therapy as having been extremely helpful and significant, and they chose to return to the same clinician because it had gone so well. After the second episode of therapy, they again felt improved and pleased with the benefits. They were also confident in the knowledge that they could always recontact "our psychologist" if the need ever arose.

As a final example of a primary care model of mental health practice, we present the case of Lance, seen by one of us at different points over a 9-year period.

When Lance first contacted the therapist, the patient was in his early 30s. He came in because Irma, the woman with whom he had lived for 9 years, was demanding that he make some "substantial changes" or else she would move out. After an initial evaluation session on his own, Lance was seen for 10 sessions with Irma. It was Irma's impression that Lance could not be direct or assertive, was cold and unfriendly toward people, and was exceptionally detached from their relationship.

Lance felt overwhelmed by Irma. He saw her as being *too* controlling in their interactions. Although it initially appeared that the couple might be able to resolve some of their differences, Irma began to feel after six visits that a resolution of their problems was unlikely. She moved out of the apartment they shared, and during the next couples visit told Lance that she saw their separation as final.

Lance was crushed. He felt terrified and sank into a deep depression. Shortly after the separation, Lance was referred to a crisis group (along the lines described in Chapter 10 of this book). Following the crisis group, which met for 4 weeks on a twice-a-week basis, Lance was seen individually for four more biweekly visits. These sessions and the crisis group seemed to help Lance "pull himself together." Although he remained somewhat depressed, he also began to function better at work and with other people.

Lance was not seen again for about 24 months, at which point he returned for more therapy because of a problem with impotence. As he had again begun to date and go out, he had at first occasionally and then with greater frequency started to have problems sustaining his erection when sexually involved with a woman. Lance wanted help in dealing with this problem, which he related to having "lost a lot of self-confidence over this whole mess with Irma." The patient was treated using some of the principles developed by Masters and Johnson (1970) and Helen Singer Kaplan (1974). The therapist also implemented a hypnotic approach to the problem. Essentially, it was recommended to Lance that he not attempt to initiate sexual intercourse with the woman he was then dating, but that he do "other things that are pleasurable to you and your partner." It was also emphasized that ejaculation need not be central and was "not the goal of your sexual interaction with Frieda." It was clarified to Lance that all men went through some brief periods of impotence and that he was obviously worried about "more failures" after his failure with Irma to make a go of their relationship. Lance also was taught to use self-hypnosis to relax himself when sexually involved with a woman. Finally, it was recommended that he read the book by Kaplan (1974), which could help him better understand his impotence problem. Once Lance was able to become more involved with "what" he was doing rather than "how" he was doing sexually, his performance began to improve. After several months, his impotence was nearly eliminated.

About 4 years later, Lance again contacted the clinician. He was at that point married to Meg, an extremely attractive woman 12 years his junior. A year after his last contact with his therapist, Lance had met Meg at a club and had been "smitten" by her. She was beautiful and bright, and had a very good job. The element that Lance had (against his own better judgment) ignored was that for many years, Meg had had a serious drug and alcohol abuse problem. Nonetheless, because she too was so enthusiastic about the relationship and appeared to love him "so much," he decided to marry her. Some months after their marriage, Lance learned about Meg's three serious suicide attempts in her late teens and early 20s. It also became clear to him that when she became angry while under the influence of alcohol or drugs, Meg could become explosive and lose control. She would punch Lance or throw things at him. He responded first with fear and withdrawal, and then with rage followed by guilt.

Meg and Lance were seen together for three visits. During the second conjoint visit, the therapist recommended to Meg that she would have to go to AA or see an alcoholism/drug abuse counselor in order for the treatment to continue. During the following visit, Meg became furious with the therapist, overtly because she felt that he was siding with Lance against her. She said that she would never see the therapist again and ran out of the office, viciously slamming the door behind her. The week after this appointment, Lance phoned and stated that he was calling at Meg's behest to say that they would be seeing someone else for additional couples treatment.

About 6 months later, Lance called the therapist for an emergency appointment. When he came in 2 days later, he explained that Meg was planning to leave him and that he was now a "two-time loser." The precipitating event in their breakup was Lance's admission to Meg that he was a transvestite, something that he had never admitted to anyone (including the therapist) before. After several months with the new couples therapist, Lance had begun to feel a bit more comfortable with Meg. This was particularly true after she began to get treatment for her substance abuse problems and things became calmer between them. In a "moment of trust," he admitted his transvestitism to her. Meg became enraged. She began to scream at Lance that he was "sick" and should be in a hospital. She also said that she could not stay married to him under these circumstances. Two days later she had moved out of their apartment and refused any further couples therapy with him.

Initially, the focus with Lance was again upon dealing with the crisis of the second loss. After several weeks, the therapist suggested that he and Lance examine what had gone on in the relationship with Meg that had led to the dissolution of the marriage. It was also recommended that they talk more about Lance's transvestitism and the implications this had for Lance's life and interaction with others. After another several weeks, Lance decided to stop therapy with the psychologist he was seeing and to seek therapy with someone who was more "analytically oriented." "Since the transvestitism has deeper roots, I want someone who can really understand this."

About a year later, Lance returned to the original clinician because "my therapist never said anything very helpful and I *really* want to deal with the transvestitism now." He was much less anxious and debilitated than he had been after the breakup with Irma, but he felt even more frightened of relating to women than he had at that time. Lance felt as though he "always chose the wrong people to get involved with." He was also able to discuss his cross-dressing with the therapist for the first time. It was something that he had begun as a teenager, and it never involved going out of his house in women's attire. He felt no interest in actually being a woman or being sexually involved with a man. He was, however, obsessed with the feeling, texture, and beauty of women's clothing and the fact that "women have it so easy in their lives."

Lance wanted to be able to rid himself of this obsession and his compulsivity regarding putting on women's clothes several times per week. In the seven individual sessions that were focused upon helping Lance deal better with this problem, a number of important issues were clarified. The cross-dressing in many ways appeared not to be a sexual act. Rather, it seemed more to be a way for Lance to reduce his fears and anxieties. His telling Meg about his "problem" was viewed as being in some ways self-destructive (because she lost control and broke up with him at that point), but it was also interpreted as a way for him to finally "put his cards on the table" and to try to deal with an aspect of his life about which he felt great shame and embarrassment. (The transvestitism, as noted, had begun in Lance's early teens; he had always wanted to work on it, but saw himself as "crazy" for having this problem.) The transvestitism was addressed by having the patient keep weekly logs of his thoughts and activities, with special emphasis upon those points at which he began to want to change into women's clothing. Initially, the therapist requested that Lance attempt to limit his cross-dressing to once a week. The following session he was asked to limit himself to once every 2 weeks. After three sessions, the cross-dressing had subsided, and by the end of the sixth session it was nearly under control. Following the sixth session, Lance threw away all of his cross-dressing paraphernalia.

In the next 12 sessions of weekly therapy, the therapist focused with Lance on his fears about relationships with women. In these visits he spoke about specific problems he was having in relating to women, asking them out, knowing what to say or how to get close to a woman, and so on. During this period of treatment Lance began to date a new woman, but agreed to focus this time with the therapist on what this relationship was like for him. Of particular interest was working with Lance on being able to express his needs to Mary Ellen, the new woman in his life. The therapist also worked with him on being clearer and more directly assertive in the therapy relationship. After these 12 visits, Lance took a break from treatment, planning to recontact the therapist periodically as things developed with Mary Ellen.

These cases are illustrative of the work that is done in brief therapy stressing the concepts of primary care, intermittent treatment, and life stage development. They demonstrate that although patients may not be definitively "cured," so that they never return for more treatment, they can be helped over significant obstacles in their lives. Often, patients may make significant and far-reaching changes; at other times, the modifications that occur are much more modest and limited.

It is most important, however, from our perspective that the patient be encouraged to view the therapist as interested, helpful, and available. It is also essential that patients understand that the desire to return for therapy does not by any means indicate a failure. We believe that it is often the case that people cannot make particular changes until the time is right. All clinicians have had patients who have been "stuck" and unable to make any significant progress; suddenly such patients may move into action and begin to modify behaviors that up to that point have seemed unchangeable. We believe that it is not always necessary for the therapist to "chip away" at a patient's defenses in order for such a significant transformation to occur. Rather, it may be that under some circumstances the therapist may plant the seeds of change, which then lie dormant until developmental or life change factors "trigger" the patient to take some steps toward growth. For example, Lance had never told the therapist, over many years of contact, his "dark secret." With the dissolution of his marriage (and, it appeared, a desire to get this problem out into the open at last), he was willing to address his transvestitism. It appeared to the therapist that Lance was at that point ready to give up his cross-dressing and to try to achieve a more honest relationship with the therapist and with others in his life. He stated that, being in his early 40s, he really hoped to finally begin relating to people in a more genuine and direct way.

People change over time, as do circumstances. It is simply unrealistic to assume that as therapists we can treat our patients in such a way that future problems can be avoided. As exemplified by Rhonda's cancer, we have no way to anticipate future illnesses, losses, changes, and so on, which play major roles in all of our lives.

The primary care model of brief therapy takes into account the basically imperfectable nature of human existence. The model assumes that people can and want to improve their lives and their interactions with others, but that it is unlikely that many of us will soon reach a state of nirvana. It is, however, clear to us that even with the limitations of time, resources, and the curative powers of psychotherapy that have been described in this book, we can still assist our patients in improving their lives in significant and indelible ways.

12

A Case Transcript

This final chapter is an edited case transcript that provides an example of our model of brief treatment.* David, the subject of this transcript, has been previously discussed in Chapter 4.

David was initially seen about 2 years after his wife Kate's untimely death from the complications of systemic lupus erythematosus, a sometimes fatal autoimmune disease. He complained about his inability to be romantically involved with women for any extended period of time, and was unaware of the relationship (which the therapist believed existed) between this problem and Kate's unmourned death.

The therapist treated David initially for five visits. During this period they discussed the patient's relationships with women at present, but focused particularly upon Kate and her death. It appeared that David made some progress in being able to express his feelings about Kate's loss, and that he gained a better sense of how these feelings were connected to his difficulties in relating to women. He also became less depressed and withdrawn.

The patient was not seen again for 2 years, at which point he returned for additional treatment. It is this episode of therapy from which the transcript is taken.

A number of points should be noted in reading the transcript. First, the patient *did* return to the same therapist for treatment. Although he came at the urging of Lisa, his current girlfriend, it is clear that he liked and trusted the therapist and that the therapeutic alliance had endured during the hiatus.

Second, the therapist, because of his prior contact with David, "knew" him. That is, he understood how what was going on at present fit in with what had transpired for David previously. The clinician could quickly determine how David's relationship with Lisa was similar to or different from his interactions with the women with whom he had been involved at the time of his prior therapeutic contact. Because of this familiarity, the

---

*The therapist was Simon Budman. The boldface commentary interspersed throughout the transcript is his, while the italicized comments are those of Alan Gurman.

clinician rapidly made a decision that he would ask David to come to a session with Lisa. Although under other circumstances (e.g., when the clinician believes a relationship to be "not very serious"), the therapist might still ask the patient to come in with the significant other (or "insignificant other"), the purposes would be different. In this particular instance, Lisa was asked in because the therapist believed that David was reluctant to be too intimate with her for fear of sustaining another major loss. Therefore, it seemed that a useful strategy would be to have David and Lisa discuss in some depth and detail Kate's death and its effects on their current relationship. This would allow David to confront his fears actively *in vivo*.

In the initial individual visits, the therapist tried to help David again examine how he had been affected by his wife's loss, and also how family-of-origin issues might have affected David's abilities to be intimate with a woman. The therapist believed that David returned for treatment because he was now ready to change. He was active in assisting David to understand the reason for his problem, but also urged him to confront the situation actively, rather than simply ruminating endlessly about it.

In our view, where possible, action as well as insight must be fostered in therapy. One of the problems most frequently encountered by the very analytically oriented clinician is client passivity. Such passivity may be a direct function of the therapist's own reluctance to take any actions that might be perceived as moving out of a "neutral" therapeutic stance (Messer, 1986). In this regard, Appelbaum (1975) quotes the analyst, Leo Rangell as having stated: "I have seen a wrongly moralistic antiaction attitude[,] which creeps into some analyses, fortify the patient's own phobic avoidance of action and lead in some cases to almost a paralysis of the latter and a taboo even against the necessary actions of life" (p. 290).

The reader will see that a variety of routes certainly could have been taken with David. Among these would probably be the alternative of continued open-ended treatment. The patient was a bright, verbal man with a significantly adverse family history and some marked characterological difficulties. The clinician chose to maintain the focus of treatment on the issues of developmental dysynchrony and loss. (David felt developmentally "ready" to be in a loving, committed relationship, but could not overcome Kate's death.) These issues were focused upon in an active, time-effective, circumscribed manner. We believe that if and when David wishes to receive additional therapy, he can always return and do another piece of productive work with the clinician.

DAVID: SESSION 1

Therapist: We spoke a little bit on the phone, but maybe you can tell me more about what is going on.

[Why now?]

Patient: Well, basically, getting back to the same things that we talked about before, I started dating someone again. I think I mentioned to you about—talked about dating Bonnie, and it didn't work out too well. Because it was just a problem she and I had, at least since New Year's. And I started seeing her with the intention that I really wanted to develop a lasting relationship together. You know, I figured it was long enough since my wife, and I just wanted to develop a lasting relationship so I could possibly get married again.

T: You started seeing other people since that?

P: Yes. Since Bonnie, I was dating around a bit and I found this woman, Lisa, who I enjoyed very much. We met skiing. She was a very good skier and we had a lot of fun. And very active athletically. So we instantly had a lot in common. You know, she liked to dance, and athletically we had a lot in common. So you know, we started seeing each other pretty regularly right away. And then I just dropped off seeing anybody else. I was very interested in her. What happened was, as I started getting a little bit serious, well, I told her right up front. I said, "Listen, I have gone through a series of problems with not just short-term relationships, but a number of relationships that did not last that long. They were not going to work out, and I am ready to meet somebody that I can have some sort of a meaningful relationship with." So, you know, we talked about that. And I think that caught her a little bit off guard. You know, this was about a month or so after we started seeing each other. And one thing that was bothering me is that I am fairly active in my Temple and she was Catholic. And you know, I was wondering if this was going to be a conflict. So, because I was fairly interested in her and I did not know if this would work out, I brought it up with her. I talked about religion a bit, and—not that I'm well educated about my own religion, my folks didn't practice at all—but I immediately found out that I knew a lot more about what I was interested in than what her religious backgrounds were. I mean, she was Catholic *because* she was Catholic. And I guess it's the same thing as, you know, you're brought up if you're Irish, you're Irish. That kind of thing. But it was the kind of thing, I said, "Well, what if we ever got married or something like that and we had kids? What would you want to do?" And she said "Well, they'd have to be Catholic." And I said "Well, that's impossible, because if I had kids I'd want them to be Jewish." So we got into this thing. And it was sort of a stalemate. You know, it was very early in the relationship to push that very far, but it was something that I said, hey, if there's going to be a stumbling block this could be one. So I did—I could see that, you know, we weren't going to resolve this. So I said, you know, well, maybe I should talk to somebody else. So I went to see one friend of mine. And we talked—we had dinner together, and we talked quite a bit. And I thought he was going to come out and say, "Hey, this just is not a good idea; it's not going to work. You're better off ending this thing." Actually, another good friend of mine who I worked with at State College, I had a long conversation with him and he basically told me, "Forget it, it's not going to work." And, you know, he was strongly influenced but he had a Jewish background. And, he just didn't see how the two could meet. And he said that it wouldn't work. And I respect this fellow's judgment quite a bit. My other friend, though, really surprised me. Basically, his attitude was if you really love somebody and you really want to make it work out, you can make it work. He said, "There's no doubt it would be very difficult. You know, you're going to have some very strained times because you're going to want to go to temple, she's not going to want to go. She's going to want to go to church, and you're not going to want to go there. And if you have children, you're going to have to basically expose them to both. And, you know, let them make their own decision." And he said, "It's not that the common beliefs are—there are a lot of commonalities that could be found," but he said, you know, that eventually children would have to make their own decision which way they wanted to go. So I thought I was kind of optimistic after talking to him. So I went back and I talked to Lisa about it. Be we just sort of let that ride. And what happened shortly after that was we went on a bicycling trip and she had a really bad accident. She tore apart her leg really bad, and broke her collarbone too. And she was in a cast for months and months. And she lost her job. She was in a job where she needed to travel—she needed to drive a car. And you can't drive a car with a full-length cast on and your collarbone broken. So she lost her job. And, you know, we continued our relationship. At first, you know, we thought it would be like 4 weeks. And then 4 weeks stretched to 8 weeks, then 12 weeks. And when the cast came off she had a brace on. And she was on crutches for a long time. Basically, it sort of drained our—you know, it just kept going on and on and on. And our activities were pretty much limited. I mean, obviously you couldn't go dancing or couldn't do any more cycling or, you know, outdoor activities which I enjoyed.

T: So then what happened?

P: Pardon?

T: Then what happened in the relationship?

P: Well, I started seeing a leveling off. And what happened is . . .

T: Did you find yourself less interested, or . . . ?

P: Yeah, Yeah, it started coming to the point where we were saying, "You know, this isn't really going to work out." And I was kind of, in my mind I was thinking this—and true to past relationships, I was not the one to bring this up and I sort of let things slide, but my actions became apparent.

T: Did you say to her, "I'm feeling less involved; there's something wrong"?

P: Not right away. No. Well we did have a conversation, you know, probably after 3 months and I said, "Listen, I'm feeling held back. I'm really kind of tired of all this, you know, with the leg." I said, "I know it's not your fault, but I've gone through this kind of thing before with people, and particularly my wife, in going through sickness, and I'm not really anxious to do it again. And I'm just a little bit, you know—well, tired isn't really the right word," but I just didn't want to wait for her, basically. And with her being out—we talked a bit, and basically what she said was "Well, if you'll hang in there, this isn't me, I'll be better when my leg gets back. And things will be fine and we can be more active. And I'll begin skiing next winter." I mean, when I think of it, I'm not sure if that was it entirely. What happened is I was starting to get to know the person a little better and I really, like, I mean she had a lot of strength to carry through this—she was very optimistic—but you know, I was finding that we didn't have a lot in common besides activities. You know, we went out to dinner a lot and stuff. Our conversations were always fairly light, limited to the point where we couldn't talk about anything. We'd read the paper on Sunday morning and she'd point out to me, "Oh, did you see *Peanuts* today?" And that would be the extent. You know, she'd read the whole paper, but that would be the extent of something that would impress her. You know?

[In the therapist's previous contacts with David, very similar issues had arisen. In David's relationships with women after his wife's death, the same pattern was often apparent. That is, he would become involved with a woman and quickly become bored or detached. Having discussed this pattern previously, and connected it with his wife's untimely death, the therapist attempted to see whether David still recalled some of their previous discussions.]

T: I remember having a conversation with you almost identical to this about Bonnie [previous girlfriend].

P: Um, um, maybe not Bonnie. Bonnie was fairly probing, intellectually. Now Helene—after my wife I started dating Helene and I think that was more true with her.

T: Bonnie was the dentist?

[The therapist must be familiar with information about patients seen on an intermittent basis.]

P: Yeah, that was Bonnie.

T: Bonnie, I remember your talking about there not being a lot to discuss between the two of you, and a certain kind of distance between the two of you. Do you remember that?

P: Oh, yeah. Well, we didn't have a lot in common. That was a little bit different, too. See, it wasn't so much like an intellectual thing. I mean, she was very—she was a really smart woman. And she was always inquisitive and probing. But the kind of thing with us was that what interested her didn't really interest me. Not completely overall. But there were a lot of things that would interest her that, you know, just didn't do anything for me. And the stuff that I was interested in she wasn't particularly interested in. You know, we did have a lot in common but there was a kind of—there was a void. I think I mentioned to you that things that struck her funny would never be funny to me, and vice versa.

T: Yeah.

P: I thought something would be funny and she just didn't see any humor in it.

T: So then what happened between you and Lisa?

P: [David then described ups and downs in his relationship with Lisa. He discussed her long recovery from her accident and his feeling that she did not make a sufficient effort to get a job once she was able to do so.] So, you know, I said she is not challenging herself. So if she's not challenging herself she's not pushing, and therefore how can she be interesting to me or challenging to me. If she's not willing to push herself?

T: So you felt the issue was her lack of being interesting?

P: Well, that's what I was putting it on at that point. Because I couldn't think of anything else. I was thinking, you know, physically we were very compatible, and she was very caring. There were some other minor issues. You know, she was kind of pushy, she was kind of aggressive. She's a little "rough around the edges." She's not a very—what I would call a sophisticated woman, from the standpoint I'd walk down the beach with her and she'd almost act like me, you know. Or a guy. Where, we'd go down the beach and she'd see a friend, "Hey, Joe, how you doin'?" You know, yell down the beach and I would be sitting there and would say, "Easy,"

T: Again, let me just ask you. If the issue is from her "roughness around the edges" or her lack of sophistication, how come you're here to see me?

[It is critical that the therapist clarify a patient's reason for seeking treatment. David's complaint was centering around Lisa's inadequacies. If he did not feel that *he* had a problem, he was probably not ready for treatment and need not have been seen at this time. A patient's readiness to see the problem as somehow related to his or her behaviors, interactions, or ways of thinking

**is essential. If this is not the case, then psychotherapy *at that point* may not
be the best course to follow.]**

P: Well, that's the thing. You know, I look at it and I say, "OK, try not to
pick on her weaknesses." Which is a thing I seem to exploit in relationships. I look at somebody and if I don't think . . .

T: With many women?

P: Yes. You know, I look at something or other. Their hair isn't right. The
skin complexion isn't right. Or they're not good enough in bed. They're
not intelligent enough. I seem to focus on those things. So, you know,
so in my mind I'm trying to think of what is basically wrong with our
relationship. There's things about her that I don't like but I overlook.
Um, you know, there were other issues. Nobody in my family—not one
member of my family, or for that matter my friends—after meeting her
for the first time, came back to me and said "Wow, you know, I really
like Lisa. You know, I think she's really great for you." Not one. As a
matter of fact, I got kind of negative feedback from my sister and my
mother. My mother actually came out and said to me, the last time I
was home, she says, "Are you going to marry Lisa?" And I said, you
know, "I don't know. I don't think so." And she goes, "Oh, thank
God." You know, she just came right out and said that. My mother's
not one for subtleties or being very smooth about things.

**[The patient did perceive that he was overly critical and distancing in
numerous circumstances with women. It was, however, not easy for him to
maintain this position. He quickly introduced the fact that his mother and
sister also had serious reservations about Lisa.]**

T: Let me just ask you again. Where do things stand at this point? What's
the situation right now?

[Why did David choose to come in at present?]

P: Well, it's sort of hot and cold. You know, if I'm not with her for a while
it's funny, and when I don't see her I think in my mind, "This thing's got
to end at some point." But when I'm with her you know, I just, I really,
when I get up the next morning after we've been together all night it's
like I really care for her a lot. And I really do. I don't know if I'm to the
point where I can honestly say to myself I love her. I think I *do* in some
respects, but I've even tried to say that to her just to see what it
conjured up in my own feeling. And it sounded kind of hollow in my
own mind. I would say "I love you" and it just didn't seem to be—I
really didn't feel it. So, you know, I don't know if I'm coming here
trying to convince myself that "Yes, you know, this is not going to work
out," or probably more importantly, to find out if I'm just preventing
myself from coming into a relationship or really fully developing a

relationship. I think I've more developed a relationship with Lisa than any of the previous women I've been with. We have more communication with each other. We actually talk about these things. We had one conversation recently where I told her basically she wasn't interesting to me. I mean, it came out a little hard because she said to me, "Well, did you think about what our problem is?" And, I said you know, well, I told her what I had said to you, which was basically, "You're not challenging yourself; you're not challenging me; you're not, you know, using your mind. You're a smart person, but you're not challenging yourself." And I gave her the example about how she reads the newspaper and the only thing she talks about is the cartoons. And she said, "Well, the only thing you talk about is sports." And I said, "Well, there's probably some truth in that." And I said, "But I know on many occasions I will talk about political issues or foreign affairs, or even social topics, or something like that, local. And I get maybe a one- or two-word response from you and that's it." And, you know, she doesn't seem to be too interested in other things other than having a good time, and, you know, intellectually we do not get into any heavy conversations other than if we talk about our own relationship. And that's the thing where I can see that, you know, that she really does think things out. After a big fight recently, she said to me, "If we're going to work this out, you should go see Simon Budman."

T: But do you feel like you're here because she told you to come and see Simon Budman?

[Obviously some of the impetus for David to come and see the clinician was coming from Lisa. However, the patient had clearly discussed his previous therapy with Lisa, and presumably had viewed it as valuable enough that she would urge him to return.]

[*At this point, David's motivation for therapy was unclear, whereas Lisa's motivation for him to change was quite clear. David might be the "patient," but since Lisa was the complainant, her inclusion in therapy would probably be essential.*

P: Partly.
T: Partly?
P: Yeah. And partly because I think it's worthwhile to do. And partly because I told her I would. Um, and I don't know if this goes back to Kate [his deceased wife] or if—you know I'm wondering if—I think I saw our relationship go down. I don't know if it's because of her leg, because she is not interesting enough to me, or if . . .
T: Let's just look for a minute about how it might be related to Kate. What do you think the relationship might be with Kate's death?

[The therapist tried to lead David back to the mourning focus, which they had discussed in his previous treatment.]

P: Well, I don't think that's the case.

T: You don't think it's the case?

P: I don't think that's the case, because when I started seeing her [Lisa] I really wanted to develop a relationship. I was being up front with her. I told her that. And I think, and I've been thinking about this since I've talked to you on the phone, that I still haven't resolved the fact of children and Judaism and Christianity. I just haven't resolved that, and I think—I think what happened, I saw a leveling off after that point. That I was always thinking in my mind, well, even though I listened to my friend and you know, he said it could work but it would take a lot of work and it's going to be a constant struggle, I'm wondering if I made up my mind, I said, you know, "Fine, it's possible, but do I really want to work at it that hard?" And I think that is where the leveling off occurred—at that point.

T: So it's not an issue of Kate's death?

P: I don't think so. I really don't think so. Because I, you know, I would really like to develop a relationship.

T: You know, you said that when Lisa had that problem with her leg, what it made you think about immediately was dealing with somebody who was sick.

P: Yeah, Well, that's my only other situation with that.

T: Having to take care of somebody who is sick. And I'm sure that for you that there was tremendous dread and real fear about what might happen at that point, having gone through that nightmare with Kate.

P: Well, what I was thinking is that her leg just took so long to heal. She developed other problems, too. I mean, right now she's suffering from other problems. She gets terrible migraine headaches all the time. They can't find the cause, but it's a terrible burden for her. But that basically has now been a lingering problem for the last 2 months. Sometimes it ends up interfering with our physical relationship as well. I have a problem because when I'm not with her I'm constantly looking around at other women.

[Although in his previous therapy with the clinician David had been able to "see" the connections between Kate's death and his problems with women, he had "pushed away" this connection. The therapist believed that these issues were related to one another. David's "insufficient" mourning of Kate had made him vulnerable to avoidant behavior with women. He was so frightened of being left and hurt again that the closer he became to an appealing woman—in this case, Lisa—the more likely he was to pull away and find fault with her. The two major foci that were emerging here were (1) a focus on Kate and her death (the loss focus), and (2) an ancillary focus

on the developmental dysynchrony David was feeling regarding his inability
to form a lasting relationship with a woman, and on how the first focus
related to this problem.]

T: How do you feel about yourself in that relationship [with Lisa]?

P: I know that it gets to a point and then I just put up all sorts of
roadblocks. And I really feel that. I just, with Lisa, basically shut her
off. Um, and almost try to—I'll be with her, but you know, I'll push her
away. And it's the kind of thing you can sense. It's not so much words,
but more like through actions. And I really feel that. It's like, you
know, I don't want to get any closer with her. And I can't really say
why. So then I start thinking of these—I'll think of anything.

T: I would think that that is almost like a visceral, physical response. This
sort of shutting down, or shutting off.

P: It's, you know, it's very apparent to her. You know, she'll say we get to a
point and it seems like we're making a breakthrough in our relationship
and then all of a sudden I'll just say, "No, that's it."

T: How are you feeling at those moments? How do you feel at those times?

P: Kind of empty. You know, I'm saying, "What am I doing this for? I'm
with someone I care about and I want to push them away."

T: Do you feel lonely at that time?

P: No, just sort of empty.

T: Empty?

P: And I don't feel anything.

T: You feel frozen.

P: Yeah!! I just feel completely—I'm not angry or sad; I just put up a block
and it's a shield and I don't feel anything. The times when I feel
something are, I am having an awful time hurting someone. Or the
concept of hurting someone. It's extremely difficult for me to say to
Lisa something—when I told her (we had a conversation about a week
or so ago about that I didn't find her very interesting), it was mechanical, and then I'm expecting her, or maybe I want her just to say, "OK,
it's over. I give up. We're not getting anywhere here." And it's almost
that's what I want to happen. But I can't say to her that's what I want. I
want it to end. I can say things to her to indicate that I'm not happy,
but I can't really say that. Because, you know, deep down inside I don't
want that to happen.

T: I think that you may care about her quite a bit.

P: I think I do. I think I *really* do.

T: But there's this barrier that you can't get beyond.

P: Yeah.

T: We have to stop in a few minutes. But let me just mention a couple of
things to you. What I think would be helpful is for us to meet maybe
four times, ourselves, you and I. And then perhaps have a meeting with

Lisa. I think that would be very helpful to you and give me a lot of information to be able to meet with both of you together, and get a better sense from her of how she sees what's going on. Um, as I said to you before, I continue to believe—you know, I don't know if it agrees with what you see—that Kate's death has a huge impact on you on a day-to-day basis. Now you may not consciously think about it as much or as frequently in the way that you used to when we met before. But I think it's there. I think it's there in the shadows. I think that you had a very close, intense, and committed relationship with Kate. And I think that every relationship that you have is held up to that as a measure.

[The therapist brought David back to the central foci again—namely, that Kate's death remained very important to him and that her death was related to the current problem he was having with Lisa.]

T: But I think you recognize this to some degree. I think you look for safety in a relationship. I think you do look for relationships that are not going to be consummated in one way or another, so you won't be left or hurt again. If religion is so central and important to you, you go out and find a *shiksa* to become involved with.

P: Well, that wasn't—Well, maybe. I don't know.

T: I think that there's some safety in that.

P: Yeah. Well, I think so . . .

T: Let's talk more about that next time. How do you think Lisa would feel about coming in?

P: I think, you know, positive.

T: OK That's fine. All right, why don't we go and set up an appointment, say, in 2 weeks? And as I said, what I'd like to do is to meet with you, you know, four more times, individually. And then to plan to have a meeting with you and Lisa together. How does that sound to you?

P: Fine.

T: Do you have any questions for me that you want to ask about this?

P: No. Basically, I'd like—I think it's important that—there's part of me that's saying, "Is it really all worthwhile doing this?" But, there's also something that—I don't want to go on the rest of my life this way. I have a lot of fun being single, to a point, and having that freedom. And I think I really enjoy that to a point. But I think what really I want, I *would* like to meet somebody and get married again. I want to have kids and a family. You know, be it a Lisa or someone. And so I think there's this kind of—it's very important that I work through this. If I've got a—still have a hangup and problem related back to Kate, you know, I think it's important that I—we ought to work on it because I'll just continue the cycle for the rest of my life. And, you know, I'll never be happy. I want to get on with my life.

T: I agree. I think that this is a good time to try to work on it and try to make some changes. I think it's a very good idea that you've come back at this point. I believe that in a fairly short period you can make some real progress on this issue. OK?

P: OK.

DAVID: SESSION 2

P: You had suggested that we meet a few times and then I bring Lisa in. That kind of makes me a little anxious. And the reason why it makes me anxious is that if I've got a basic problem to deal with, you know (it would be the same with any woman, regardless if it was Lisa or anybody else), I have to resolve that. And my feeling is that, you know, if I bring her in here it may be valuable in some respects, but on the other hand, then I'm going through this sharing process with her and she's helping me overcome my problems. And then I would feel a dependency on her or a need for her as a result of that. You know, if she is going through this process, I almost picture it like marriage counseling or something.

[Patients often worry that bringing someone into treatment with them implies too great a commitment to another person, is too demanding or too needy, or makes them too vulnerable.]

T: So you would be beholden to her?

P: Yeah, and plus that it says something from me to her that I really want our relationship to work out. And that in order for it to work out we have to go through this thing. If we go through it successfully, does it tie me in? I was going to say "commit me to her." You know, that makes me uncomfortable, I guess. And I told her about this kind of thing. And she said, oh—she thought that was really positive. I mean she's really encouraged that I'm doing this, and she thinks this is great. And, you know, I'm just, I guess, a little anxious about it. I'm not sure that I really want to, you know, I want to find out about myself more. But I'm not sure if I want, if I'm able to bring her in on it, I guess. That's the thing. And where will that lead to? You know, that's kind of scary.

[The patient was feeling increasingly ambivalent at the thought of taking a step that would move him closer to Lisa.]

T: Well, I wonder if part of you wants to find out more about yourself, but you're not as sure about whether you want to change.

P: Maybe. I thought about that this week, too. And I said, "What am I doing this for?" It's almost—it's work, basically. "Why are you just starting up something that is causing anxieties and, you know, new emotions?" And I said, "Maybe I was just happy to let the things go the way they were," and I did think about that this week. You know, just coming over here this morning I was thinking about a couple of excuses. I said, "Well, maybe I can call in today because I'm really busy at work." And those thoughts were racing through my mind, too. And then you just say, "The heck with it." I guess the overriding thing is that I want to follow through with this to see where it leads to, if it will help.

T: Or *part* of you wants to follow through?

P: [David proceeded to talk about his reluctance to commit himself to "anything" recently. Members of his temple group wanted him to work on the temple's 40th anniversary celebration, but he was hesitant about doing so. He then began to describe how hard it was for him to say "no" to people and how he ended up feeling guilty when he could not meet others' demands.]

T: Well, you know, in terms of the issue of saying "no" to somebody, saying "no" to people, I wonder if you're worried about getting into a relationship, getting committed in a relationship, and getting swallowed up in that relationship. Not being able to say "no." That if you get involved with Lisa or something, something's going to go wrong down the way. And then you lose the freedom, you lose the possibility of making choices, because you're so much of a "yes" man.

P: Yeah. I think that's very true. I think that's what I look at as one of my biggest weaknesses. I find it very difficult to say "no" to anybody or anything.

T: What was the situation with you and Kate? When Kate was living, did you feel like this was an issue in the marriage? Did you feel like in your relationship with her that you were imposed upon? Or that she put pressure on you? Or put demands on you that you couldn't say "no" to?

[The therapist again turned to the focus on Kate.]

P: No. She wouldn't really ask me for anything.

T: She was not a demanding person?

P: I mean she was demanding, sort of, because of her condition later on. But, she wasn't demanding of me, saying, like, "I want you to do this," or "I think we should go here." She—you know, I think things seemed to be pretty natural between us, where we would do things. I can't remember ever feeling pressured to do something because of her—that I didn't want to do—that I would say "yes" to and really feel "no." I can't remember that. And then, even when it came down to the point when she found out that, you know, that she had lupus pretty bad, and when it came to the issue of marriage, I'm the one that pursued that. I mean, she allowed me every opportunity to say, "Hey, listen. You know, this is bad news. This is really bad stuff. You know, no hard feelings if you say "no" and get out of this. There really isn't." And I never really felt any regret about that. And that's one thing that I just think I was acting on my heart a lot. I wasn't certainly thinking about it—a lot of things that logically follow it through. But I never felt that with her.

T: So you never perceived of her or felt like she was controlling or demanding?

P: No. I mean, at times I felt really burdened by what was happening. I felt overwhelmed about, you know, her condition. I was going to school at nights. I was working and my job was very demanding. And I was spending all of my free time in the hospital. What free time I had was very little. And, um, but I didn't feel like, "Oh, I'd rather be going to the ball game. I don't want to go to the hospital. I don't want to see Kate." I really wanted to see her. There was something that drew me to her that I really—she was uplifing to me. Even though in a bad situation, you know, I really felt really good being with her. And I was proud to be with her. I can't remember ever being with a—very seldom being with a woman that I just felt proud to be with her.

T: What was the pride? Why did you feel proud of her?

P: I don't know. I just thought that she was such a heroic person and that she exemplified so many characteristics of strength and being able to deal with major problems in such an upbeat way. She was never demanding. She was never—I mean, she would get down; everybody would get down. And there's that kind of situation, you know, when she'd ask "why" and she'd cry and stuff like that. But, you know, she was just so strong all the time. She had this real uncanny knack about making people comfortable about her. You know, she might have been in a wheelchair and some people would come over and say—you know, I could sense it right away, they didn't know what to say: "How are you today?" Or "How's everything going?" You know, they would stumble with it. And she would just smile and in a few minutes you could see the guard would drop down and the people would start to relax and they would just feel very comfortable about her. And that's the kind of thing I just—she just had this uncanny ability to do that, and to meet these challenges. And she would always say that, I think, part of the thing is that she really needed me. Um, I would look at her and see a lot of strength, and she would look at herself, saying, "I don't have the strength to do this. But you help me. You give me that strength." And I guess I felt really needed by her and that made me feel important. But I never felt like she was making me do something I didn't want to do.

T: So these issues about control and commitment, or not being able to say "no," just didn't come up in the same way with her? You didn't feel that in the same way?

P: No. I mean, anything we did I think we did mutually. I felt really strong about doing things with her or being with her. I mean, she'd never—she would say, "Hey, you've been with me the last couple of weeks when it's been really tough; I really think you should get away this weekend. Why don't you go out to your parents' house and just be with them?" And I'd say, "Do you really mean that?" And she'd say, "Yeah, I really do." And she would constantly think about me as far as how I was faring. And I would. I would take off for a weekend. I would go visit with my folks or do something with my friends. And she was always encouraging from that standpoint. I mean, she was very sensitive to how well I was doing. She seemed to be in tune. She knew when I was getting overwhelmed, maybe. And she seemed to sense it, and before anything would happen she would say, "Hey, you know it's time to get away. Take a breather. You know, my brother or my parents are gonna be down this weekend. I don't need you to help me out." Um, or even, she wasn't demanding-like. Her presence was demanding but she didn't verbally make demands at me, I guess. There were times I felt resentful because I was really tired and stuff like that. But not very often. You know, I would get sometimes to the point and say, "Why is this happening to me? It's not normal married life." But that would go away and I wouldn't feel that way very long.

T: Your memories of Kate are really of her being an extraordinary person. And I think that the diary which you gave me is really exceptional. It sounds like she faced a terrible situation with extraordinary courage and strength. I think that it's hard to find people like that. She was unusual.

[In the earlier course of therapy, David had shared with the therapist Kate's diary documenting her last year. It was an extremely powerful and profound exposition of her struggle with her disease.]

P: Well, when I first met her, I mean, I didn't think of her as that kind of person. I mean, I liked her, I loved her for what she was. I just thought she was a very good match for me. And we had a lot in common. She was extremely hard-working and, I thought, a very intelligent woman and loved to learn. And she loved life. And if nothing had happened to her and that didn't occur, I think we would probably have led a very normal life. We would have had plenty of fights, and I think I always am the kind of guy who has an eye for an attractive woman, you know. And I would have always been looking around saying, "Gee, what would happen if I, you know, I had met somebody a little more attractive," or something like that. But I don't know if that's unusual, but overall I think, you know, we would have had a pretty good relationship because the strong point between us that had never occurred with any other woman was her real drive to make me communicate. Or to open communications up, because she really wanted our relationship to work. And she was the first person ever to really try to open me up. And try to make me talk. And try to make me verbalize what I was thinking about when I was happy, or sad, or when there was a problem. You know, if there was something bothering her she would bring it up and want to talk about it. I mean, I have always hated to talk. I just have always been—I don't like that. I just don't like—I am not good at it. Um, I think that maybe inside I want to, you know, when I'm by myself I'll think of things that I should be saying, you know, to Lisa or anyone I'm dating. I try to be honest and open. I can think those thoughts, but then when I get with the person they don't come out. But with Kate, she made them come out. At first it was very, very difficult, but she didn't give up. She kept working at it, working at it up to a point. You know, then it came easier, where we would, we could tell each other basically everything.

T: So she pushed you for a commitment to communicate?

[*And for this overcontrolled and controlling obsessive man, Kate's success in this way was probably the most therapeutic (change-inducing) experience of his life. In a sense, David felt he owed Kate his emotional life. Perhaps for this reason, David could not allow himself to acknowledge anything at all negative about her. If this aspect of mourning was not addressed at some point (though perhaps not now), Lisa might never measure up to Kate. At this point, David's critical attitude toward Lisa protected his idealized image of Kate, and this well-defended image was as much a part of his relationship with Lisa as anything on an overt level in their interaction.*]

P: Yeah, Yeah. She really did. And after she died, I just went through a couple of relationships, you know, with Helene and Bonnie. And we didn't talk at all. I mean, I fell back into my old self, not expressing myself when I was unhappy. And they were afraid to say something for fear that the relationship would end—because I know that they were unhappy—so we just let it die. You know, we just sort of let it go without—I didn't express my unhappiness, but I showed it in my actions. I didn't, you know, treat them the way they wanted to be treated, or show them the affection that they wanted. And they were afraid to verbalize until what would happen is that there would come a point where they'd say, you know, "The hell with this. This is it. I'm knocking my head against the wall for the last 2 years and this guy isn't going to give in," so they would either force the issue and say, "Hey, make a commitment to me or get out, or let's stop this." And so I'd say, "Well, I don't want to make a commitment to you," and the relationship would end. And that was identical with both of them. And Lisa is the first person I've dated since Kate who wants to work at this communication thing. She pushes that. When something's bothering her, she's reluctant to talk about it, but she finally will bring it up. And she'll say, "Hey, listen, you know, something's not right here. I'm not really happy with what's going on. And why are you being this way? How come you don't like to make plans with me? Every time I suggest, 'Let's go some place next month,' you always hedge. You always say, 'Well we'll see,' or 'I'll think about it.' And you never say 'yes' to me." That really bothers her. Um, she brings it up and she forces me to talk, and I've talked more with her in probably a couple of months than I did with the two previous women I dated altogether. And I think that's probably why I'm closer to her than I was to the other two. I really didn't care as much about them.

T: Did you feel scared with Kate about the communication? I mean, did you feel frightened when she pushed you to communicate? Would that make you scared or worried?

P: It made me anxious, yeah.

T: It did?

P: Yeah.

T: And how would you handle the anxiety? What would you do?

P: Well, when she would ask me something I would sit there dumb. But she would patiently wait until I would come out and would mumble something. You know, I'm thinking thoughts and I said, "Well, here's what I'm really thinking. But can I really say it? What if I really say that?" And so I'd be thinking of three or four different ways how to say something. So something stupid would come out of my mouth, like "Dah, you know," or nothing. And gradually, very, very slowly, words will start to come out and she would patiently say, "Well, how do you feel? What do you mean by that?" And not say anything, just wait for me to talk. And I would gradually—words would come out. And I'd be around about and around about and then finally I would, after maybe a long time, maybe an hour, get to the point. Um, it was hard for me, I guess, just to be honest.

T: Did it get to the point with Kate where you were much more able to do that? Where you could really start to communicate with her—start to be open, spontaneously yourself? Did that ever happen over the course of the marriage?

P: Yeah. I think so. I was able to talk to her. You know, I can't think—it's hard for me to remember. I don't remember, you know, when you put it that way, I don't remember ever expressing to her my fears about our marriage and her health.

T: You never really spoke to her about it?

P: I spoke to my friends, but I can't remember. I remember talking to her about it. You know, she would say, you know, "I'm really scared. You know, I might die in this stupid bed." And I would remember kind of being encouraging for her. And trying to give her strength. But when she was like that I would never say, you know, "Yeah, I'm really kind of worried you're going to die, too." And this is really getting to me. I don't remember saying that. I remember talking to maybe her brother or my friends, and I would be pretty open about that. But I don't recall, you know, I just didn't want to get her down. I was there to try to support her. But I think about our relationship—as far as our relationship goes, you know, what was going on in my mind—I think I was probably pretty open. Um, especially before she got ill. I mean, I was able to—she was able to pull it out of me, and then I would later on—when we would start these conversations it wouldn't take so long for me to get going. It would come out a little quicker.

T: Let me just comment on something, which is that it's striking to me that for a guy who can't talk about his feelings or has a hard time doing so, or is scared to do so, you seem to me to do at least reasonably well since you came back to start to see me again. And, I think—I'm just trying to recall what you were like, you know, 2 years ago when we met. And I don't think that you were as able to talk about things, or bring things up spontaneously, as you are now. I think that there have been some changes over the last few years. Do you experience any of that? Do you feel any of that yourself?

[The therapist used his previous knowledge of David to reinforce the patient's progress since he had first been seen in treatment. At that time, his constriction had been even greater than it appeared to be at present.]

P: I feel a desire to. See, it's easier for me to talk to you than if Lisa was sitting here, although I've been more honest with her than I had been with the previous two women I had dated. And when she confronts me now with things I tell her more closely what's on my mind. [The patient went into a long explanation regarding his continued reservations about Lisa. During this discussion, he also brought up the fact that there were also many things about her that he found attractive and appealing.]

T: As you describe this, though, it certainly sounds to me that this is a much more involved relationship than some of these other relationships that you've been part of since Kate's death.

P: Yeah, I think it is.

T: You're involved in a variety of ways. Even though it's hard and unpleasant, sometimes you've, on some occasions at least, tried to be frank with her and tried to be open about your feelings. You've tried to be helpful to her on certain things. And I think that even your coming here, in part, does have to do with her encouragement for you to do that.

P: Yeah, in part, I think that's very true.

T: I mean, obviously it's not the whole story. And if you didn't want to come she couldn't have made you come. But there's something about that relationship that certainly sounds to be more involving for you than some of the other relationships that have happened in the recent past.

P: No, I think that's true. I think that's very true. But it gets back to something I was bringing up before. When I'm making plans with her and doing things, I still have this reluctance because I keep thinking that there's something else that's going to be out there that I'd really rather do. That I'm going to meet somebody else that I could do something else with that weekend who would be more fascinating or interesting to me. Um, and I keep hedging those things. And what I'm finding is . . .

T: I think it also has to do with what you said a few minutes ago about getting sort of stuck, or caught, or committed. Maybe in part it's that something else exciting or interesting will come up. But I think you have some real fears about—aside from that, aside from the most beautiful or the most intelligent woman in the world coming across your path—I think you're also afraid about what can happen in a committed relationship. Because you said before with Kate that, sure, you thought about the possibility that you might always have an eye for attractive women, or that you might always kind of keep an eye open for somebody else coming across your path. But it didn't sound like it was a most central concern. I think that, as I said to you last time, I think that there is a real fear about getting involved in a relationship, getting committed to a relationship, and getting hurt again. Getting hurt very badly again. I think that what went on with Kate was extraordinarily painful. When I saw you, what was it, 2 years after it happened—when I saw you 2 years after her death, I think at that point in some ways you were still numb. And still in some ways in a state of shock from her death. And I think, you know, I think more recently, in more recent years you've come out of that to a great degree. But I think that that enormous loss is still present as a factor in relationships with other women. How could it not be?

[That Kate's death followed a prolonged and painful illness, and that it was developmentally "off time," certainly made for more long-term complications for David. While it was not addressed here, it might be that peers were avoiding him because being with David required them to think about their own mortality. Kate's off-time death also seemed to be generating a good deal of conflict (submerged) between David and his parents, who apparently still idealized Kate as much as David did, and did not approve of their son's current lover.]

P: You know, I'm sure it is. When I committed myself to her [Kate], I did it very freely. I just felt very comfortable about it. You know, I woke up and I said, "Hey, this is what I want to do." I felt good about this. And I never had any fears about commitment at that time. I never did. The woman who I had dated before Kate, I dated for a long time—through college, and we went out for about 6 years; we lived together for a while. I was very committed to her. She wasn't so committed to me at that point. But I had no problems about throwing myself into that relationship. She went through some tragedies with her family. Her mother and brother died in a very close time period. And she had to move to Florida to take care of her brother's child. I moved down to Florida to help her out. Because I really felt committed to her. And that, you know, she needed my help and that it was important for me to be there. So I quit my job and moved down there.

T: Wow. That's a lot.

P: And for those relationships, I didn't feel any problem throwing myself into a relationship. Later on in that particular relationship, I started feeling it wasn't going anywhere. And she didn't want to get married and, you know, I just felt like we were living together and it would work out. And then, when she finally said she was unhappy with the relationship, I said "Good, I'm out of here." And I left very quickly and felt very comfortable about it. Other than having become attached to the child that she was raising at that point. [David then described his relationship with this other woman, Linda, with whom he had lived just prior to Kate. He was left by her for another man, and although he stated that he was relieved by that ending, he clearly expressed hurt and a sense of betrayal.]

T: I think that the more you talk about this, the clearer it becomes to me, at least, that here are these two relationships with Kate and Linda that were very, very significant relationships, very significant commitments, which were extremely painful to you, for obviously different reasons— very different reasons. Linda and Kate sound like very different people, and the relationships were very different. But the consequences were the same. The consequences were that you were left and hurt. You know, I think that there is tremendous pain—tremendous fear and anxiety on your part that that could happen again. And it's better to be safe than sorry. If you don't get into a committed situation with Lisa, if you just stay far away enough to keep things tentative, maybe you won't get injured in some way.

P: Perhaps I think about that, you know. Sometimes I say, what happens if, OK, I just said, "That's it, I'll just commit myself to Lisa. Right. I'll go the full route and I'll just be really open with her and spend as much time with her as I can." Um, I guess what I'm thinking is that once I do that, then it's all over. You know, that means marriage. But, I guess what I was thinking about . . .

T: I think to you it means possible loss. It means getting involved with somebody, loving that person, caring about that person, feeling committed, and then in one way or another you get shafted at the end of the story. With Linda, she left in, you know, sort of a hostile and malicious way. With Kate, she left through dying. But nonetheless the consequences are the same: You're left. You're looking pretty sad; what are you feeling?

P: Being left is pretty, you know, uncomfortable for me. I hate the thought of that happening again.

T: Let me just say a couple of things before we end in a few minutes. One is that I think it would be helpful to get together with Lisa after our next meeting. Not because I know that this is the right relationship for you and you ought to get married to Lisa, but because I think that whether or not you continue with the relationship, it will be helpful to you to meet with her. I think that it will be useful for the three of us to talk here together and to get some sense from her about how she sees you in the relationship, and how you interact with her, and how she interacts with you and feels about you in the relationship. This may be a problem that you would have with most anybody that you felt particularly close to, or cared about, or who cared about you. But the person who's there now is Lisa. And I think that it gives you an opportunity to really examine this issue and work on this issue in a live situation. We can talk a lot in the abstract about the relationship with Lisa and what that's like, and what she's like toward you, and what you're like toward her. I don't think that any of that becomes as clear until we sit down together, the three of us, and we look at the situation—look at how some of the sort of distancing or fearfulness is actually played out in that relationship. You know, my hope is that you don't say to her, "I'd like you to come in and meet with Budman, and we're going to get married right after that." Because that's not the situation. What you're doing is, you're coming here to talk a little bit about what's going on right now in this relationship. And there's no long-term commitment being made. You're not signing on the dotted line.

P: Well, maybe I ought to talk to her about that. You know, just to express—after we met last time I did talk to her, and I told her more or less what we had talked about. Um, and I mean she was pretty encouraged that I had done this. And you know, I think I can tell her that. I think that I wouldn't have a problem telling her that. You know, "This is something I'm thinking of that we're going through this thing, and if we do this I'm fearing that I have to commit myself to you because you helped me through this thing." And I think I should talk to her about it.

T: I agree. Um, let's set up a time to get together in 2 weeks. And if you can talk further with Lisa, that would be good. It would be helpful. And we can plan about the three of us getting together afterwards.

P: OK.

T: All right?

P: All right.

DAVID: SESSION 3

T: How are things going?

P: OK. Nothing too exciting. I think this week has been kind of frantic. I spent last weekend with Lisa, and it was an OK weekend. It was her birthday. And we went out to dinner and we had a nice evening. And you know, the weekend was OK overall. She took off for Seattle, Washington, starting her new job this week. So she's been gone a whole week.

T: How long will she be gone?

P: She's gone until Saturday. But then I'm taking off Saturday morning, and I won't be back until Monday night. And she's going to be with her folks, so I probably won't see her until sometime next week. When I'm away from her I really start convincing myself that I should start seeing somebody else. And I don't know why. You know, it's not like I have this—what I was feeling this week is that I like Lisa a lot. I care for her. But I can't see myself married to her for some reason or another. I just can't picture it. And I keep thinking to myself whether—I really have this strong urge that I wanted to meet somebody and settle down with that person. And I don't know if I'm kidding myself or what. But I had this feeling that there's somebody else out there that I would meet and that things would click with better.

T: The "ideal woman"?

P: You know, I think about Lisa. When I'm with her I guess I pretty much I enjoy myself. I enjoy being with her. You know, I'm not sure if I'm entirely satisfied with the relationship. And I keep thinking that this, you know, getting back to it, that there's this kind of settling for someone that I'm not sure that I would be ultimately happy with. And I keep thinking to myself, "Well, gee, maybe I should just give in and, you know, tell Lisa, 'Let's get married.'" And then I was thinking, I said "Well, and you can get divorced in a few years." And I thought, "What am I thinking that for? That sounds crazy." Um, it's almost like a defeatist attitude. You know, I'm tired of arguing with her, not arguing with her, or putting up a battle with her. You know, I just want to give in and try it out and see what would happen.

T: You said that when you're not with her you feel distant. You feel like there's somebody better out there for you. What happens when you are with her?

P: Well, I'm pretty much—when I'm with her, for the most part I'm pretty happy, I'd say. You know, it's hard to explain. If we're doing something together, you know, I'm pretty much happy. Like that weekend we were together. We went fishing for the day. I had this really strong urge I didn't want to be with her. And I was really kind of standoffish. We went out on the beach and I brought my fishing equipment. We went

out there and she was sitting there, and I didn't think she was really—
you know, I think she was kind of bored, but I really wanted to—it
wasn't because I didn't want to do something with her, I just wanted, I
love to fish. And so she was sitting there. And she wanted to go to
Gloucester. And she was wanting to "hang out" there. And that didn't
interest me much. So then she went and picked up a fishing pole and
she started fishing. And she was getting into it. Or at least she said she
was. And she seemed to enjoy it. And I started feeling pretty good. You
know, I was watching her throw it out, and I was kind of—it made me
feel good, I guess that she was starting to enjoy that. Um, but for some
reason, I just don't have this feeling about her. This warm feeling, the
feeling of love for her, you know. And I know there's a very strong
physical attraction with her. And I think that is a very, probably the
strongest part of our relationship—the physical aspect of it. And you
know, that's very satisfying. But I question, I guess, the rest of our
relationship. As far as you know, after 10 years or something, or
whatever number of years, that's going to start to wear off and that
becomes less important. And then what happens with us trying to
communicate and being partners from that standpoint? And I just don't
know about that. Um, you know, I try to look in her eyes and I think
she would be very protective of me. And she would be good from the
standpoint of—she would care for my interests. I mean she would be
really totally devoted to me. I can sense that. I mean, she'd be a good
person like that. And I have no doubts about that aspect. I think she
would be terrific in that respect. I guess what it comes back to is that,
you know, will we have an interesting relationship? Getting back to
what I said earlier, would she challenge me? Keep me interested in her,
beyond the physical aspect of it?

T: Did you have those kinds of doubts with Kate? Did you feel the same
kind of doubts or questions? Did those things ever come up?

P: No. I don't recall.

T: You never had doubts with Kate?

P: No. Well, we split up once. When I started going out with her it was—I
was seeing many women and I kept looking for this other woman that I
would say that was better than Kate.

T: "Ideal."

P: Yeah, the "ideal woman." But I'd go through the week and I'd try to line
up dates with these great-looking women or something like that, and
things would fall through. Or else I'd go out with them once or twice
and find out they weren't really interesting. They might be good-
looking but not interesting, or whatever. And I'd inevitably end up
going back with Kate. I'd see her at least once a week and it would be
the last-minute kind of thing. I would call her up—if nothing else better
had developed, I would call her up—and I'd say, "You want to get

together tomorrow night?" or something like that. And she'd always say she'd be there. And then after a while I got to know her better. And as a person I got to appreciate her more with time. And I started being less and less interested in other people. And she, you know, fascinated me as a person to talk to. I enjoyed talking with her. And she challenged me. She'd push me. I think that was one thing. She really pushed me into things that, you know, I wasn't at first blush—I wouldn't be particularly interested in.

T: Like what?

P: Oh, just going to the theater or going to the symphony, or just doing things that are a little different. Taking advantage of what was in the city. If there was something going on she would always be on top of it and say, "Hey, there's something interesting here." And my first reaction—oh, I'm pretty much like this. I don't expand my horizons without a little nudging, usually. And she was always into that kind of thing. And I found that usually when I tried something, I liked it. And we did a number of things—or she got me involved in them—just exposed me to different things that I wouldn't normally do by myself. She was active like that. Um, and I liked that. It was something that I would kind of be interested in doing but I wouldn't take the initiative to start something myself. And so, you know, I might give her a hard time about it if she came up with the idea, but then I'd go along with it and then enjoy myself. And she, you know, she, as I say, sort of pushed me and challenged me to get me going into things like that. Um, and that's the thing I miss. I really, you know, you can find somebody. It's easy to find somebody that's physically compatible, I think. And just, you know, you can—you know, physical relationships are easier to come by. But to develop the mental side of it, or the sharing and the interesting side of it, I think takes a little something. I don't know if it can be there with Lisa.

T: So why are you staying with her?

[*The therapist had tried hard to leave openings for David to acknowledge something less than "ideal" about Kate, even to push for such thoughts, but David would not let such feelings into consciousness. It was not surprising, then, that it was at this moment that the therapist switched the focus to David's feelings about Lisa. Although David would probably need to confront a deidealized Kate at some time, now did not seem to be the time to push the matter any further. In brief therapy, the therapist must often be content to work only with what is available at a given point in time, lest he or she increase resistance, and thereby possibly lengthen treatment.*]

P: I don't know. I keep thinking things—do I have this tremendous, you know, physical dependency on her now? You know, I've got somebody that really loves me and wants me a lot, and that's hard to give up, even though I'm not completely satisfied. It's hard to say, to push that aside and say, "I can't, you know, I don't want to see you any more." I just, I find that's probably the hardest thing for me to say to someone—that "I can't see you any more." You know, I always wait for them to get tired of the situation and initiate the ending. And then it's easy to say, "Oh, yeah, I'll go along with that."

T: Might there be any other reason for that? Why you stick with her?

P: Well I think there's a really strong urge in me right now to sort of settle down and be with somebody. And she's providing some stability. And I haven't had this—a few years ago when I was seeing somebody else I would just, I would have been out a night or two a week trying to date other people, too. With Lisa I haven't been doing that. I just really don't have the energy for it, or I just don't want to put up with that hassle. Um, and I guess I'm basically torn. I see a lot of—Lisa is probably the best person I've gone out with since Kate, from the standpoint I feel more close to her than anyone else. But I keep having this gnawing feeling that she's still not "the" person. And you know, it's just hard for me. It's like the candy shop thing. Looking around, I see other people and I say, "I wonder what it would be like to meet that person?" What they would be like. And I've been really thinking about signing up with a dating service, that kind of thing. I have no—I used to go to bars a lot, and I just don't feel like doing that any more. And I used to go out by myself a lot and just go out and hang out at a bar and have a few drinks and meet somebody. And I guess I just don't have the energy for that. Or I just—it never goes anywhere. So, the only time I meet somebody is if I'm—through a friend. That's how I met Lisa. Um, or at a party or something like that.

[The patient clearly described the developmental dysynchrony issue here when he talked about the "strong urge" he was having to "settle down" and be with somebody. He was growing tired of going out with many different people. This developmental thrust, although he obviously felt continued ambivalence at the same time, was viewed by the therapist as an important force moving David toward allowing himself greater intimacy with Lisa.]

[*And, at this point in time, this forward-moving developmental urge was stronger than David's capacity to deal with any ambivalent feelings toward Kate, including his probable anger at being "left" by her. Therefore, the therapist went with this thrust.*]

P: I'm really torn about this situation with Lisa. I wanted to talk to her this weekend. She was saying to me, "I'm really crazy about you," and I just find it very hard for me to reciprocate.

T: So how did you respond? What do you say?

P: I don't say anything. I'll say something like "I care about you a lot." But I just don't feel it to say "I love you." I even tried it before, to say it. It just sounded so—I mean, there was no feeling behind it. I really don't have that feeling.

T: Last time, at the end of the session, you started saying something to me about how your family fit into this. What were you saying?

[After the preceding session had ended, as David walked with the therapist to another area to make his next appointment, he had begun to talk about his family and its "coldness."]

P: Well, the thing I mentioned to you about my mother talking about my father and saying that he never says anything positive to her. Never says he loves her, never touches her, never kisses her. He's very aloof toward her. As a matter of fact, as I grew up, it's hard for me to remember him ever ever kissing her or touching her or showing some affection to her, ever, that I can remember. Even at special occasions like a wedding, anniversaries, that kind of thing. And she was describing him—my mother was describing my father to me, and as she was doing it, I was seeing, hearing, what she was saying: "Gee, I would like it if he would just once in a while touch me or tell me that he cared about me or just said something nice about me," she says, "I don't ask for much." And it sort of made me cringe to hear this. It almost sounded to me like some of the things that somebody like Lisa would say to me: "You're cold; you never like to touch me in public," or "you're not affectionate," or something. It really kind of struck home that I'm very much that same way. I think the worst part of it is that I used to be much worse. I remember relationships where I would never in public show any affection. I think the first relationships I had, I mean when I was at least old enough to realize what was going on, I wanted to be able to hold hands and touch and kiss and stuff like that. I guess when I—it's not that I don't want to do that; when I see Lisa I have this wall built up before she comes over there. And when she gets over there I just have this wall built up: "I don't want you to enter my world." And I try to keep her out. You know how magnets have reverse polarization, or whatever it's called where if you turn the magnets a certain way they just sort of bounce off each other. Well, that's the way I feel. Even if I want to, I don't. There's just something there that forces me not to touch her or kiss her, or if I do it's not with much warmth.

T: What is that like for you? What does that feel like?

P: Well, I know it's happening, and it usually takes me a little while to warm up to Lisa. When she first comes over I have this wall up, and then if we talk and she's around me for a while, then I sort of back off and those barriers get reduced after a while. A lot of times we'll have a drink or something like that. I don't know if it's the drink or if it's just time starting to relax and accept her being there. You know it's uncomfortable. I realize that it's happening, and I know she senses it.

T: You're scared of something?

P: You mean I'm afraid to show? I don't know. To me, I would really feel good if I was able just to see her and to feel like I really wanted to give her a hug and a kiss. I think that would make me feel very good.

T: You said that that's a general problem. It doesn't sound like it's just with Lisa. And it's a general problem in your family.

P: Yeah, that's true.

T: What do you feel like it would be like to have Lisa in here [i.e., in the therapy session] with you? How would that go?

[David had just clearly and poignantly detailed the multigenerational heritage that was now being expressed in his generation. This was a crucial decision-making point for the therapist: He could have chosen to explore David's family issues further, and perhaps even to try to bring them into the therapy, but he chose to stay with what appeared more immediate. He also judged from his knowledge of David's family that they would not be easy people to engage on such loaded issues as death, maintenance, and loving; also, he switched to talking about bringing Lisa in, since she seemed to be much more open to change at this time.]

P: I don't know. That's why I wanted to talk to her about it, and I was very afraid to talk to her about this. That scared me. I wanted to say to her, "listen"—I can think these words in my head, but when it comes down to actually verbalizing to someone, I have trouble. You know I was thinking, "Well, listen, Lisa, if we do this, this isn't a marriage counseling thing to necessarily better our relationship. I'm trying to work out a problem, and you would be doing this to help me do this. And in the long run, if it came about that I'd be understanding my problems better or dealing with my problems better that our relationship would improve, that's one thing. But I didn't want you to view this as I wanted our relationship to work; I'm trying to overcome a problem." And I couldn't say that. I just thought about it over the weekend a couple of times and, you know, I'm always waiting for the right situation, but those situations never come up; you have to really go to the issue.

T: Why couldn't you tell her? What were you afraid to tell her?

P: I don't know.

T: You see it as a problem with marriage?

P: I'm sorry?

T: You're afraid she'd see it as a marriage problem, even though you told her otherwise?

P: Maybe. I still have a hard time in engaging in a conversation that's dealing with feelings. I avoid that kind of conflict or confrontation as much as possible. It's easier not to say those things. It's easier not to talk about them. I know she'd be upset or she would start probing me, and that always makes me uncomfortable. It makes me nervous, or "anxious" I guess is the term. I guess maybe you can't separate the two. I would just like to be able to deal with me by myself and work through this thing. Maybe I'm just spinning my wheels and going nowhere because I'm not facing the person who causes this anxiety or causes these feelings. It's easy for me to come in here and talk to you, because I know I'm going to leave here in an hour, and this doesn't make me anxious.

T: I think that you are very able to intellectualize about the problem, but I think it would be much more difficult for you to consider your feelings about Lisa directly with her here. Are you willing to deal with the discomfort of trying to do some work with her here?

[*In brief therapy, the therapist cannot patiently wait for matters to unfold. With an obsessive patient like David, waiting for him to do something other than intellectualize about his problem could take a very long time. Bringing Lisa into therapy would not only make David's problem real; it would also keep the therapy focused and moving ahead.*]

P: I can say "yes." But I know that that would be very difficult for me.

T: That's good. I think it's good that it would be difficult for you, but I think that if you don't challenge yourself you're not going to get very far with this problem. You can go on as long as you want to, dealing with relationships with women this way. I think you could do it for quite a while. The option on the one side is that you "play the field" for a while and see how things go—see what happens with other relationships with women. And then come back and talk to me in a year or two and see if you have found the person that you are looking for yet. I would guess that that's not going to happen, but one never knows. The relationship with Lisa may not be ideal. It may not be the perfect relationship, and she may not the person that you are going to get married to. But I think that the problem is broader. The problem has to do with a difficulty in letting yourself move into a closer relationship with somebody right now. I think that has to do with, in part, the terrible loss that you went through with Kate, which I think can't be underestimated in terms of its long-term effects. It has a major effect, I think, on you and your life. And the other thing is in terms of your family situation. I'm sure that your family situation is one that was not very conducive to really being able to talk about feelings or express yourself or get very close in a realtionship.

P: I think I spent my whole life trying to overcome that. I've always, and my brother's the same way, you have this tremendous urge—well, I should just speak for myself—to be accepted, to be needed, I guess. My father, particularly, no matter what accomplishments we made, would never say, "Hey, I'm really proud of you guys, you really done good," or anything like that. He would always be quick to criticize. If we did one thing wrong he would beat the hell out of us or tell us how stupid we were or how—"stupid," I always remember that word "stupid."

T: He's a really violent guy?

P: Pretty much, yes. I mean, never really hurt any of us too badly. No broken bones or any of that stuff. But he'd bang us around pretty good, and we were always "stupid." And I think particularly my brother really had it tough going. I mean, he was labeled worse than I was. I sort of slid through. And I was, seems to me, I never wanted to get caught. If I did anything wrong I didn't want to get caught at it. And I was pretty good, I guess. My brother wasn't as lucky and he'd always get caught. But we'd always have this thing. We'd have to show off. We'd have to do something. We'd have to be a little more daredevil. We'd have to be a little more crazy in anything we did. My brother barely made it through school. Well, I didn't do much better, but I got through high school all right. We couldn't prove to him [their father] the ways that we were good. Although he wanted us—he kept saying, "You guys got to go to college. You don't want to be digging ditches like me and that kind of thing."

T: That's what he did?

P: Well he never dug ditches but he worked manual labor, a welder. And, you know, we would really screw off in school. We never got his attention, so we knew one way to get his attention, I guess, would be to do badly in school and that would really piss him off. And he'd punish us. We'd do—you know, my brother threw a rock at a train one time, and our punishment was that we had to stay in our yard a whole summer. We could not leave our yard. It was summer! We couldn't leave it. One time we did and he beat the shit out of us. This is how we started our whole life. He got married, he left home as soon as he could, and I left home as soon as I could. I eventually got into a small community college. I didn't get accepted at any other colleges and I got this on my own and I didn't have anybody telling me that I had to do good. I was just sort of there. And also my grades went up. I just got on the dean's list and I did really well. And I remember getting that first grade. I was on the dean's list and I showed it to him. He just sort of nodded and I was so proud to do that and . . . (*Becomes sad and starts welling up with tears*)

[*This was probably the multigenerational context in which David learned to inhibit his aggression, and that was now what was stopping him from experiencing any anger toward Kate.*]

T: What are you feeling?

P: It's hard for me to talk, but he really just never acknowledged anything good we've done. So after that I said, "Well, I'm going to do it for myself." (*Crying softly*)

T: What are your tears about?

P: You know, I just—it's something I missed.

T: Getting that kind of support.

P: Yes. I know my brother is the same way. I think he had it much worse. We never had any positive support.

T: Where does your brother live?

P: He's out in Maine. And he has a wife and three kids.

T: How's he doing with his life?

P: He's doing good. I'm real proud of him. He married someone who—they're a great pair. I mean, they argue a lot and they've had a tough marriage on and off, but he's got great kids and he just loves his family. And she believes in him and is supportive of him and has allowed him to make something of himself. (*Begins crying again*)

[*The multigenerational pattern of men in David's family feeling unloved by their parents and, therefore, seeking very supportive nurturant women emerged for David's brother as well.*]

T: Why do you cry as you say that? What does it mean to you?

P: Well, it's hard because my parents should be the ones to do that.

T: Support him or support you?

P: Well, I mean to—he [the brother] just started building a house, and he [the father] gave him nothing but grief. He said, "You're stupid to do that." My brother was living in a tiny little home, and his wife pushed it and said, "Listen, we need a bigger place. We have no place for the kids to play." And they said, "Let's sell the house while the market's good and buy some land and build a new house that we could really enjoy." My parents didn't support him one bit. And I say "my parents"—my father particularly. And my mother told me about this and it really disturbed her, but he needed money. He needed financial support. He needed to make a down payment on the land. Her parents—Vera, my brother's wife's parents—loaned him $10,000 to buy the land, with the agreement that they would pay them back when they sold their house and they'd have the extra money. And Phil also needed money to clear the land and put the foundation in before he would get the construction. He went to my parents and they wouldn't give him a nickel. And my mother told me that my father said that—my mother really wanted to give him money, but my father said, "If you give him any money from our account I'll leave you."

T: What do you think?

P: It's a pretty shitty thing to do. I have spent all my life trying to prove to him that I was worth loving. (*Crying*)

T: And with Kate what you had was somebody who really believed that. Who really believed in you.

P: And she needed me.

T: And she needed you. She was really supportive. She loved you. She needed you. Let me just ask you before we stop: How do you see this tying in with the situation with Lisa? What's the connection?

P: I don't know. I feel bad that I can't make a connection right now. I think that part of it is not being able to show emotions. I don't know if that's just by example or what, but . . .

T: You've been taught that it's pretty risky to show emotions.

P: Well, you know there's another thing, too—that our relationship went downhill pretty quickly when, you see, when I brought Lisa home. My parents weren't very impressed with her. As a matter of fact, even my mother said to me the last time I was home, "Are you going to marry Lisa?" And I said "I don't know, Ma. I don't see it happening right now." She goes, "Well, that's good." And I just went, "Holy shit, that's my mother." I got negative feedback from my sister as well, although I think my sister regretted saying that after she did. Lisa sort of turned her off in some ways, and I guess, you know, Lisa is kind of assertive. My mother calls her "pushy." My sister sort of has that same thing. I guess they'd like to see me with someone very feminine and whatever, caring in different ways. And so they didn't like Lisa. So I got all this negative feedback from my family, and I know when that happened, especially, it came first from my sister and later from my mother.

T: That influenced you.

P: I think it really did. And I thought about that. "Why are you letting that influence you?" But I cooled off to Lisa. I think that was the point when our relationship leveled off.

T: You're still trying to please them.

P: Yes, being my own family.

[*David's mother was intimidated by Lisa's assertiveness, and David, grasping at any chance he saw to get parental approval, was wavering about Lisa.*]

T: We have to stop. Let me just propose two things to you. One is that you talk to Lisa about coming in and that the three of us have a meeting together. But what I'd like to do before that is to see if the next meeting that we have—what I'd like to do is for the two of us to be together one more time, because I feel like we're just sort of starting to get into some things.

P: Sure.

T: All right. Let's do that. Let's you and I do that in a few weeks, and hopefully you can talk to Lisa in the meantime and see about her coming in with you the time after that.

P: OK. I'll see her early next week and I'll talk to her then.

T: My plan is not necessarily to meet with both of you over an extended period of time together, but I would like to see what the situation is like between the two of you and what input she can make about what's going on.

P: OK.

DAVID: SESSION 4

T: Can I ask you about what you remember in regard to our last session?

P: I remember it, but, um, we started talking about my parents and my relationship with them and some of the things I felt. That my brother and my sister and myself were always trying to impress or get our parents attention, and it probably still goes on. [David then described, at some length, his father's hostility and abusiveness toward him and his brother. As he mentioned in the preceding session, the father rarely showed any support or caring, and seemed unable to allow any free expression of affect in the family. In response to a question from the therapist, David stated that his father did really "adore" Kate and tried to be helpful to David in uncharacteristic ways after her death.]

T: What are you thinking right at this moment?

P: I don't know. I'm thinking about Kate's death. I miss her. I'm talking about her right now. I feel sad that she's gone. I feel sad that, about my father, I think he really cared about me for what I went through. I think that he saw—I don't know if this makes sense, but I think he saw what I had with Kate and he knows how much that meant to me. I think it meant a lot to him too. I think maybe he, I don't know, maybe he wished he was as lucky as I was to have Kate, I don't know.

T: But you lost a tremendous amount in that death.

[*From a systems perspective, David lost not only Kate, but also perhaps his only connection to his father. Her death, then, brought about a marked shift in an already long-standing, tenuous set of family relationships. While this shift could very reasonably have served as a focus for psychotherapy, it was not David's central current concern ("Why now?"), and so it received selective attention from the therapist.*]

P: Yes, with somebody who I loved very much. It was very important to me.

T: And with such a sharp contrast with your family situation.

P: Yes for myself. Her family was very open, very loving, and very generous. And I liked that. I liked that feeling. I liked that environment. She and her family filled a big void in my life. She helped me talk. She helped me open up. Her family showed me love and kindness, and it was really important to me. In her death, I really didn't want to lose the Browns. And I told them that I really cared a lot about them and no matter what happened in my life after that, they were still going to be my second parents. Even when I write them I address the letters "Mom and Dad." I do it partly because I really feel that way about them and partly because I think it makes them feel good too.

T: I think—as I said before, I think that the loss of Kate was extraordinary. I think that it's extremely difficult for anybody to lose a spouse. But what you lost was really tremendous. You had somebody that you cared about and felt close to and was so supportive and encouraging.

[*Again, the therapist could have chosen to give as much emphasis to David's loss of hope for getting closer to his father, but stayed with David's loss of Kate, in order to intensify the focus of therapy.*]

P: The thing is that she's gone and there's nothing I can do about that.

T: I think part of the problem for you, and I said this to you before, is that you didn't really allow yourself the opportunity, because I don't think you really knew how, to really mourn as much as you need to.

P: I think I can remember crying a few times after she died. You know, when I was by myself. I think I was in bed at night and I just really missed her. What I did at that time, I sort of put all of my energies into work, and I started running. I was trying to run a marathon like months after that. I remember I would be out on the street at 5:00 in the morning trying to run. It was really stupid—I mean, I hadn't run since I was in high school. Within a few weeks I was doing 6 or 7 miles a day. I hurt my feet, my legs, and I was running and I was thinking to myself, "Kate lived through a lot more pain than this. You can do this." I would think of her any time I felt pain. And I said, "Gee, she would just laugh at this," you know, and "You can do this." I was pushing myself for the wrong reasons. For about 4 months I was running; I got to the point where I was doing about 50 miles a week, and finally my legs just gave out. I mean I couldn't walk. I gave up the idea of running. I couldn't. I could barely walk. I couldn't even run the marathon. So I took a vacation. I went to Vermont with some friends. I didn't start running again for a while, but then I backed off. I started running because I wanted to run. I was a little bit weird then. I still run now, but I do it because it is a release for me.

T: You had to find some way to push away those painful feelings.

P: Well, I had to do something and I think work was the thing. After that I just really threw myself into work. I met Judy, I don't know, just a short while after Kate died. I started dating right away and I started jumping into things, you know, with Judy. But it was mostly a physical thing. Somebody to be with. Somebody to do things with. But I never opened any emotions to her. And she's the one that, when things didn't go well, she's the one that talked me into coming to see you the first time. She said, "Hey, you got a lot of hangups about you." You know, she was the one who was kind of convinced that that was the case.

T: So each time you've come in, it was at the urging of a different woman?

P: Yes.

T: One time you came in because of Judy, and one time you came in because of Lisa. But your own tendency, I think, is to run away from these feelings as much possible.

P: Yes, ignore them, they go away. (*Laughs*)

T: Do they? Have they?

P: I don't know. I think maybe they just get suppressed. The only time I really think about Kate is when I'm here talking with you. You know, I don't really think about her when I'm by myself or doing things. I think that's been the kind of attitude or feeling with my family. I know my parents think that going to therapy or something like that as "You're sick." They think of it as a negative thing. They're like, "You can deal with your own problems."

T: Do you feel that way about being here now?

P: No. I think it's positive. At times I'm a little reluctant to come. It would be very easy for me *not* to come—let me put it that way. I could think of 10 different excuses for not coming. I think it's something I sort of have to force myself to do. It's like any time I have to communicate with anyone, I have to force myself to do it—with Lisa, you know, and coming here. And it's not natural for me. It's not comfortable for me. I just don't come from a family that talks about their own problems. And I realize that a lot. And I think I mentioned to you when I talked with my mother and she was saying how she just doesn't get any affection from my father and he takes her for granted and it's very difficult living with him. I said to her, "Why don't you ever say something to him? Talk to him about it?" She sort of shrugged her shoulder and said, "I can't." I go with that pretty much. That's the way I always saw it. We just don't talk about feelings or emotions or showing things.

T: So you took all those feelings about Kate and ran away from them, and then, lo and behold, your father's prophecy came true.

P: That what?

T: "You'll never find anyone like her again."

P: Yes, I think, I mean he's right. I think when he says that, he says that in a gentle way, or compassionate way. It's also sort of pre-empting me; you see, he really wants to see me get married again. I think he does more so than my mother. I think he really feels the loss of Kate and what I went through. I mean, he never really verbalized it to me, but I sensed that it hit home with him very hard and he would really like to see me happy.

T: Have you spoken with Lisa about coming in with you?

P: Yes, I spoke to her a couple of weeks ago. We were talking and things were going so well, and she started saying that every time we get close I back off. I guess we were talking about coming in here, and I said, "I don't know how to say this to you, but I asked you if you want to come in here and you said 'yes,' I'm kind of anxious about that." I said, "I don't want you to think that this is some sort of vehicle or mechanism to get us married or something like that, that this is a marriage counseling situation. I'm going here because I'm trying to work out a problem, and if you want to help me work out that problem, I appreciate that and I think that's great, but you've got to go under those conditions— that this is for me and it's not to try to square things with us, because I want to look at you for you and not go through the situation and feel I'm dependent upon you to solve these problems." So she said, "That's exactly right." I said, "Well, why would you want to do that?" She said that she thought I was a good person and that it was worthwhile helping me out of these problems, so we started talking some more and I don't know how this happened or the sequence, but what it came down to, we were talking about our relationship and I said, "Well, basically, the way I see it right now is that I enjoy being with you, I like your company, but I can never see me getting married to you. I see us going through a time for a while and having some good times, but I don't see us getting married."

T: So you're feeling closer to her or not?

P: Yes, so then I punch her [figuratively].

T: Throw her down the stairs [as David's father did to him].

P: Yes, well, she said the same thing to me. She says, "Well, I can't imagine getting married to you either."

T: Because of the way that you were acting?

P: Yes. You know sometimes I'm not real cool about the way these things come out of my mouth. She said the same thing. She said, "I have some real doubts about that happening anyway. I see some real problems." She said, "I really can't see us getting married either." So I looked at her. I said, "Gee, that takes a big load off my shoulders. That makes me feel a lot more comfortable." I always have these suspicions that women say things that they don't mean. Not that guys don't say things that they don't mean, but my feeling with her is that she'll say things that are appropriate at the time, but I don't necessarily believe her entirely. Although she's pretty honest. She's pretty open.

T: What's your feeling about coming in here with her?

P: I think I can do that. Actually, I'm feeling pretty good about Lisa these days. That was about 2 weeks ago. It was right after I saw you last time. It's funny, I go in these really weird cycles. Last weekend I went home to see my folks because they were leaving for a trip. I didn't ask Lisa to go with me; I just went out there by myself. I didn't talk about it with her. I just left. You know, I could have taken her with me and asked her to come, but I didn't. And I was just trying to keep my distance from her. And I was out there over the weekend and I started thinking about her. I was sort of missing her. I got home Sunday and I told her before I left, "Well, I'll get back at a reasonable hour and I'll give you a call. We'll do something Sunday night." Well, I got back at 6:00 and I sort of forced myself *not* to call her. I just didn't call her. Well, I called her at 10:00 that night and she was kind of mad at me that I hadn't called before. She said, "You said we were going to get together and you never called." I just made some dumb excuse up. I said, "Well, I got sidetracked or something." So I saw her the next night and I kind of kept my distance. It was a funny night. I just felt weird being with her, I guess. I don't know if I was tired or what, but then we said we'd get together on Wednesday and I didn't call her Tuesday night, and then Wednesday when I got up I said, well, I was really thinking about her and I just wanted to see her. I just kind of missed her. So I called her up at work. I had never called her up at work. And I said, "You know, I want to make sure we get together tonight and do something." You know we had a nice evening together and we had a good time. This may have something to do with it. She told me that she was going away for the weekend. It's usually me that does that. I'm usually the one that says, "Here are my plans. This is what I'm doing, and if you're included in, fine; if you're not, too bad."

T: But when you're able to get her sufficiently far away from you, then it's OK to start getting together again.

P: Yeah, it's like a yo-yo almost, going back and forth. You know when she said she was leaving this weekend, I got attracted to her and I wanted to do something and we got together last night and we had a nice evening. It's almost like I know there is distance there and I feel comfortable with that. And if she puts the distance there, I like her more that way. If I do it I don't feel as comfortable.

T: So maybe that's what you need right now. Maybe you need a distant relationship.

[The therapist challenged the patient's readiness for change.]

[*This is an excellent illustration of how "reframing" a patient's problem can force a clearer focus in brief therapy, as discussed in Chapter 6 on marital and family conflicts.*]

P: That's what I've had for the last 3 years or 4 years or something, distant relationships.

T: So you don't want that?

P: Well, I feel I have this really strong feeling that I would like to get married. I would really like that to happen. And in the last weeks I keep thinking that I'm going to meet this wonderful person, but I don't take any initiative to go find this person because I'm seeing Lisa. So I'm sort of in this crazy situation, but I think of her and I think, "Could I get married to her?", you know, "What are the problems?" And sometimes

I could sort of say, "Yeah, it could happen." And then I could see that being OK. I almost see myself saying "All right, I give in, I give up, let's try it with Lisa and see how it will work."

T: Your father said it all. I mean I think it's absolutely clear. Your father told you, "You'll never meet anybody like Kate again." So your fate is sealed. How can you hope to ever meet anybody as good and as giving and as caring as she was?

[*While the therapist did not physically bring David's father into the therapy, he brought him in symbolically by expressing the father's feelings.*]

P: Well, I can't. I guess I can't. I guess I'm looking for someone who is good and caring and will make me happy, I guess. And I guess I would just like to get on with my life.

T: But I think the other part of the problem here is that, even if you settle for somebody who wasn't as good as Kate or wasn't as wonderful as she was but was nice or positive in her own way, then the problem that you have to face is the problem of loss again.

P: How do you mean?

T: Well if you get involved with somebody, and committed to somebody, and let yourself care about somebody, you could be devastated again.

P: Yes, I suppose that's possible.

T: They could die or leave you, or you could break up in some way. So it's a much, much, much safer position, the position that you're in right now.

P: So it's a comfortable or safe position. But what about these feelings that I have that I would really like to get married, that I would really like to be in love with somebody? I have really strong feelings about that. I would like to share my life more with someone.

T: In part, I think that that's true. In part, I think that that is not true. There's part of you that would like very much to love somebody, to be with somebody, to start a family with somebody. All those things that you were anticipating with Kate. There's part of you that I think is simply *terrified* about doing that.

P: Well, there's a very strong part of me that fights that. So what do I do about that? Or do I do anything?

T: I think the question for you is "Can you bear the risk of really letting yourself love someone again and be committed to someone again? Can you take that risk?" That's the question.

P: I think about energy level in a relationship. When I first meet somebody, I put a bit of energy into a relationship and I want that person to get attracted to me, but after I get to know somebody a bit, then I sort of back off and I do sort of the bare minimum—sort of the maintenance level and that's it. I remember, with one woman before Kate, I used to get flowers and I used to send cards all the time. You know, Valentines, birthdays, any other special occasion. I could really send cards that said—you know, were real mushy, sweetheart cards. I have not been able to do that. Any time I get a birthday card or a Valentine card, it's got to be a joke one. I cannot pick up one and feel comfortable about one of those cards that are real sentimental or something like that, to a woman I've been out with.

T: This is since Kate.

P: Yes. I know I am capable of doing that. I think I want to do that. I think it would be kind of neat. I think it would be great. But somehow I need to be really attracted. I don't know, maybe it doesn't happen. It seemed like, with Kate, our relationship, I wasn't really gung-ho about our relationship at first with her, but it sort of grew and developed and I grew to love her sort of gradually.

T: I think the situation for you has been one where you grew up with a tremendous amount of emotional deprivation, with not very much support or an open, loving family. And then you got involved with Kate, who was a very giving, warm, and caring person. And that all got ripped away from you. And I think that you're extremely reluctant to risk it again. It's like you show a starving man food and allow him to start eating it and then you pull the plate away, or somebody who needs water, you give them a little drop of water and then take it away.

P: I don't know. Maybe. I don't know if time does anything about that. Talking to you, talking to Lisa.

T: What are you feeling now?

P: Well, I think what you said sort of describes my feelings.

T: Well, what do you feel?

P: I feel sort of hollow. I don't feel any emotion. Just sort of blank. My mind is thinking, but I don't feel good or bad or anything or happy or sad. I don't feel anything.

T: Why are you pushing away your feelings right now?

P: I don't think I'm trying to. I'm trying to think about what you said and think about that for me because I feel . . .

T: But you're determined not to feel about it.

P: No. I think, if anything, what I feel is a little bit of sadness, if you will, if that's going to be my fate. I think that would make me sad if I was not able to ever meet someone that would make me happy, that I really want to develop a relationship with. Because I think I would really like to have a family. I would really like to have kids and I think I have a lot to offer from that standpoint. I think I'd be a good father, and a good husband, or whatever, and I think if I wasn't able to do that I could deal with that, but I think that would make me sad. I think I would be really missing something in life if I wasn't able to do that again.

T: It's enormously important for you to continually push away the feelings about Kate. Always to keep them at arm's length, especially when there is something powerful welling up.

P: You mean any time I get into a relationship I try to push them off?

T: Let me get back to the beginning. What are you pushing away right now?

P: I don't feel like I'm pushing away anything.

T: When I made that analogy, you started to look very sad.

P: Well, it's almost like you've sort of reached the point where you're saying that the way things are going right now, there's very little hope that I'm going to develop into a relationship because of the way I am, my needs, or whatever. And I think . . .

T: Did I say that?

P: Well, that's the feeling I'm getting. That's what I'm hearing.

T: Huh? What did you hear me say about it?

P: I guess your description of what I'm doing is that I'm agreeing that that is what I'm doing. You know, I'm pushing—when I'm involved with a woman I want, I push her away.

T: My description before was about your feelings. And the feelings of enormous deprivation, the feelings of having started to get something and then losing it.

P: I don't feel—I never had this conscious sense that I'm afraid to love someone. I think it's on the contrary, I feel like I want to love someone.

T: So you want to punch them in the nose?

P: You know, I guess I do that but I can't figure out why I act that way, figuring that someone like Lisa would say, "The hell with you, I don't need this punch in the nose," or something like that—"Get out of my life." But she just absorbs it. It just sort of deflects off her, I guess.

T: It's reassuring?

P: Well, I think she's wearing me down. She's slowly but surely wearing me down to where I get that sense—it's almost like the point where I'm ready to give up, give in, and stop being a bum or whatever, and stop punching her in the nose. "I give up, I love you," you know, that kind of thing. I said to her, "Why do you"—about a month ago when we were having dinner, I said something to her that there were things that I didn't like about her or whatever, then I finally said to her, "Why do you put up with me saying these things to you?" "You know why?" she said, "Because I care about you a lot." And I just looked at her and I said, "Boy, you are the most stubborn person I ever met." I mean, doesn't she understand I'm doing this to push her away and she's staying there fighting me back? I guess in a sense that's the way Kate was because she wouldn't take "no" for an answer. She just wouldn't give up.

T: She wouldn't let you *not* love her.

P: Yes, she said to her brother—I found this out later—that she wasn't going to let me go. She said, "You know, I really don't like the way he's handling this relationship. He calls me up at the last minute to go out and things like this, but I'm not going to let this guy get away. I'll put up with all this for a while." And she did. I was like that for, I mean, we went on for a year that way. I would just take her for granted, and finally I got to the point where I said, "I really like, I love this woman." I'm almost sensing that happening with Lisa, and last night when I was with her I almost found myself telling her I loved her. I was actually feeling it and I was saying, "I can't believe these words are going to come out of my mouth," and I didn't say it. I guess I was afraid to. I was saying to myself, "Is this a moment of weakness or is it everything you are really feeling?" I think our relationship sort of reached a low point a couple of weeks ago and maybe it went over the weekend. I see this sort of transition happening where I'm starting to feel closer to her than I felt to anyone before. She's going away this weekend and I'll see her in the next week. Before, I was anxious in a negative sense about her coming in here and talking but I'm kind of anxious in a positive sense to want to hear what she has to say.

T: What do you think that will be like? What do you think will go on?

P: I don't know. She's pretty honest. She's pretty open. She says what is on her mind.

T: So she'll be pretty frank about it, about you, and about your relationship?

P: Yes, I think so. I think I'll be defensive at least initially. I can sense that, but I think it will be good to see because I really feel that, like I say, I don't know if Lisa is the right person. Things are happening a little bit better for us, but I really feel that I really want to be able to love somebody. I think that what you said about taking that risk is something I've been thinking about. I've been saying it in a negative sense, so I've been saying "giving up." Giving up would be taking that risk. I was thinking, "Gee, I've never gone on a trip with Lisa." I don't do anything that people who are in love would do together. You know, really go away someplace together and really spend some time alone instead of with your friends. I haven't purposely avoided that with her. I mean, we may go someplace for a weekend, go skiing, but with other people. I don't think I've ever gone anywhere with her for more than a day or so with just the two of us. So I was thinking about that. That might be something we could do that could be positive.

T: Maybe taking a little risk with her?

P: Yes.

T: I think coming in here with her is taking a risk. Because I think you know that I'm going to ask you some tough questions and I'm going to ask her some tough questions, and it will mean getting a little bit more open, a little bit closer. I think that's a risk for you. I think that you've been scared to do that with anyone.

[*While this was undoubtedly going to be a major risk for David, it was probably a smaller risk than the one that would be involved in a confrontation with his parents. Thus, the therapist chose work with that part of David's interpersonal system that had the greatest motivation and capacity for change, as discussed in Chapter 6 on marital and family conflicts.*]

DAVID AND LISA: SESSION 5

David came to the fifth session with his girlfriend, Lisa. After some initial conversation about what David had explained to Lisa in regard to the meeting, the therapist asked Lisa, "How do you see things in the relationship right now?" She explained that things seemed to go "up and down." She went on to indicate that during "bad times" David was extremely critical of her. Lisa cited several examples of David's seemingly making harsh comparisons between her and his deceased wife, Kate. Throughout much of this session, David was far more emotional and forthcoming than in individual sessions. The fact of Lisa's presence and the examination of the problems between them *in vivo*, as well as the clinician's thrust toward constantly weaving the two themes together (i.e., his emphasis that the problems with Lisa and Kate's death were related), appeared to have great impact. It has often been our experience, even with very resistant or low-affect patients, that a conjoint meeting with a lover, friend, parent, or sibling has a surprisingly potent effect. In this session, Lisa's presence was significant. She was expressing caring for David just by coming to the visit. Furthermore, in their discussion their problems clearly displayed themselves (as in David's criticism of Lisa's handling of her accident). However, rather than the usual cycle of withdrawal on David's part, the therapist's efforts to relate David's criticism of Lisa to the issue of Kate's death were very fruitful. David was able to do some mourning with Lisa, as well as to continue to communicate with her instead of locking her out. As for Lisa, she attempted to reach a better understanding of David's pain and conflict, and of how these were connected to the troubles in their relationship. The transcript begins at a point about 10 minutes into the visit.

Lisa: Maybe those are the times that you say, unconsciously, "I wish that you were—well, Kate didn't do that," or "I wish that you were more like her in this way," or "This is what she would have done." And subconsciously I think I was feeling that when Dave said that his friends say, "I'm looking for the perfect woman. That's why I'll never get married." We had that conversation a while ago, about when he was telling me things about myself that he wasn't happy with, and I said, "Dave, nobody's perfect." And you're right, we all have our faults, but if you're looking for the perfect person that's a good defense, because you'll never find that person, and therefore you'll never get that involved, and therefore you won't get married. With Kate, I always was under the impression that Dave really never grieved her and never went through that whole process of talking with somebody at that time, a psychiatrist or a psychologist, and going through that. You can't put it aside, but you can certainly start moving on with your life again after you've gone through that grieving phase.

Therapist: (*To David*) I think you have done pieces of it, but I think it's very, very hard to do. I think, as I said to you many times, I think that that was an enormous loss for you. What are some of the feelings that you really haven't shared with Lisa about it?

David: What I was feeling as a result of her dying?

T: And during her [Kate's] dying?

D: I don't think I've told her [Lisa]—I think she senses, but I don't think I've told her how hard it was. I didn't think about it until after she died, you know, like what I went through. I was going to school. I was working full-time. I wasn't going to school full-time. I was taking two or three courses a quarter and I was working full-time. And soon as I got out of school I would go up to the hospital and spend the rest of the night up there, or go home and spend it with her and sort of relieve her brother. And spend all this time together. I almost didn't have an ounce of free time at that time. I'd get up in the morning and just throw myself into everything. I was studying and working and spending time with her, and there wasn't any time when I wasn't doing something. I would try to spend as much time with her as I could. I look back and I don't think I could go through that again. I don't know how. I think I was sort of like a robot then. I was living through it. I was doing everything but I wasn't really, I guess I sort of tuned out what was really happening. I really loved her a lot and I really cared about her, but it was just like accepting everything and jumping into it and not really thinking about how hard it was.

T: And not feeling a lot better. You were going through the motions; you were doing what you had to do.

D: Yes, I was taking on a responsibility and doing it because I felt like I had to. I wanted to do it, but I think it was a little bit overwhelming.

T: Maybe a lot overwhelming.

D: I didn't give myself a chance to think about it. Because I was always doing something—"now I got to study, now I got to go to school, now I got to work, now I got to go to the hospital." But I would be there with her, I mean, we would be very close. It wasn't like when I was with her it was like, "Oh, now I'm here I've done my duty," or something like that. You know, we would talk. We would really talk a lot. We would talk about her and us, and she would try to focus on what I was going through.

T: Would she talk about her dying?

D: She would talk about that—not all the time, but sometimes she would talk about there was a good chance she was going to die and she wasn't going to make it through this. That would be the time that I would try to bolster her up. (*Begins to well up with tears*)

T: Why do you make yourself *not* cry about this?

D: I don't know.

T: You don't feel like you should cry?

D: Yeah, I guess. (*Choking up*)

T: I think what you went through was really horrible, terrible pain. What you went through was awful.

L: When Dave talks about, or the few times that he has talked about Kate, I get very upset at just feeling what he went through and the feelings that he had and how strong they were. And I feel that. I feel that for him, and, like you said, not crying, that's just an emotion that—it feels good to cry, it feels good to get that out, let it out, because it's a relief after that happens.

T: The diary is incredible. [The therapist is referring to Kate's diary, which David had shared with him in their previous therapy.] The strength that she had during this whole thing is just unbelievable. And I think also that the role you played, so much you did for her, is also just remarkable, what she writes about you there. It was an extraordinary time.

L: (*To David*) When you said that there was the responsibility and commitment that you had to Kate at that time that you'd do this like a robot, you'd go to work, you'd go to school, you'd go to the hospital, and you had a commitment and a responsibility, do you ever see that in relationships? Like, that's how that relationship was, and do you perceive other relationships to be like that too, that it's a sense of obligation or a need to have to do that?

T: (*To Lisa*) Are you asking about you?

L: No. Well, I'm asking about relationships generally. After the commitment that you had to Kate and the responsibility, do you feel that that also carries over into other relationships? Do you feel that there is a responsibility, a commitment, a dependency, so to speak?

T: (*To Lisa*) Let me go over that question a little bit, because I think it's clear that *your* accident had an impact on Dave. I think that when you got into that biking accident and hurt your legs (*turning to David*) I think that the impact in terms of your feelings about dependency and Lisa needing you were very great, and I think that there really was a reminiscence about the situation with Kate, somebody being sick and being dependent and you had to feel that. Not surprisingly. (*Turning back to Lisa*) How did you feel during that time? What was that time like for you?

L: It was awful. I had a broken leg and collarbone. I was out of work; I was dependent upon other people; I couldn't drive. And it was a time of my self-esteem slipping, my feelings about Dave—I thought about Dave an awful lot, and that was the time that he felt I was dependent upon him and he'd pull back and go forward and go back, so it was a confusing time for me because I really felt that I was in an eggshell. Not working was difficult. Not being free to just go out and enjoy and to be doing my physical activities—I was very physically active and I couldn't do those. I was very frustrated, and it was probably the most difficult time in my life, going through that. I was unemployed for 7 months, and looking for a job and having a bad leg at the same time was very frustrating. What I'd usually do when I was frustrated [before the accident] was go swimming or go work out at the gym, and I couldn't do that. And then to compound it, what was happening with Dave, where I really didn't know what was happening because I really didn't know what was happening with myself.

T: (*To Dave*) Did you recognize some of the feelings from Kate's death?

D: It was just the attitude of getting over the injury. She [Lisa] dealt with it pretty well. She was very optimistic. She worked very hard at it, getting it back, keeping her life going on, and so forth. I think we talked about this a bit and we got to a point where she sort of went neutral, at least from my perception. She wasn't really working at it as hard as she could have been working, and sort of letting events take control rather than taking charge. And I was really kind of unhappy at that time, because I would say, unless she took charge, this thing would go on forever like this. And I was getting more and more unhappy about our relationship and I didn't like the dependency thing. The whole thing about her getting a job and turning her life around a little bit and sort of getting into things and being aggressive about life, I guess—that was really important to me, and I think that's why I kept pushing and saying, "Go for it," you know, "Try to get this job." In that kind of thing I compare her to Kate.

T: Do you think about how Kate would have handled something like that?

D: Yes.

T: And where did Lisa come out?

D: Well it's difficult to compare. She [Kate] was the strongest person I ever met. (*Begins to sob*)

T: I think it's good that you cry about that, because I think that it's been years—you know, when we spoke a couple of years ago I think that you were able to shed a few tears and talk about it, but I don't think that you were able to get into it as much as you're getting into it now.

D: It's hard for me to talk about her because I do feel a lot of emotion, and it's not fair to Lisa for me to compare the two of them because I can't.

T: You can't *not* compare either.

D: Well, I feel that, but I can't say to Lisa, "Gee, Kate would have done this." She was just too unbelievably strong and I said to myself, when we were together, I would look at her and think, "God, if she can be strong, I can be strong too." And we would feed off each other that way, and we got stronger together, because I'm sure she felt weakness and there were times where she cried and she was down. But most of the time she kept picking herself up and forcing herself ahead to do things. She was amazing. I was thinking about the time, Christ, she [Kate] was out there playing tennis in terrible pain. That's why it's hard when you say to me, "I'm not going to ski this winter, or I can't bike in the fall; I'm afraid that I'm going to hurt my knee again." It's just hard for me to accept that. I understand it and I'd probably be the same way, but I think that it's just an attitude and you can do anything that you want to do if you believe in it.

T: Lisa, how are you feeling right now?

L: I'm feeling a little angry. I'm not that strong. That's just me.

D: I don't—it's hard for me—I don't say to you, "Kate did this and that," but I feel this, but I understand you and it is difficult for me to not compare you at times. I'm just being honest. And that's why I don't do it. I don't think it's fair to do that, because I think that was just an unusual circumstance, but you have to deal with this whole thing.

L: Well, I want you to be honest with me, but that doesn't mean that I may not get angry about it either. I'd rather you be honest with me so that I can come back to you and say, "Well, you're not being fair to me. That's not me. That's not who I am." And not looking at me for my attributes but just looking at the negative side. Right now my leg is at 69% of what my other leg is, and right now I'm not thinking about downhill skiing. I'd love to be downhill skiing. I'd also love to go back to bicycling, but at the same time I'm not going to risk messing up my leg again. I just couldn't go through that. It's not to say that I'm not going to do those things again. I'm going to work hard at doing it. But it's not going to be for a few more months.

T: Something which is significant to me, though, is that I think you [David] must trust Lisa quite a bit because this is one of the first times that I've seen you really let yourself feel as much, express as much, about Kate over the years that I've known you. (*To Lisa*) And that says to me that he has a lot of trust in you.

D: She is the only one that tries to make me talk about things. She works at it and I feel good about that.

T: I think that you know that some of these things are not rational or reasonable to expect—that Kate was really extraordinary in some ways, an exceptional person in some ways—but I think nonetheless you have some of these feelings, and I think that the fact that you can talk about them together is very important for this relationship. And I think that you are right (*to Lisa*). If you can talk about it then you can say,

"But I'm not that way," or "This is what I'm feeling," or "This is what I'm thinking." If it's not spoken about, then it festers inside of you.

L: (*To David*) And I don't know where you're coming from. Your actions speak very loudly, but I don't know what they are saying to me. And it's difficult sometimes for me to be the initiator of the conversations, or "What's going on here?" or "What are you feeling?" "Why are you doing this?" Sometimes I feel those ways and I get very frustrated and I'd like for Dave to say, "What's wrong with you today?" or Why are you acting like this?" or "What are you angry about?", so I can bring it out. I think it's always more difficult for me to say, "Well, I'm feeling angry today because of this." It's easier if somebody says, "Why are you feeling angry?"

D: I think I'm pretty bad at that because, you know, I sense that at times when you're angry or upset I usually know why and it has something to do with me, I'm sure, and I'm afraid to say—it's like setting yourself up for something by saying, "What's the matter today?" And then knowing that the person is going to come back and know that you're going to come back and beat me in the head, you know, sort of figuratively.

L: Yes, but it's not always you, David. I mean there are other factors in my life—there are frustrations and anxieties and anger, and it's not just you—and sometimes I may use you as a sounding board if I'm with you after something has happened. And sometimes it is you, but I would like you to be able to say to me, "What is it?" I take risks all the time when I say that to you, and I have to be ready for you to say to me, "Well, it's this that you're doing," or "I feel that we are getting too close. I need some space." You know those are very difficult things for me to accept and to hear, but I need to know. Maybe that's where we're different. I need to know what's going on.

D: Well, that's why I think we've gotten this far, because you're the only person I've been seeing that will do that. Regardless of the risk, you're not afraid to do that. I'm afraid to do that. And when it usually happens I'm with someone who is afraid to do that, and so it's comfortable then and things just meander along, and it has happened before where things have died because it would just be very frustrating.

L: But does that scare you that we talk and you feel very close to me?

D: Yes.

T: (*To David*) It's terribly frightening to you, for sure.

L: What's scaring you?

D: It scares me to talk about emotions, to talk about what I'm feeling. Remember, I said that when I go for a run I think about things I want to say to you. But when it comes right down to it, when I see you that night or the next day, I just can't say anything. I freeze up. The words just don't come out. I put it off and I say to myself, "This isn't a good time. It will be better some other time." I mean, it's never a good time, and the only time it happens is when you get to the point when you say, "I've got to talk about this. What's going on?" And then I start to be able to say some of the things that I wanted to say, but I have never been able to do that. Kate was the only person who could, who just wouldn't take "no" for an answer. She would just say, "Listen, there is something wrong here. This is bothering me. I want to talk about it." She would sit there and stare at me for 15 minutes when I would say nothing. I would think about things I wanted to say, and not a word would come out, nothing. She would just wait. She was extraordinarily patient and very extremely persistent. I feel kind of vulnerable just saying this to you now. It's like giving keys. This is one way. You know, it's like giving away secrets, and that makes me nervous.

T: I think that you've always had a fear about talking about feelings, expressing feelings. I don't think it happened very much in your family. I think at the same time it's something that at some level you want to do. I think you responded well to your relationship with Kate, and I think that that's something that you respond well to here [with Lisa]. I think that's something that's attractive to you about Lisa is the fact that Lisa is persistent. That Lisa wants to talk about feelings. I think that's very important to you. So I think that it's a two-sided thing. On the one hand, it's very hard for you to do. On the other hand you really want it.

L: And Dave always tells me after we talk or after we have an emotional conversation how much better he feels.

T: Let me say a few things, then ask you something. Something which is clear to me is that at least for right now I think that there's a third party in this relationship, and that's Kate. (*Both Dave and Lisa nod*) I think that maybe it would be better if it wasn't that way, or it shouldn't be that way, or it should be that way, I don't know. But in any case that's the way that it is. It's very clear to me. It's what I've been feeling for quite a while. When we first started talking again, I said to you [Dave] that I thought that the event of Kate's death was very important in terms of your relationships with women, and I'm *sure* of it as we talk today. But I think that the best way to deal with it is by talking about it. And it may be something that ends up making you angry or upsetting you, but I think that it's got to be discussed because it is there.

L: I agree. Like I said, I may get angry, but I'd rather it be discussed. I don't like being in the dark and I don't like not knowing where these emotions are coming from. I think I want to know and if it does make me angry, that's OK.

[*Lisa was quite comfortable with acknowledging and expressing her anger. She also gave David "permission" to show his anger. If Lisa could sustain this support, David might be able to learn to express his anger directly to Lisa instead of being so critical of her, and this might offer a foundation for dealing with his anger toward Kate.*]

T: Let me ask both of you how you felt about our meeting today.

D: Me? Well, it started off kind of like I was having trouble not laughing, just sort of smiling, thinking about what we're doing, and I guess I feel pretty good because I think you hit one thing on the head. I get embarrassed when I cry. I get really embarrassed. I'm not supposed to do that. That's how I feel. I feel better. I feel pretty good right now. I wasn't anxious about this meeting. I was sort of, "Well, we'll wing it and see what happens." I had no expectations, really, one way or another. I guess this kind of thing, I think I would have admitted this— I mean, I think it's something I need, and I don't realize how difficult it is for me to talk about Kate before I start talking about her. I may think about her occasionally, but to actually talk about what happened during that time and what things I went through and things about her, I just get tremendously emotional and I guess I need to do that more.

T: The impact upon you is enormous and the effect is enormous, and I think that lots of times you push that away or don't acknowledge it. But I think that you were very, very much involved with Kate. I think you were very much in love with Kate, and I think that her death and the way that she died were enormously painful to you and *continue* to affect you. And I think that your style of trying not really to deal with or express feelings closes that over, and I think that you can't close it over forever. I think that you really need to talk about it. Something that I would recommend strongly is that the two of you talk about it more. You can't *not* talk about it, because it's there. I think that after Kate, the relationship with Lisa is the most important relationship with a woman that you've had, and I think that this brings up a lot of the feelings from Kate and Kate's death for you. And I think that those feelings need to be acknowledged. What was this like for you, Lisa?

L: I was pretty uneasy at the beginning, nervous, anxious. And as we got into it I felt more comfortable. I was pleased with how it went. I've never done this before. It really shed a lot of light on issues that are very important to both of us, and hopefully this will allow us to be able to deal with them more easily. And for me it's very important for Dave to be able to acknowledge what he's feeling and how he's feeling about things and to be able to want to talk about them and want to be emotional, and I think he will understand it himself—it will help him to do that, you know. I'm really pleased with that.

T: Let me ask you about this. What if the three of us have one or two more of these meetings together? How would you feel about that?

L: I'm comfortable with that.

T: What do you think?

D: Yeah, that's fine.

T: We can set that up right after this. We can do it in 3 weeks from now. Again, what I would say to you, and I think is very important, is that what you try to do between now and then is to continue talking about some of these issues that we raised, especially about the issue of Kate and Kate's death and some of what that was like. Dave, if you felt comfortable with it—I'm certainly not saying that this is something that you *have* to do, but if you felt comfortable with it—I would also suggest that Lisa take a look at the diary. How would you feel about that?

D: That's fine.

T: How would you feel about that?

L: I don't know. It's very personal.

T: It's a very moving kind of thing. But again, I think in terms of understanding Dave and in terms of understanding his relationship with Kate, I think it's something that could be very valuable. It would be painful. It really was painful to read it but I think it's also very powerful. OK? See you then.

DAVID AND LISA: SESSION 6

D: We've been seeing quite a bit of each other and talked a bit about Kate the other day, and I don't even know how we got started on it, but it was kind of me relating to her some of the things that happened.

T: Did you bring it up?

D: I don't know. Did I?

L: We were talking about Kate's mother, and we talked about some of the health problems she was having, and I asked if it was related to what Kate had. Then we started talking about Kate.

D: Yes, I started describing to Lisa what her problem was. What kind of disease lupus is and the treatment she had to go through and just going through that whole thing, and, as usual, talking about that sort of thing I just sort of get welled up with emotion. It was difficult for me to talk about that.

T: It becomes painful when you start talking about it?

D: Yes. And we talked a little bit about Lisa reading Kate's diary. Well, I don't know if it's a diary or a recap of events. I think there's probably a little bit of reluctance on both parts for her to read this. I sort of—I said, you know, "Do you want to read the diary?" I didn't sort of, like, give it to her and say, "Here read it." But I think the reluctance on my part was kind of forcing something on a relationship that you don't want to do. And I think she was saying to me that she felt funny wanting to read it because she didn't know if she should. That kind of thing. So we're both a little uncomfortable about doing that. I was just reading it over last night a little bit. I had started writing my recap of what I saw that happened at that time, you know, sort of filling in how I met Kate and what attracted me to her and how our relationship went, and I never finished that.

[During Kate's illness David had also begun to keep a diary, which he never completed.]

D: I got to the point when, just before she got sick, I just stopped it there. It's like one of the projects that you start and you stop it. Lisa was asking me, "Did you not finish it because you couldn't? Was it one more thing that was sort of left hanging that you didn't deal with?" I didn't think so. I thought it was something that took a lot of time to do to sit down and go through and write this kind of thing.

T: What did you feel, David, in reading the diary again?

D: I didn't read the whole thing. I just read parts of it. I didn't feel anything bad or anything. I just felt sort of a little bit of accomplishment in saying that I had it all redone. I read mostly what I had written and just a little bit of what she had written. I was trying to fill in the gaps in the sequence of events. It didn't feel painful or anything like that.

T: Lisa, what did you feel when David was telling you something about Kate's illness?

L: What did I . . . ?

T: Feel?

L: Um, I have mixed feelings. I want David to talk about it because I feel it is important for him to express his feelings and emotions with Kate in a way of feeling more comfortable talking about it. And you (*to David*) weren't as upset as I've seen you in the past talking about Kate this time.

T: What are your mixed feelings?

L: I was talking to David about this last night. You know Kate made it very difficult for women in David's life because she was his, you know, hero. And it makes it difficult for someone to come against somebody's hero and try to—you could never try to replace them, but try to become a part of their life, and you're confronted with this steel wall that's really hard to break through. Sometimes I see her as—you know, like David is still involved with her.

T: He is.

L: Yes, so it's almost, it's a jealousy. It's not a good feeling to feel jealous about somebody who is not living and is not present, but it's still somebody who David is involved with.

T: It's kind of an impossible competition for you.

L: I don't see it as impossible, because I think that David is still at the point of wanting to work it out and . . .

T: And letting it go.

L: And letting it go. That's what I think. I see that he's working toward that.

T: (*To David*) Do you see it as an impossible competition?

D: No. You see, if I start to look at it in the context that we have been talking about, and if I'm trying to find somebody who is just like her, then it is impossible, but I don't think I am. I don't think I have been using Kate as a gauge. Especially with Lisa, I don't think I've used her in my mind and said, "Kate did this and you do this," and that kind of thing. I don't see it as impossible because I think I really want to get through this thing. I don't want to continue it on and make it impossible. I just don't feel that way.

T: You want to be able to love someone else?

D: Yes. And I think that in my own mind if I feel that way, if I feel that desire that I want to be in love with someone else, then it can happen and it's just a matter of time and exercise, and this is one way of working through that quicker.

T: Exercise?

D: Well, I mean just sort of talking about it and going through the motions.

T: Like *The Exorcist*?

D: Yeah, but not quite like that. (*Laughs*)

L: (*To David*) Maybe we should perform an exorcism on you?

D: Lisa was over at the house last night and we were in bed watching the TV, um, and just talking, and all of a sudden a light on the wall came on. It's one of these old-fashioned sconces with bulbs on it. There was nothing, then all of a sudden the light came on.

L: That was after we heard noises downstairs.

D: And she said to me, she goes, "What did that?" And I said, "It always does that. Without turning the switch, it just goes on by itself." And she asked me if there were ghosts in the house.

L: I said, "I've never seen that happen, ever."

T: What did you say about the ghosts?

D: I didn't.

L: Are there persons in the house? Is there something that I don't know about?

T: Well, I said to you before that I think that Kate's ghost is very significant here in terms of relationships with women. And I think that's an important aspect, and it's real.

L: (*Laughs*) I like the way you tied that together.

T: Thank you.

L: So she was in the room last night!

T: How do you (*to David*) see things, and how do you (*to Lisa*) see things? Between the two of you? What's been going on between the two of you?

D: Things have been pretty good. I've tried to be more open and sort of trying to work at not putting up a wall. Trying to let things flow a little easier.

T: What have you done specifically?

D: I don't know. I think this past weekend was something where I think—normally I'd probably just stay down at your folks' house for the day and take off. I just hung around with her parents and the whole family for the weekend, really. And kind of relaxed and just did basically what you and your family wanted to do. I didn't say, "I have to be here. I have to do this." You know, at the end of the weekend, I had to take off Sunday but . . .

T: You didn't try to get away?

D: No, I didn't try to get away. I just tried to enjoy their company and I felt pretty good about that. I think it was a nice weekend. And just talking about making plans. I usually wait to the last minute and things. My office Christmas party and going down to Washington for a weekend, you know—instead of waiting until the last minute, I at least gave Lisa a little advance notice.

L: Well, the Christmas party was a little bit like a last-minute thing. We were taking a walk after dinner one night, and David just casually mentions it: "Oh, my office Christmas party is next weekend."

D: I told you before that.

L: No, you didn't.

T: How do you feel about that?

L: Well, that's natural. That's how our relationship has been. That's been very normal for us.

T: To what?

L: For David to just say, "Oh, by the way, this weekend we're doing this, or next weekend." It's usually "*this* weekend." Yeah, I did have a week in advance, but it's usually been last-minute.

D: I told you before. I know I did. I told you at least the weekend before then.

L: Well, I don't remember. You may have. But I don't remember. And I remember dates and things.

T: (*To Lisa*) Well, if it does happen at the last minute, what is that like for you?

L: It depends on what it is. Sometimes I may have made plans for that weekend, or I may have just made plans that weekend. You know, weekends, especially when you're in the working world, they are precious because you are very busy during the week. It's something that I want to go to and I didn't have something else that I had plans for. I like planning in advance. I just like planning in advance. That's just the type of animal I am, and David likes to do things at the last minute.

T: Do you think that's a distancing kind of thing?

L: Um, in a way, yeah.

T: How does it distance you?

L: Well, we've talked about that before. It's like waiting for the last minute to see the best offer that comes up and not wanting to commit to anything until you've had many offers to select from. So when it is a last-minute situation—not often, but there have been times when I felt like, well since nothing else has come up, or you couldn't get away with somebody this weekend to go skiing or to do this or that, then you want to make plans with me. I haven't felt that that often, but I feel that that is just a measure of wanting to get it all in and not wanting to miss out on anything. I think that also comes with commitment.

T: Did you (*to David*) feel that that happens?

D: Well, I know that's what I do normally. I just wait until the last minute. Like I could, and these things would come up that I know about in advance and I just sort of store them in my mind and don't say anything to Lisa and then sort of at the last minute, tell her, you know, "This is going on this weekend; do you want to go?" I've always been that way. I never—you know, I think 3 days' notice is a long time.

L: Yes but I feel bad when you do that.

D: I know.

L: Because I could have had an opportunity to make other plans at the same time, and then, you know, it may be something that I would really like to do with you, but you didn't give me the option of choosing whether I wanted to do it with you. It was at your convenience that you decided to let me know. And like you've said, you've known weeks in advance, or in advance, whatever.

D: Well, sometimes, yes.

L: Well, not all the time.

T: I remember you talking about that with Kate as well, that when you first started going together you would do something similar.

D: I'd wait until the last minute and call her up and say, "Hey, do you want to do something tonight or tomorrow night?" or something.

T: What does that do for you? What do you get out of that?

D: I don't know what I get out of it. I know—going back to Lisa, and I've talked about this with Lisa before—it always seems like I have a lot of options on social activities, either a number of different things to choose from or even people to choose with who I do it with, and it seems like I need to have a whole bunch of choices and then I want to choose the best one. That's why I wait until the last minute to see everything that could happen, anything that could come up, and then say, "OK, this is what I want to do." Like I don't want to miss anything.

T: Well, it's the same thing that keeps you ambivalent about this relationship, because maybe something better will come up.

D: The same thing happened with Kate, too. That's what I was reading last night. Something that I wrote myself when we started getting close. I said, "No, no, this is it. I'm losing my freedom and I don't want to do this." And I brought it up with her and she basically said the same thing, and we said, "Well, we don't want to lose our freedom," so we stopped seeing each other.

T: You and Kate did?

D: Yes.

T: How long did that go on for?

D: About a week.

T: Six days? (*Laughs*)

D: Six days, yeah. That's what I was reading last night, and the thing that when I wasn't with her I was very miserable. I remember that I was working out in the country and I was staying with my parents and I was just in a lousy mood all week, and my mother said, "What's wrong with you?", you know, "You're a real pain in the butt." And you know, I told her what happened and I said, you know, that I missed Kate a lot and she said, "Why don't you just call her up and tell her what you told me?" So I did, and when I called her she felt the same way. I mean, we both did something we really didn't want to do, and then when we got back together, you know, that was the commitment. I was afraid to make a commitment to her and she was too to me, and we backed off and we realized that it was worse not being together, so that's why we got back together again. So I don't think this is anything I've started just because of Kate. I think this is the way I've always been.

T: Right. So you (*to Lisa*) don't have to take it personally. (*All laugh*)

L: I don't take it personally. I really don't take that personally. He's told me this before and I understand the type of person he is but, you know . . .

T: It still hurts.

L: Yes, because I don't see it that you lose your freedom when you're with somebody you want to be with. You either want to be with them or you don't want to be with them. Because being with them can create as much freedom or more freedom for you, because you have a companion to do things with. Certainly you can do things on your own as well.

T: Lisa, let me ask you, have you felt at all over the last few weeks that David has been more open to you?

L: Yes, I do.

T: In what way?

L: We spent a lot of time together, and it's been very natural time. We get together during the week, have dinner, we may watch TV, we may both be reading something, but it's been very natural time. It hasn't been— um, it's been less of a strain. It's been very comfortable, and I didn't expect him to be there all weekend. I expected him to stay there Thursday night. I worked all day Friday and I didn't say to him, "I want you to stay, please." You know, I just left it up to him and, you know, he was with my family, and it was really pleasant. It was really nice.

T: The strain that you talk about before was what? What was happening or how was it happening that there was a strain?

L: Well I find that when there's a lack of communication or feelings that aren't being expressed, for me that's a strain. It's very difficult for me if somebody has something on their mind and doesn't say it, you know. And I think that's something that David is becoming more comfortable with.

T: So before, what was happening is that you were spending time together, but you sensed that there was something on his mind that he was not talking about.

L: Yes, and that created tension. For me it did. I think David just had a way of blocking it out.

T: How would that show itself? What would happen?

L: Well we talked about that last time a bit. Um, avoidance or just coldness, isolation.

T: So he'd be distant from you and that would be painful for you?

L: Yes. I get very frustrated and then mad.

T: What do you (*to David*) think is allowing you to start being more open?

D: You know, part of it is just by talking. These meetings with you have been helpful. It's sort of like a catalyst to get things going and making me more conscious of it. I guess my feeling is that I do want to work things through, and Lisa's been very good about talking about things. She's been very receptive to opening things up, and she doesn't seem to be afraid to talk about things, and so that makes it more comfortable. It makes it easier for me to talk. I sort of look at it as venturing out a little bit. I feel like I'm doing something I haven't. It just feels really strange to say, "Lisa, let's do something 3 weeks from now." That's not me to make plans like that.

T: How else are you venturing out?

D: Well, I guess we're seeing each other a little more often. I would always, I think in the past, keep my distance that way by saying, you know, we could see each other maybe twice a week, you know, once on the weekend and once during the week, and not get any closer than that. Now it's sort of like on the spur of the moment. If I'm not doing something at night, or something like that, I'll give her a call or . . .

L: And I'm not doing something that night.

D: . . . to see you if you're not doing something that night.

L: And I feel comfortable doing that too. Just find him and say, "Do you want to go to dinner?"

D: And that's something that I normally wouldn't do.

T: So you're (*to Lisa*) feeling safer in the relationship too?

L: You know I just think, well, "What the hell, I got nothing to lose," you know. I think I'm being more of myself. You know, if I want to call him I call him. And David and I've talked about this, and I'm not into the games of "Oh, should I call? Shouldn't I call?" Just doing what I want to do as opposed to what I feel like I should be doing. If I want to call him, I call him. I don't wait to have him call me.

T: Are you (*to David*) feeling less frightened?

D: Yes, I guess that's true. I don't really think about it. I sort of have the same attitude, or I'm trying to develop the same attitude as Lisa, where you let yourself go a little bit and see where it takes you. I'm still not really completely open, but more so than I have been. You know, what I think would be a big deal, she would think would be normal, that kind of thing. (*Reaches out to hold Lisa's hand*)

T: Like what?

D: Like making plans in advance. That kind of thing. I'm trying to relax with that or get more comfortable with that. I don't think it's making me frightened or anything.

T: Can you tell me a little bit about how you are feeling toward Lisa these days?

D: I think comfortable. I feel more relaxed by talking. I don't feel like—I think it's just basically more relaxed. I feel like our relationship is real good. I feel like when we're talking more, our relationship is better. We've been talking a bit in the last few weeks, and I think things have been going pretty well, and I feel good about being with her and I look forward to seeing her. I think sometimes in the past, if we got together midweek or something like that, I would go over there and say, "Oh, I shouldn't have done this."

T: Afterwards you'd feel . . .

D: Well, I'd get over to her place and be very cool, very casual. I don't think I'm doing that as much.

T: You'd want to come over and at the same time you'd not want to be there.

D: Yeah. There would be something in me that would say, "You can't do this, this is wrong." And be there in mind but wanting to be someplace else. There would be kind of a confusion, because I wouldn't be very warm or very friendly to be with.

T: How are you doing with your ambivalence toward this caring about her, but at the same time having millions of questions about whether she's enough in this area, enough in that area? What has that been like?

D: I don't know. I think I'm still picking at her. I think I am awful at—um, there's always something that I bring up, and I just have this nasty tendency to do that.

T: It just sort of leaps out of your mouth.

D: What?

T: It leaps out of your mouth?

D: Yeah, kind of.

L: What's the latest criticism (*of her*)?

D: I don't know. I say things that are on my mind that I probably shouldn't say. They just seem to roll off her back somehow, which is amazing to me. Or she'll give me a smart answer, like "This is the way I am, so forget it!"

L: Like what?

D: If I talk about anything, if I say anything to you that indicates that you're not perfect. I was saying that you had wrinkles on your face, and, you know, I think some women would really get bulled or really get upset, but she laughs at me basically.

T: Do you feel picked on with him? (*Lisa nods*) You do?

L: Oh yes. But things don't, you know—I remember, I remember small things. I remember details and I remember small comments more than I remember the larger picture. I remember what happened within that large picture. I remember all these things. It's not that they just roll, but sometimes I just find them so ridiculous and say, "I can't believe you, you know? So what? Who cares?" I have wrinkles because I smile a lot. If you don't smile a lot you don't have wrinkles, right? You have wrinkles, you smile a lot. You know, so I don't let them phase me. I think that's ridiculous to get upset or agitated over.

D: It's just me, the thing coming out where I'm—you know, I have this, what I talked about before, I was looking for the "perfect woman." She can't have any skin with any wrinkles and it has to be just perfect, and I'll pick at the smallest things, which will be ridiculous.

T: You see it as ridiculous as well?

D: Well, yes, after I do. But in my mind, I'm thinking, "Oh, this is only going to get worse. This is going to be bad." Or something like this.

L: Like wrinkles? Because you did mention wrinkles the other night. They only get worse. And I said, "No problem, I'll just have a face lift."

D: That's the kind of answer she would give me, and I would laugh about it, you know, because then I would feel ridiculous.

L: Yes, but I like when he says those things because that's just a part of him, and I'd rather have him say them and it's humorous to me, and it's good when you can humor each other.

D: But there's a part of me that it's somewhat serious, you know. I say these things because I'm thinking of them and as negative things, and if I don't talk about them I sort of store them up and say, "OK, here's one for this side and here's one for this side. Here's another one for the bad side," or something like that. And if I don't talk about them I just store them up.

L: As long as you balance them out with good things, you can.

D: You do have many more good things than bad things.

T: You feel that way?

D: Yeah, I do.

L: And that was something which was difficult for David to express to me.

You know, and this happened a couple of weeks ago, you know, I really spent a lot of time getting dressed and doing my hair and putting my makeup on, and I thought I looked great. And I was leaving and a friend of mine, Danielle, said, "You look great tonight. Oh, wait until you see David!" I was all excited to see David. I'm always excited to see David, you know, I always get twinges when I know I'm going to see him, and I just walked in his house and I got a "Hi!" And I was hurt. I had just a nice new dress and I really liked the way it looked, and he didn't even notice me. I just crept into a shell and then I couldn't talk. I got really upset about that one thing, that he didn't make a comment or notice how nice I looked, notice that I got a brand-new dress, and then I felt badly about that. I said to him, "It may sound really bratty but it's really nice to be complimented, it's nice to be noticed, especially when you put time and energy into wanting to look nice for somebody."

T: So you felt really deflated?

L: Yes.

D: That wasn't an intentional thing. I mean, that wasn't like, "Oh, she looks good, but I can't tell her that."

L: No, that wasn't intentional. You didn't even realize it.

D: I probably had 10 different things in my mind. Sometimes she will come over and we'll be in a rush, or sometimes I'll be busy or something like this and nothing registers. Usually what happens is I'll be with her for half an hour, and all of a sudden I'll look and I'll really look at her and I'll say, "Oh, you look good tonight," and then it's too late.

L: Or "Is that a new sweater?" And by that time I already feel shitty. It's like, "Yeah, it's about time you noticed."

T: I think you do care a lot about Lisa, though. When you were talking a few minutes ago and held her hand, and then you put your arm around her. I think you feel a lot of tenderness toward her. But I think that it's hard for you to show that for some reason.

D: Yeah. I think you're right.

T: What are you feeling right now?

D: I think I do care a lot about Lisa. And I feel bad for the kinds of things that she has put up with. You know, she's really a terrific person and even—I really, I don't think I would hurt her intentionally, you know, and I'm sure I have over the last several months have been mean or nasty or whatever, and I just . . . (*Turns to Lisa*) I guess I love you for . . . (*Begins to cry. Puts his face into his hands and sobs. There is a long silence*)

T: For what?

D: You know, I appreciate that. I think what makes me sad is that I can't say these kinds of things normally. I don't feel comfortable with it when my feelings just come out naturally, and I don't—I try to either control them too much, or there is something there that doesn't let things happen normally or naturally. I wish it would happen a little more naturally, because I think I miss a lot because of that.

T: I think you take a big risk in talking like that and opening up this way. I think you took a big risk in first coming in here a few weeks ago with Lisa together, because I think that was something that was very scary for you and very frightening, and I think you just took a big risk in talking about how you feel toward her. And I think what's happened for you was—and we spoke about this before—I think that you came from a family where people just didn't talk about their feelings, or emotions weren't expressed, or things were kept back from one another. I think you got involved in a relationship with Kate and found out that this was very, very different from your relationships with your family. And then you lost that, and then I think you pulled back into a shell, in a way, and I think that you're just starting to come out now in this relationship with Lisa. I think that you've done a lot of things with her that you haven't been able to do in years. That's a big step. I think it takes a lot of courage to take that step.

[This interpretation by the therapist again captured the core themes of David's treatment: first, that Kate's death had had a major impact upon his relationships with women; second, that his family history also tied in to this problem; third, that there was a difference in the relationship with Lisa. He *did* care about her (albeit with a sense of fear and trepidation), and he felt ready to change his troubled interactions with women. Finally, the therapist was supportive and encouraging regarding the changes David had already begun to make and the chances and risks he was taking in the treatment, a very good example of the latter being his ability to express his emotions with Lisa just minutes before.]

[*This session also demonstrates that working through developmental deprivation in one's family of origin can occur in healing relationships in adulthood. Harnessing the power of such naturally occurring relationships certainly provides a broader route for many patients to change than does relying on the traditional therapist–patient relationships.*]

D: It's something I want to work out, and I think it's going to take time too. You know, I can say something this morning and it's maybe just one little crack in the wall, and I think it's something that I have to work at constantly.

T: When you've lived your life a certain way, it's very unlikely that it will happen like that, that things will change all at once. But I think what you're starting to do is you're starting to take some risks and starting to make some changes which are very important and which go a long way in terms of making an overall change. (*Turning to Lisa*) And how are you feeling, Lisa, in terms of what's being said?

L: I think that, you know, this weekend, spending it with my family, David can better understand me too. And I came from a very warm and very open family. You know, we all hug, we all kiss, we all tell each other we love each other, and that's a very important thing for me. And David and I have talked about that and I need that, I need that affection and the warm lovingness. That's just a part of me, and without that I just don't feel whole. And it's true. I think David is starting to feel more comfortable with that. I've always been like that with him, and when we first started seeing each other I said, "Do you mind if I kiss you or hug you in public? Does it bother you that I always want to hold your hand?" He said, "No, I like it." And I just kept doing it. It wasn't so much returned to me and I'd say to him 2 months later, "Does it bother you when I hug you or kiss you in public?" He said, "No, I like it." So he's getting more comfortable with it too, and, you know, just holding my hand here in front of you or, you know, with my family, putting his arms around me, you know, it makes me feel wonderful.

T: That's terrific.

L: Because David knows that I love him and that he can trust me and I'm not going to take advantage of his feelings or emotions or him as a person in any way.

T: So what you feel right now is what?

L: It's a sense of accomplishment that David is feeling more comfortable with that.

T: That's terrific. We have to stop in a few minutes, but what I'd like to do is I'd like to have one more meeting between the three of us, because I think that these are helpful and useful—to talk here together like this and then be able to start to make some of these cracks in terms of what you're able to express, what you're able to say. And I think you really do feel like you want to get out of this sort of straightjacket that you've been in for so long in terms of expressing your feelings, in terms of being able to love somebody and express that love. I think this is helpful in doing that. How do you feel about it?

D: If Lisa can get some time from work to do that, that will be fine.

T: All right, I'll go with you in just a minute and we'll set it up in a few weeks. (*To Lisa*) What do you think?

L: I want to find out what role I play in all of this after a while.

T: What do you mean, "what role you play"?

L: You know, as of last week, after I left, you know, I just felt like, I don't know, it was a good feeling and I was wondering, "What am I doing here? What's the expectation here? What role do I play? Where does David see me in another year? Where is this going to leave us, basically?"

T: Well, I hope that you can do some talking about that between one another between now and when we meet again, because I do think that you have some questions, and I think that there are things that you need to talk about together.

L: And I have a question for you. Um, I know that David is seeing you less than weekly. He started seeing you every week and then he started seeing you every other week or so. Why don't you see him every week?

T: Well, what I planned to do and what I will do with David is to see him for some brief period of time. I think that our meetings together are part of that, and I think that what's most important really is not that so much that David just talk with me about his ambivalence or his uncertainty about relating to women, but I think that the thing that's really important is starting to make some changes in the world and starting to do some things differently. The kind of thing that has been going on today and what went on last week. I think that David and I—I think (*to David*) that you and I could talk together a long time about ambivalence and about uncertainty, and it wouldn't mean a thing if you weren't doing some things to really change the way that you're interacting outside the therapy.

D: Sort of like doing my homework?

L: Yeah, but David has said how helpful and beneficial that those meetings with you have been.

T: And I plan to have some more meetings with him in the future, but also to have some period of time during which, hopefully, what you're doing (*to David*) is practicing your homework, and then we would meet again and see where things were at that point.

D: I guess what Lisa is saying is that she thinks I should be meeting more often with you instead of less often.

L: Yeah, I'd like to see him meeting with you on a regular basis as opposed to once every other week and once every month, because when I was seeing a therapist for a while she basically wouldn't want to see me every other week. You know, I'd suggest, "Well, why don't I see you every other week?" She said, "No, because a lot happens in a week and after you leave a session you have a lot that comes up that filters through your week, and by the time 7 days are up there are a lot of other issues to be discussed."

T: I think that's a good question. My view of therapy is somewhat different than her view of therapy, and I think that it's a matter of "different strokes for different folks." Different people needing different things from therapy. But I think that what's really most significant is that what gets started for you here gets taken outside.

[This is an important interchange about the nature of psychotherapy. At times, patients or significant others come to treatment who are "friends and supporters" of long-term traditional psychotherapy. That is, they feel that

psychotherapy must be continuous, weekly (or twice-weekly), and ongoing. In a time-effective therapy context, it may be necessary to clarify that the brief therapist's view of the process of treatment is different from the patient's or significant other's. Some patients may accept the restraints upon treatment indigenous to this model, while others may feel angry, unhappy, or deprived, because they cannot get the type of therapy they view as ideal. One certainly must make every effort to be flexible and to appreciate the patient's or significant other's concerns. However, occasionally a patient views his or her idealized therapeutic format as inviolable, in which case the patient may be dissatisfied with the treatment. Fortunately, in our experience, this is quite rare.]

T: We can talk more about this when we meet again, but what I would like to do, and what I feel would be helpful, is for us to meet for a short period of time. And then for us to take a break for a period of time, and then to get together again and see where things are at that point and what's been going on during that period.

L: I just don't agree with that. I just don't.

T: There are different ways to work and different ways to operate. I think that what can be helpful is to get things started, then for things to take their course after that and then to meet again afterwards. I think that what happened before in terms of David and I is that some things began, some things got triggered, some things got started, a couple of years ago. I think that you moved some distance with that and used that, and I think that at this point you were ready to do some more work and I think that that's what happened now. But again, we can talk more.

D: OK.

[*The therapist wisely and successfully resisted Lisa's attempts to put David's welfare squarely back in the therapist's lap. The therapist did something very therapeutic by turning aside Lisa's request for more individual therapy for David: He forced David to continue to make his problems real, by containing them in the relationship with Lisa, rather than diluting them in a series of obsessive individual therapy sessions.*]

DAVID AND LISA: SESSION 7

This session occurred 1 month after Session 6.

T: Where do things stand between the two of you? How have things been?

L: Oh, just wonderful.

T: Is that facetiously? Is it seriously?

L: No. Things have been very good. They really have.

T: (*To David*) What has it been like? What's been happening?

D: Like Lisa says, things have been going pretty well. We spent some time together in Maine.

T: Did it go well?

D: Yes. We stayed at the hotel up there and it was kind of nice. It was very pleasant. We had a nice weekend. The weather was lousy, but we had a nice time. We did a little sightseeing. They have some tours out there. It was good. I think that's the first time we had actually gone away and done something together like that.

T: Did you get "antsy" or uncomfortable over the weekend? Was it hard for you?

D: No, I didn't get uncomfortable. I didn't want to spend much time in the hotel. I didn't particularly enjoy that. Some of the things that—I like to do things, you know, I wanted to get out of the hotel as early as I could. I think it was a nice weekend overall. We wanted to do some jogging and we couldn't. Lisa's leg was acting up.

T: How has your leg been recently?

L: It's been good. We jogged yesterday.

T: Oh, you did?

L: Yes, but last week it was really bothering me. Fortunately, David got into some running on his own.

T: But you're better for the most part?

L: Yes. It has its ups and downs.

T: How have communications been between the two of you? Talking? Communicating about things?

D: I think OK. Since the last time we saw you I think we've probably talked a couple of times—you know, had some, what I call "heavy-duty-type" talks.

T: Initiated by whom?

D: Lisa. For the most part.

T: Was it hard for you to talk?

D: I don't think it was as much hemming and hawing as I usually do. You know, I didn't feel really uncomfortable. And it's getting to the point where it's predictable when she wants to talk. She doesn't try to hide it.

T: Are you being more outspoken about that?

L: Yeah, but what I'm finding is that I really don't have a difficult time spilling my guts and saying how I feel about David and our relationship. And I wish he would do the same. He doesn't really—well, I just don't have a difficult time doing that, so . . .

T: Do you think he's getting any better at it?

L: Yeah, I do.

T: What is he doing differently? How is he being more able to do that?

[*In brief therapy in general, and especially as treatment nears the end, it is essential that the therapist emphasize the patient's strengths and his or her positive movements toward change objectives.*]

L: Well, like he said, he's not hemming and hawing. He'll just say what's on his mind as opposed to procrastinating. So I think it's getting a little bit easier. I still would like for him to just spill what he feels as opposed to having to be cautious about what he says.

T: That may take a while. I mean, that's something that has been a lifelong pattern for you (*to David*). It sounds like doing something different is not all that easy, but it seems like you're trying.

D: Well, yeah. I may not be initiating something, but I sort of pick up on it a little bit quicker and, you know, sort of get myself ready to talk, because I can sense when it's a time when we should discuss something.

L: But it still comes back to me: "What's on *your* mind?" "I know *you* want to talk about something." So than it's put over to me.

T: What were the "heavy-duty" conversations about? Do you remember?

D: Just our relationship. Where we are going and that kind of thing.

T: These were recent?

D: In the last couple of weeks. Being through a couple of things—my best friend and my roommate got married. Lisa's best friend is getting married. I think that was what sort of prompted or at least was a catalyst to discussion. The woman that's getting married is one of Lisa's best friends. It's like—doing things together for ages and ages, and I think part of the discussion was, I think, Lisa was sensing a loss from her friend and questioned where we were going. I kind of—we just talked about our relationship and, you know, "Are we going in any particular direction or are we sort of just passing time?" and that kind of thing.

T: (*To Lisa*) These are questions that you asked?

L: Yes.

T: And what did you say afterwards?

L: Well, I thought that our relationship was getting better. I mean, we've been spending more time together. Really, we hadn't done that before. We are seeing a lot more of each other.

T: How frequently are you together?

L: At least 4 days a week, anyway.

D: Four or five nights. For the holidays, we've been spending Wednesday through Monday morning together. Previously I would never commit myself to that much time. Any relationships I've had since Kate, I just—when I get to that point, I just back off and say, "That's it, that's it." So I say I think it's getting better. I'm consciously aware of that, and I have the sense of hitting this danger, panic button, but I'm recognizing that. And so I'm saying, "OK, don't worry about those things and just let yourself go." I think that's helped a bit, just going through these kinds of things and being able to recognize that, you know, why I'm like that. And I felt more comfortable with it.

T: So you realize when you start to get frightened, you just sort of calm yourself down in a way.

[*Again, the therapist took advantage of a good opportunity to reinforce the patient's self-healing capacities.*]

D: Well, at least I recognize it. You know it for what it is, rather than this mysterious feeling of "Oh, I've got to get out of here. I've got to escape. I've got to get away." And just, you know, get very cool and distant. I don't think I've been that way.

L: No, you haven't, because I can sense when he feels like that. He gets very cool and then he turns himself off to me. That's the syndrome that we've talked about before. And then I get uptight and defensive. I think I haven't been feeling that either. I get to a point when I feel like that also.

T: Like?

L: "We're spending a lot of time together. Maybe we shouldn't be together tonight." Now it's like, "Why not? Why fight that?" Basically.

T: Do you feel satisfied with where the conversations have gone? What are you (*to David*) saying about the direction of your relationship?

D: A couple of times that we did talk, I think it's been very late at night and I'll be really tired, and it seems like that's when the conversation starts. And I'm about ready to go to sleep, and, you know, she wants to talk. A lot of times when that happens, I just don't have the energy to get into that kind of discussion or just opening up. I'm just—it's the kind of thing where I think there's never a good time, but for me, that's the worst time, when I'm really tired. And it seems like that's when the conversation starts. You know I can look, and her eyes will be wide awake and she'll be looking at me or something like this, and I'm going "Uh-oh." I'm dying to go to sleep and she wants to talk. And actually there might be a method to the madness, because I know I won't be able to go to sleep until we've sort of resolved this thing, so I'll say, you know, "What's the matter?" or "What's on your mind?" or something. I think that's the way the last one started. She was just sort of looking at me, and I knew exactly, she wanted to talk about something. I said, "OK, what is it?" Actually, I thought that was pretty good. Usually I wouldn't even say that. I would just sort of ignore it and say "Good night," or something.

L: And I won't sleep well. I just don't sleep. I'm up and down and up and down.

T: Just thinking about what?

L: Yeah, that I really had something on my mind and he knew that I did and didn't bring it out of me.

T: (*To David*) Let me ask you something. Are you wide awake now?

D: Yes. (*Laughs*) I'm a morning person.

T: Is this a good time to talk?

D: Yes. (*Laughter from both*)

T: (*To Lisa*) What's the question that you have? What are the questions that you have about the direction of the relationship?

L: What I was just going to say, you know, what I would like David to do then in the morning is say, "Why don't we talk about what we started talking about last night?" or "Why don't we continue that conversation?" It's always *me* again who will have to bring up the conversation that maybe really didn't get finished. You won't bring it up again. And then it comes back to me saying, "David, I've got to talk about this again."

T: (*To Lisa*) Well, let me just tell you that I don't think it's going to change all at once. I mean, I think that it's unlikely that in the very near future—it's not to say that it won't happen at some point—but I think that it's unlikely in the very near future (*turning to David*) that you're going to rapidly change from the person who had a hard time talking about feelings or issues at all, to the person who brings everything up. But I think that it's progress for you to be responsive and to engage in the conversations, you know, once you (*to Lisa*) do bring it up. But just in terms of now, what are the things that you (*to Lisa*) are wondering about? You mentioned this before too, that you have some questions or thoughts in your mind about the future of the relationship. Is it about whether you're going to get married, or what specifically do you think about?

[*The therapist's intent in the middle of this segment was not to parodoxically restrain change by suggesting that David go slowly, but to remind both David and Lisa of the importance of setting reasonable goals for change and a realistic "timetable" for such changes. He did not discourage them from seeking further change, but highlighted what he saw as important and achievable at this time.*]

L: I have questions in my own mind whether I want to spend my life with David. What that would be like and what it would be like to have kids, and how we would bring them up. And I'm not sure myself. I'd like to talk about it to get more clarity on just how I'm feeling.

D: Well, those are the kind of things I'll think about too. I'll open up and I'll spend time with you and do things and sort of give that kind of commitment. If it happens that I feel everything is working out fine and, you know, we can talk about marriage. Right now, to me, that doesn't—you know I think about it, but I don't—I mean, it's not the primary thing in my mind. I think that's still an issue we haven't really resolved. You know we talked about kids and religion and things like that. We talk about it a little bit and we sort of don't really resolve anything. We sort of put it off and really haven't dealt with that issue.

T: What is that issue as you see it? [David and Lisa then talked more about their religious differences and how these would have to be resolved in order for them to marry. This was followed by a discussion of some of their other differences. David appeared in this part of the conversation to be hopeful that these differences could be adequately resolved.]

T: What are the good things that you see going on in the relationship?

D: We care about each other a lot, and I think we enjoy spending time together. (*Lisa nods*) Lisa does a lot of things very well. She's organized and she takes charge of a lot of things that are good, you know, like just in shopping and doing anything when we are together and I don't have the time to do it or I don't have the energy, and she'll say, "Oh, we ought to go do that and take care of it right now." You know, to think about it, and she's right. And she sort of pushes me to get things done. So I think that with her I think I accomplish more than I would without her. And I think, you know, we just enjoy each other's company. Yesterday we had a great time. We went jogging and I just enjoyed the whole day. I got up early and played basketball and that was fine. She doesn't give me any grief about those kinds of things that I need to do with friends, and I think she recognizes my needs I have outside our relationship. And we spent the rest of the day doing things together, cooking dinner, and I think we can spend a lot of time together and enjoy each other very much in whatever we are doing, if it's just sitting around reading or talking about music or whatever. Those certainly outweigh the problem issues. I think those couple of things I mention, you know, things that we have to talk about.

L: Yeah, and, like, I'm glad you brought some of this stuff up. You really should do it more.

D: Well, I don't think I really thought how to say them, but I think we had this type of discussion and it came out in a very awkward way. We were sitting at the dining room table and we talked about how I felt you weren't very interesting, and that's what I think I told you. Just the way it came out, it was like I stuck both feet in my mouth and it just didn't come out very well. I think, just talking today, I can more clearly see what it is. That her interests are different from mine in some respects, the intellectual interests, and it's not that she's not an interesting person. It's that certain things motivate her over others, and we had talked about this before, and that's sort of the discussion and it sort of fell down miserably because of the way it came out. It's sort of like a body slam or something that shouldn't have come out that way. I feel badly about that conversation.

T: (*To Lisa*) That must have been very uncomfortable for you.

L: Well, David is—and he realizes this and says this to me—he's very hard on me. He's extremely hard on me. And that's hard for me. I mean I'm only a person, too, and everybody has their weaknesses about when they are picked on and it hurts me. I feel miserable. What about all the good things about me? Why are you just picking this one thing out of 10 that you may see as a weakness? Do something to strengthen it or help me to strengthen that weakness.

T: Well, part of that critical nature, I think, had to do with Kate. (*To David*) It related to your ambivalence about getting into a relationship with another woman and your fears about that. Something has happened over the last few months since we started to meet, and that is that you may have some continued ambivalence, but you seem to be a lot less ambivalent than when you started out here. That's my feeling about it.

D: I think that's absolutely right. I think just by talking about it and bringing it out, I recognized what the problem was. Because I didn't know what it was before and I felt very uncomfortable. I felt angry or unhappy. I didn't know what it was, so I would focus it all to Lisa. I would say, "It must be you. You're the only person I'm with, so it's got to be you," instead of saying, "Well, it's with me or inside of me," and addressing those issues. I think by talking about it, it has helped me a lot, a whole lot. So anyway when I do feel those kinds of things, at least I can say, "OK, I have to work with that," and when I recognize it, it doesn't feel so uncomfortable.

T: I see you as really handling that ambivalence differently now. I think you are trying to handle it differently. (*To Lisa*) I think you feel that as well.

L: Yes, I do.

T: (*To David*) That your pain or anger or fear is not just sort of coming out and slamming Lisa when you feel uncomfortable in yourself. If you're confused in yourself about this relationship and how this relationship compares with the relationship with Kate, and if you're having feelings of fear and anxiety about getting involved with somebody, you're not attacking her in the same way. I think at this point, though, the issue as I see it is really as much more between the two of you and has to do with how the both of you are going to work out this relationship. How you are going to work out the things that you (*to Lisa*) value and the things that you (*to David*) value and the things that are important to both of you on the religion issue, the interest issue, and so forth is central. And I can't tell you how that's going to work out. Nobody knows how it's going to work out, but I think that what's important and what's centrally important is that you both be talking about these things. It's certainly not going to work out if you don't talk about it. Under those circumstances, it's doomed to failure if you are not discussing these things with one another and if you are not sharing with one another and if you're keeping a lot of feelings and uncertainties in yourselves. I think what's essential is that these things be brought out and spoken about. I don't know, maybe for a while it will have to be you (*to Lisa*) that brings it out. You know, bringing up issues for discussion may not be the thing that you (*to David*) are most comfortable with, but hopefully you can start doing that as well. And start thinking about that, keeping in mind when you (*to David*) are feeling something that it would be useful to talk about. I think at least at this point you are being more responsive and are willing to engage in conversation when Lisa brings something out, which is important.

D: I think you're right.

T: But I do think that the work that has to be done at this point really lies with the two of you. (*To David*) My view is not that it's you as the patient now. I think that you're at least thinking about and are more aware about how your past and how Kate's death and other things in your past have affected you. And I think that the work that lies ahead lies with the two of you. If this relationship is going to work out, it would require some hard work on both your parts, I think. But it sounds to me as though you really care about one another. I think there's a real sense of commitment that I hear on both your parts. I don't think that you (*to David*) would have been as interested in really dealing with this problem [of commitment] now if you hadn't felt some strong feelings toward Lisa. And I think you were very ready and interested in coming in and working on things. So I think that there's a real caring and real involvement, and you have to see where that goes right now. (*To Lisa*) What are you thinking about?

[*Again, the therapist emphasized, in effect, that life is to be lived in living, not in interminable psychotherapy—a key value position of the brief therapist, as discussed in Chapter 1.*]

L: I agree. I mean I feel very strongly for David, and I mentioned that before, and I'm willing to work at it. It's going to take work, but I want to do that. And it's hard for me sometimes to talk, because it comes back to initiating the conversations and wanting David to become more comfortable with that too.

T: Yes. We have to stop soon. Let me suggest this to you. What I think would be helpful is for the two of you to plan now to really be doing some work together over the next several months, and continuing to talk with one another and continuing to discuss the relationship and what's going on in the relationship, and keeping that active and keeping that alive rather than letting it fall to the background. And what I would like to do is to set up a time to meet with you [both] in the spring [5 months later]. I'd like to meet with the two of you again. I'll set up the time and see where things are at that point. Hopefully, what you will have done over that time is been able to keep up the work that got started here and move forward. Hopefully, there will be some progress.

D: That sounds real good.

L: Fine with me.

[This episode of the treatment ended with substantial progress made by David. It was clear that he remained ambivalent to some degree, and there was no certainty as to where David and Lisa would go as a couple. However, David's interactions with Lisa appeared to be much less dominated by Kate's death. There was substantial change but no "cure," which was (and is) highly unlikely ever to occur. David and Lisa were to return in the future after an opportunity for *them* to work on their relationship during a treatment-free period.]

[*Note that this for-now-final session ended with the clear implication by the therapist that change is a continuous process, and that the therapist would remain available to David and Lisa as their lives unfolded.*]

References

Adler, G. (1986). Psychotherapy of the narcissistic personality disorder patient: Two contrasting approaches. *American Journal of Psychiatry, 143,* 430–436.

Ahrons, C. R. (1979). The binuclear family: Two households, one family. *Alternative Lifestyles, 2,* 499–515.

Ahrons, C. R. (1981). The continuing co-parental relationship between divorced spouses. *American Journal of Orthopsychiatry, 51,* 415–428.

Alexander, F., & French, T. M. (1974). *Psychoanalytic therapy: Principles and application.* Lincoln: University of Nebraska Press. (Original work published 1946)

American Psychiatric Association. (1980). *Diagnostic and statistical manual of mental disorders* (3rd ed.). Washington, DC: Author.

Anderson, C. M., Reiss, D. J., & Hogarty, G. E. (1986). *Schizophrenia in the family: A practitioner's guide to psychoeducation and management.* New York: Guilford Press.

Anderson, J. A. D., Basker, M. A., & Dalton, R. (1975). Migraine and hypnotherapy. *International Journal of Clinical and Experimental Hypnosis, 13,* 48–58.

Andrews, G., & Harvey, R. (1981). Does psychotherapy benefit neurotic patients? A re-analysis of the Smith, Glass and Miller data. *Archives of General Psychiatry, 38,* 1203–1508.

Appelbaum, S. A. (1977). *The anatomy of change: A Menninger Foundation report on testing the effects of psychotherapy.* New York: Plenum Press.

Appelbaum, S. A. (1975). The idealization of insight. *International Journal of Psychoanalytic Psychotherapy, 4,* 272–302.

Appelbaum, S. A. (1981). *Effective change in psychotherapy.* New York: Jason Aronson.

Araoz, D. L. (1985). *The new hypnosis.* New York: Brunner/Mazel.

Atchley, R. (1975). Dimensions of widowhood in late life. *Gerontologist, 15,* 176–178.

Bagarozzi, D. A., & Giddings, C. W. (1984). The role of cognitive constructs and attributional processes in family therapy: Integrating intrapersonal, interpersonal and systems dynamics. In L. Wolberg & M. Aronson (Eds.), *Group and family therapy 1983* (pp. 207–219). New York: Brunner/Mazel.

Baker, O. V., Druckman, J. M., & Flagle, J. E. (1980). *Helping youth and families of separation, divorce and remarriage.* Palo Alto, CA: American Institutes for Research.

Balint, M., Ornstein, P. H., & Balint, E. (1972). *Focal psychotherapy.* London: Tavistock.

Bandura, A. (1977). Self-efficacy: Toward a unifying theory of behavioral change. *Psychological Review, 84,* 191–215.

Bandura, A. (1982). The psychology of chance encounters and life paths. *American Psychologist, 37,* 747–755.

Barber, T. X. (1984a). Changing "unchangeable" bodily processes by (hypnotic) suggestions: A new look at hypnosis, cognitions, imagining and the mind–body problem. In A. A. Sheikh (Ed.), *Imagination and healing* (pp. 69–127). New York: Baywood.

Barber, T. X. (1984b). Hypnosis, deep relaxation, and active relaxation: Data, theory and clinical applications. In R. L. Woolfolk & P. M. Lehrer (Eds.), *Principles and practice of stress management* (pp. 142–187). New York: Guilford Press.

Barber, T. X., Spanos, N. P., & Chaves, J. F. (1974). *Hypnosis, imagination and human potentialities.* New York: Pergamon Press.

Barber, T. X., & Wilson, S. C. (1977). Hypnosis, suggestions and altered states of consciousness: Experimental evaluation of the new cognitive–behavioral theory and traditional trance state of hypnosis. *Annals of the New York Academy of Sciences, 296,* 34–47.

Barlow, D. H., O'Brien, G. T., & Last, C. (1984). Couples therapy of agoraphobia. *Behavior Therapy, 15,* 41–58.

Barrett, J. E. (1979). The relationship of life events to the onset of neurotic disorders. In J. E. Barrett (Ed.), *Stress and mental disorder* (pp. 87–109). New York: Raven Press.

Bassis, M. S., Gelles, R. J., & Levine, A. (1984). *Sociology: An introduction.* New York: Random House.

Beal, E. W. (1980). Separation, divorce, and single-parent families. In E. A. Carter & M. McGoldrick (Eds.), *The family life cycle: Framework for family therapy* (pp. 241–264). New York: Gardner Press.

Beck, A. T., Emery, G., & Greenberg, R. L. (1985). *Anxiety disorders and phobias.* New York: Basic Books.

Beck, A. T., Rush, J. A., Shaw, B. F., & Emery, G. (1979). *Cognitive therapy of depression.* New York: Guilford Press.

Bennett, M. J. (1983). Focal psychotherapy—terminable and interminable. *American Journal of Psychotherapy, 37,* 365–375.

Bennett, M. J., & Feldstein, M. L. (1986). Correlates of patient satisfaction with mental health services in a health maintenance organization. *American Journal of Preventive Medicine, 2,* 155–162.

Bennett, M. J., & Wisneski, M. J. (1979). Continuous psychotherapy within an HMO. *American Journal of Psychiatry, 136,* 1283–1287.

Benson, H., Greenwood, M. M., & Klemchuck, H. (1975). The relaxation response: Psychophysiologic aspects and clinical applications. *International Journal of Psychiatry in Medicine, 6,* 87–97.

Bergin, A. E. (1971). The evaluation of therapeutic outcome. In A. E. Bergin & S. L. Garfield (Eds.), *Handbook of psychotherapy and behavior change* (pp. 217–270). New York: Wiley.

Bergin, A. E., & Garfield, S. L. (Eds.). (1971). *Handbook of psychotherapy and behavior change.* New York: Wiley.

Bergin, A. E., & Lambert, M. J. (1978). The evaluation of therapeutic outcomes. In S. L. Garfield & A. E. Bergin (Eds.), *Handbook of psychotherapy and behavior change* (2nd ed., pp. 139–190). New York: Wiley.

Berman, E. M. (1982). The individual interview as a treatment technique in conjoint therapy. *American Journal of Family Therapy, 10,* 27–37.

Beutler, L. E. (1983). *Eclectic psychotherapy: A systematic approach.* New York: Pergamon Press.

Beutler, L. E., Crago, M., & Arizmendi, T. G. (1986). Research on therapist variables in psychotherapy. In S. L. Garfield & A. E. Bergin (Eds.), *Handbook of psychotherapy and behavior change* (3rd ed., pp. 257–310). New York: Wiley.

Bloch, D. A. (1980). Divorcing: Clinical notes. In M. Andolfi & I. Zwerling (Eds.), *Dimensions of family therapy* (pp. 91–108). New York: Guilford Press.

Block, J., & Haan, N. (1971). *Lives through time.* Berkeley: Brancroft Books.

Bloom, B. L. (1981). Focused single-session therapy: Initial development and evaluation. In S. H. Budman (Ed.), *Forms of brief therapy* (pp. 167–218). New York: Guilford Press.

Bloom, B. L., Asher, S. J., & White, S. F. (1978). Marital disruption as a stressor: A review and analysis. *Psychological Bulletin, 85,* 867–894.

Bogdan, J. (1984). Family organization as an ecology of ideas: An alternative to the reification of family systems. *Family Process, 23,* 375–388.

Bordin, E. S. (1979). The generalizability of the psychoanalytic concept of the working alliance. *Psychotherapy: Theory, Research, and Practice, 16,* 252–260.

Bowers, K. S. (1976). *Hypnosis for the seriously curious.* New York: Norton.

Bowlby, J. (1969). *Attachment and loss: Vol. 1. Attachment.* New York: Basic Books.

Bowlby, J. (1973). *Attachment and loss: Vol. 2. Separation: Anxiety and anger.* New York: Basic Books.

Bremer, J. (1951). A social psychiatric investigation of a small community in northern Norway. *Acta Psychiatrica et Neurologica Scandinavica,* (Suppl. 62), 1–166.

Brewster, F., & Montie, K. (1987). A double life: What do family therapists really do in private practice? *The Family Therapy Networker, 11*(1), 33–35, 37.

Brown, B. B. (1978). Social and psychological correlates of help-seeking behavior among urban adults. *American Journal of Community Psychology, 6,* 425–439.

Brown, G. W., & Birley, J. L. T. (1968). Crises and life changes and the outset of schizophrenia. *Journal of Health and Social Behavior, 9,* 203–214.

Brown, G. W., & Harris, T. (1978). *Social origins of depression: A study of psychiatric disorder in women.* New York: Free Press.

Brown, H. C. (1980). From little acorns to tall oaks: From boranes through organoboranes. *Science, 210,* 485–492.

Budman, S. H. (1981a). Avoiding dropouts in couples group therapy. In A. S. Gurman (Ed.), *Questions and answers in the practice of family therapy* (pp. 71–73). New York: Brunner/Mazel.

Budman, S. H. (1981b). Significant treatment factors in short-term group psychotherapy. *Group, 5*(4), 25–31.

Budman, S. H. (1985). Psychotherapeutic services in the HMO: Zen and the art of mental health maintenance. *Professional Psychology: Research and Practice, 16,* 798–809.

Budman, S. H., & Bennett, M. J. (1983). Short-term group psychotherapy. In H. Kaplan & B. Sadock (Eds.), *Comprehensive group psychotherapy* (rev. ed., pp. 138–144). Baltimore: Williams & Wilkins.

Budman, S. H., Bennett, M. J., & Wisneski, M. J. (1981). An adult developmental model of group psychotherapy. In S. H. Budman (Ed.), *Forms of brief therapy* (pp. 305–342). New York: Guilford Press.

Budman, S. H., & Clifford, M. (1979). Short-term group therapy for couples in a health maintenance organization. *Professional Psychology: Research and Practice, 10,* 419–429.

Budman, S. H., Clifford, M., Bader, L., & Bader, B. (1981). Experiential pre-group preparation and screening. *Group, 5*(1), 19–26.

Budman, S. H., Demby, A., Feldstein, M., Redondo, J., Scherz, B., Bennett, M. J., Koppenaal, G., Daley, B. S., Hunter, M., & Ellis, J. (1987). Preliminary findings on a new instrument to measure cohesion in group psychotherapy. *International Journal of Group Psychotherapy, 37,* 75–94.

Budman, S. H., Demby, A., & Randall, M. (1980). Short-term group psychotherapy: Who succeeds and who fails? *Group, 4,* 3–16.

Budman, S. H., Demby, A., & Randall, M. (1982). Psychotherapeutic outcome and reduction in medical utilization: A cautionary tale. *Professional Psychology: Research and Practice, 13,* 200–207.

Budman, S. H., Demby, A., Redondo, J. P., Hannan, M., Feldstein, M., and Ring, J. (in press). Comparative outcome in time limited individual and group psychotherapy. *International Journal of Group Psychotherapy.*

Budman, S. H., & Gurman, A. S. (1983). The practice of brief therapy. *Professional Psychology: Research and Practice, 14,* 277–292.

Budman, S. H., & Springer, T. (in press). Treatment delay, outcome and satisfaction in time-limited group and individual psychotherapy. *Professional Psychology: Research and Practice.*

Burdick, D. (1975). Rehabilitation of breast cancer patients. *Cancer, 36,* 645–648.

Burgess, A., & Holstrom, L. (1974). Rape trauma syndrome. *American Journal of Psychiatry, 131,* 981–985.

Butcher, J. N., & Koss, M. P. (1978). Research on brief and crisis-oriented therapies. In S. Garfield & A. E. Bergin (Eds.), *Handbook of psychotherapy and behavior change* (2nd ed., pp. 725–768). New York: Wiley.

Butler, T., & Fuhriman, A. (1983). Curative factors in group therapy: A review of the recent literature. *Small Group Behavior, 4,* 131–142.

Carson, R. C. (1982). Self-fulfilling prophecy, maladaptive behavior, and psychotherapy. In J. C. Anchin & D. J. Kiesler (Eds.), *Handbook of interpersonal psychotherapy* (pp. 64–77). NY: Pergamon Press.

Carter, E. A., & McGoldrick, M. (Eds.). (1980). *The family life cycle: Framework for family therapy.* New York: Gardner Press.

Cautela, J. R. (1975). The use of covert conditioning in hypnotherapy. *International Journal of Clinical and Experimental Hypnosis, 23,* 15–27.

Chaves, J. F. (1980). *Hypnotic control of surgical bleeding.* Paper presented at the annual meeting of the American Psychological Association, Montreal.

Clarkin, J. F., Widiger, T., Frances, A. J., Hurt, S. W., & Gilmore, M. (1983). Prototypic typology and the borderline personality disorder. *Journal of Abnormal Psychology, 92,* 263–273.

Clausen, J. A., & Yarrow, M. R. (1955). Paths to the mental hospital. *Journal of Social Issues, 11,* 25–32.

Coates, D., & Winston, T. (1983). Counteracting the deviance of depression. *Journal of Social Issues, 39,* 171–196.

Cochrane, G., & Friesen, J. (1986). Hypnotherapy in weight loss treatment. *Journal of Consulting and Clinical Psychology, 54,* 489–492.

Cohen, S., & Wills, T. A. (1985). Stress, social support, and the buffering hypothesis. *Psychological Bulletin, 98,* 310–357.

Cohler, B. (1981a). Adult developmental psychology and reconstruction in psychoanalysis. In S. I. Greenspan & G. H. Pollock (Eds.), *The course of life: Psychoanalytic contributions toward understanding personality development. Volume 3. Adulthood and the aging process* (DHHS Publication No. ADM 81-1000, pp. 149–199). Washington, DC: U.S. Government Printing Office.

Cohler, B. (1981b). Personal narrative and life-course. In P. Baltes & O. G. Brim, Jr. (Eds.), *Life-span development and behavior* (Vol. 4, pp. 206–243). New York: Academic Press.

Cohler, B. J., & Boxer, A. M. (1984). Middle adulthood: Settling into the world—person, time, and context. In D. Offer and M. Sabshin (Eds.), *Normality and the life cycle* (pp. 145–203). New York: Basic Books.

Coleman, R. M. (1983). Diagnosis, treatment, and follow-up of about 8,000 sleep/wake disorder patients. In C. Guilleminault & E. Lugaresi (Eds.), *Sleep/wake disorders: Natural history of epidemiology, and long-term evolution* (pp. 87–97). New York: Raven Press.

Conn, J. H. (1972). Is hypnosis really dangerous? *International Journal of Clinical and Experimental Hypnosis, 20,* 61–79.

Constantine, L. L. (1986). *Family paradigms: The practice of theory in family therapy.* New York: Guilford Press.

Cooper, L., & Erickson, M. H. (1959). *Time distortion in hypnosis.* Baltimore: Williams & Wilkins.

Coyne, J. C. (1987). Depression, biology, marriage and marital therapy. *Journal of Marital and Family Therapy, 13,* 393–407.

Crosbie-Burnett, M., & Ahrons, C. R. (1985). From divorce to remarriage: Implications for therapy with families in transition. In D. H. Sprenkle (Ed.), *Divorce therapy* (pp. 121–138). New York: Haworth Press.

Cummings, N. A. (1977). Prolonged (ideal) versus short-term (realistic) psychotherapy. *Professional Psychology: Research and Practice, 8,* 491–501.

Cummings, N. A., & VandenBos, G. (1979). The general practice of psychology. *Professional Psychology: Research and Practice, 10,* 430–440.

Davanloo, H. (Ed.). (1978a). *Basic principles and techniques in short-term dynamic psychotherapy.* New York: Spectrum.

Davanloo, H. (1978b). Evaluation criteria for selection of patients for short-term dynamic psychotherapy: A metapsychological approach. In H. Davanloo (Ed.), *Basic principles and techniques in short-term dynamic psychotherapy* (pp. 9–34). New York: Spectrum.

Davanloo, H. (1980). A method of short-term dynamic psychotherapy. In H. Davanloo (Ed.), *Short-term dynamic psychotherapy* (pp. 43–71). New York: Jason Aronson.

Dengrove, E. (Ed.). (1976). *Hypnosis and behavior therapy.* Springfield, IL: Charles C Thomas.

DePiano, F. A., & Salzberg, H. C. (1979). Clinical applications of hypnosis in three psychosomatic disorders. *Psychological Bulletin, 86,* 1223–1235.

De Shazer, S. (1982). *Patterns of brief therapy.* New York: Guilford Press.

De Shazer, S. (1985). *Keys to solution in brief therapy.* New York: Norton.

Diamond, M. J. (1972). The use of observationally presented information to modify hypnotic susceptibility. *Journal of Abnormal Psychology, 79,* 174–180.

Diamond, M. J. (1977). Hypnotizability is modifiable: An alternative approach. *International Journal of Clinical and Experimental Hypnosis, 25,* 147–166.

Docherty, J. P., Fiester, S. J., & Shea, T. (1986). Syndrome diagnosis and personality disorder. In A. J. Frances & R. E. Hales (Eds.), *Psychiatry update: American Psychiatric Association annual review* (Vol. 5, pp. 315–355). Washington, DC: American Psychiatric Association.

Dohrenwend, B. P., Dohrenwend, B. S., Gould, M. S., Link, B., Neugebauer, R., & Wunsch-Hitzig, R. (1980). *Mental Illness in the United States: Epidemiological estimates.* New York: Praeger.

Donovan, J., Bennett, M. J., & McElroy, C. M. (1981). The crisis group: Its rationale, format, and outcome. In S. H. Budman (Ed.), *Forms of brief therapy* (pp. 283–304). New York: Guilford Press.

Duhl, B., & Duhl, F. (1981). Integrative family therapy. In A. Gurman & D. Kniskern (Eds.), *Handbook of family therapy* (pp. 483–513). New York: Brunner/Mazel.

Edelson, M. (1963). *The termination of intensive psychotherapy.* Springfield, IL: Charles C Thomas.

Edelstien, M. G. (1981). *Trauma, trance and transformation.* New York: Brunner/Mazel.

Elder, G. H. (1974). *Children of the Great Depression.* Chicago: University of Chicago Press.

Elder, G. H., & Rockwell, R. (1978). Economic depression and postwar opportunity: A study of life patterns and health. In R. Simmons (Ed.), *Research in community and mental health* (pp. 249–304). Greenwich, CT: JAI Press.

Elkin, I. (1986, June 19). *NIMH Treatment of Depression Collaborative Research Program.* Paper presented at the annual meeting of the Society for Psychotherapy Research, Wellesley, MA.

Ellenberger, H. F. (1970). *Discovery of the unconscious.* New York: Basic Books.

Emde, R. N., & Sorce, J. F. (1984). Infancy: Perspectives on normality. In D. Offer & M. Sabshin (Eds.), *Normality and the life cycle* (pp. 3–29). New York: Basic Books.

Epstein, N. B., & Bishop, D. S. (1981). Problem-centered systems therapy of the family. In A. S. Gurman & D. P. Kniskern (Eds.), *Handbook of family therapy* (pp. 444–482). New York: Brunner/Mazel.

Erickson, M. H. (1964). The confusion technique in hypnosis. *American Journal of Clinical Hypnosis, 6,* 183–207.

Erickson, M. H. (1980). An introduction to the study and application of hypnosis for pain control. In E. L. Rossi (Ed.), *Innovative hypnotherapy: Collected papers of Milton H. Erickson on hypnosis* (Vol. 4, pp. 237–245). New York: Irvington. (Original work published 1967)

Erickson, M. H. (1980). *Innovative hypnotherapy: Collected papers of Milton H. Erickson and hypnosis* (Vol. 4, E. L. Rossi, Ed.). New York: Irvington.

Erickson, M. H., & Rossi, E. L. (1979). *Hypnotherapy: An exploratory casebook.* New York: Irvington.

Erickson, M. H., & Rossi, E. L. (1981). *Experiencing hypnosis.* New York: Irvington.

Erickson, M. H., Rossi, E. L., & Rossi, S. I. (1976). *Hypnotic realities.* New York: Irvington.

Erikson, E. H. (1959). Identity and the life cycle. *Psychological Issues, 1*(1, Monograph 1).

Erikson, E. H. (1963). *Childhood and society.* New York: Norton.

Essen-Moller, E. (1956). Individual traits and morbidity in a Swedish rural population. *Acta Psychiatrica et Neurologica Scandinavica,* (Suppl. 100), 1–160.

Ewin, D. M. (1978). Clinical use of hypnosis for the attenuation of burn depth. In F. H. Frankel & H. S. Zamansky (Eds.), *Hypnosis at its bicentennial* (pp. 155–162). New York: Plenum.

Falloon, I. R. H., Boyd, J. L., & McGill, C. W. (1984). *Family care of schizophrenia.* New York: Guilford Press.

Feldman, L. B., & Pinsof, W. M. (1982). Problem maintenance in family systems: An integrative model. *Journal of Marital and Family Therapy, 8,* 295–308.

Ferenczi, S., & Rank, O. (1925). *The development of psychoanalysis.* (C. Newton, trans.). New York: Nervous and Mental Disease Publishing.

Ferster, C. B., & Perrott, M. C. (1968). *Behavior principles.* New York: New Century.

Festinger, L., Schacter, S., & Back, K. (1963). *Social pressures in informal groups* (rev. ed.). Palo Alto, CA: Stanford University Press.

Fierman, L. B. (Ed.). (1965). *Effective psychotherapy: The contributions of Hellmuth Kaiser.* New York: Free Press.

Figley, C. R. (1985). From victim to survivor: Social responsibility in the wake of catastrophe. In C. R. Figley (Ed.), *Trauma and its wake* (pp. 398–415). New York: Brunner/Mazel.

Firestein, S. K. (1978). *Termination in psychoanalysis.* New York: International Universities Press.

Fisch, R., Weakland, J. H., & Segal, L. (1982). *The tactics of change: Doing therapy briefly.* San Francisco: Jossey-Bass.

Flegenheimer, W. V. (1982). *Techniques of brief psychotherapy.* New York: Jason Aronson.

Folkins, C. H., & Sime, W. E. (1981). Physical fitness training and mental health. *American Psychologist, 36,* 373–389.

Foreman, S. A., & Marmar, C. R. (1985). Therapist actions that address initially poor therapeutic alliances in psychotherapy. *American Journal of Psychiatry, 142,* 922–926.

Frances, A. J., & Clarkin, J. F. (1981). No treatment as the prescription of choice. *Archives of General Psychiatry, 38,* 542–545.

Frances, A. J., & Widiger, T. (1986). The classification of personality disorders: An overview of problems and situations. In A. J. Frances & R. E. Hales (Eds.), *Psychiatry update: American Psychiatric Association annual review* (Vol. 5, pp. 240–257). Washington, DC: American Psychiatric Association.

Frank, J. D. (1973). *Persuasion and healing: A comparative study of psychotherapy* (2nd ed.). Baltimore: Johns Hopkins University Press.

Frankel, F. H. (1976). *Hypnosis: Trance as a coping mechanism.* New York: Plenum.

Frankl, V. (1969). *The will to meaning.* Cleveland, OH: New American Library.

Freud, A. (1965). *Normality and pathology in childhood: Assessments of development.* New York: International Universities Press.

Freud, S. (1949). Turnings in the ways of psychoanalytic therapy. In E. Jones (Ed.), *The collected works of Sigmund Freud* (Vol. 34, pp. 392–402). London: Hogarth Press. (Original work published 1919)

Freud, S. (1961). Introductory lectures on psychoanalysis, Parts I and II. In J. Strachey (Ed. and Trans.), *The standard edition of the complete psychological works of Sigmund Freud* (Vol. 15, complete). London: Hogarth Press. (Original work published 1916)

Freud, S. (1963). Introductory lectures on psychoanalysis, Part III. In J. Strachey (Ed. and Trans.), *The standard edition of the complete psychological works of Sigmund Freud* (Vol. 16, complete). London: Hogarth Press. (Original work published 1917)

Freud, S. (1964). Analysis terminable and interminable. In J. Strachey (Ed. and Trans.), *The standard edition of the complete psychological works of Sigmund Freud* (Vol. 23, pp. 209–253). London: Hogarth Press. (Original work published 1937)

Frost, P., & Weinstein, G. D. (1971). Ichthyosiform dermatoses. In T. B. Fitzpatrick (Ed.), *Dermatology in general medicine* (pp. 249–265). New York: McGraw-Hill.

Fuhriman, A., Drescher, S., Hanson, E., Henrie, R., & Rybicki, W. (1986). Refining the measurement of curativeness: An empirical approach. *Small Group Behavior, 17,* 186–201.

Gardner, R. A. (1971). *The boys and girls book about divorce.* New York: Bantam.

Gardner, R. A. (1978). *The boys and girls book about one-parent families.* New York: Bantam.

Garfield, S. L. (1971). Research on client variables in psychotherapy. In A. E. Bergin & S. Garfield (Eds.), *Handbook of psychotherapy and behavior change* (pp. 271–298). New York: Wiley.

Garfield, S. L. (1978). Research on client variables in psychotherapy. In S. L. Garfield & A. E. Bergin (Eds.), *Handbook of psychotherapy and behavior change* (2nd ed., pp. 191–232). New York: Wiley.

Garfield, S. L. (1980). *Psychotherapy: An eclectic approach.* New York: Wiley.

Garfield, S. L. (1986). Research on client variables in psychotherapy. In S. L. Garfield & A. E. Bergin (Eds.), *Handbook of psychotherapy and behavior change* (3rd ed., pp. 213–256). New York: Wiley.

Garfield, S. L., & Bergin, A. E. (Eds.) (1978). *Handbook of psychotherapy and behavior change* (2nd ed.). New York: Wiley.

Garfield, S. L., & Bergin, A. E. (Eds.) (1986). *Handbook of psychotherapy and behavior change* (3rd ed.). New York: Wiley.

Gartrell, N., Herman, J., Olarte, S., Feldstein, M., & Localio, R. (1986). Sexual contact: Results of a national survey, psychiatrist–patient contact. Part I: Prevalence. *American Journal of Psychiatry, 43,* 1126–1131.

Gedo, J., & Goldberg, A. (1973). *Models of the mind.* Chicago: University of Chicago Press.

Gergen, K. J. (1980). The emerging crisis in life-span developmental theory. In P. Baltes & O. G. Brim, Jr. (Eds.), *Life-span development and behavior* (Vol. 3, pp. 32–63). New York: Academic Press.

Gilligan, C. (1982). *In a different voice.* Cambridge, MA: Harvard University Press.

Glick, I. D., & Clarkin, J. F. (1985). *Inpatient family intervention for affective disorders.* Unpublished manuscript, Cornell University Medical Center.

Glick, P. C. (1979). *The future of the family* (Current Population Reports, Special Studies Series P-23, No. 78). Washington, DC: U.S. Government Printing Office.

Glick, P. C. (1984). Marriage, divorce and living arrangements: Prospective changes. *Journal of Family Issues, 5,* 7–26.

Glick, P. C., & Norton, A. J. (1976, October). *Number, timing and duration of marriages and divorces in the U.S.: June, 1975* (Current Population Reports, Series P-20, No. 65). U.S. Government Printing Office.

Glick, P. C., & Norton, A. J. (1977). Marrying, divorcing and living together in the U.S. today. *Population Bulletin, 32*(5).

Goldensohn, S. S. (1977). Graduate evaluation of psychoanalytic training. *Journal of the American Academy of Psychoanalysis, 5*, 51–64.

Goldsmith, J. (1982). The postdivorce family system. In F. Walsh (Ed.), *Normal family processes* (pp. 297–330). New York: Guilford Press.

Goodman, S. H., Sewell, D. R., & Jampol, R. C. (1984). On going to the counselor: Contributions of life stress and social supports to the decision to seek psychological counseling. *Journal of Counseling Psychology, 31*, 306–313.

Gordon, K. S., & Zax, M. (1981). Once more into the breach dear friends . . . A reconsideration of the literature on symptom substitution. *Clinical Psychology Review, 1*, 33–47.

Gould, R. L. (1978). *Transformations.* New York: Simon & Schuster.

Granvold, D. K. (1983). Structured separation for marital treatment and decision-making. *Journal of Marital and Family Therapy, 9*, 403–412.

Granvold, D. K., & Tarrant, R. (1983). Structured marital separation as a marital treatment method. *Journal of Marital and Family Therapy, 9*, 189–198.

Greene, B. L., Lee, R. R., & Lustig, N. (1974, September). Conscious and unconscious factors in marital infidelity. *Medical Aspects of Human Sexuality,* pp. 87–105.

Gregory, J., & Diamond, M. J. (1973). Increasing hypnotic susceptibility by means of positive expectancies and written instructions. *Journal of Abnormal Psychology, 82*, 363–367.

Grinder, J., & Bandler, R. (1981). *Trance-formations: Neuro-linguistic programming and the structure of hypnosis.* Moab, UT: Real People Press.

Grinker, R. R., & Spiegel, J. P. (1944). Brief psychotherapy in war neuroses. *Psychosomatic Medicine, 6*, 123–131.

Grunebaum, H. (1983). A study of therapists' choice of a therapist. *American Journal of Psychiatry, 140*, 1336–1339.

Gunderson, J. G., Siever, L. J., & Spaulding, E. (1983). The search for a schizotype: Crossing the border again. *Archives of General Psychiatry, 40*, 15–22.

Gurin, E., Veroff, J., & Feld, S. (1960). *Americans view their mental health.* New York: Basic Books.

Gurman, A. S. (1978). Contemporary marital therapies: A critique and comparative analysis of psychodynamic, behavioral and systems theory approaches. In T. Paolino & B. McCrady ((Eds.), *Marriage and marital therapy* (pp. 445–566). New York: Brunner/Mazel.

Gurman, A. S. (1981). Integrative marital therapy: Toward the development of an interpersonal approach. In S. H. Budman (Ed.), *Forms of brief therapy* (pp. 415–457). New York: Guilford Press.

Gurman, A. S. (Ed.). (1985a). *Casebook of marital therapy.* New York: Guilford Press.

Gurman, A. S. (1985b). The therapist's role when couples divorce. *The Family Therapy Networker, 9*(2), 17–18.

Gurman, A. S. (1985c). Tradition and transition: A rural marriage in crisis. In A. S. Gurman (Ed.), *Casebook of marital therapy* (pp. 303–336). New York: Guilford Press.

Gurman, A. S. (1987). Case commentary: The risky business of marriage saving. *The Family Therapy Networker, 11*(1), 57.

Gurman, A. S., & Jacobson, N. S. (1986). Marital therapy: From technique to theory, back again, and beyond. In N. S. Jacobson & A. S. Gurman (Eds.), *Clinical handbook of marital therapy* (pp. 1–12). New York: Guilford Press.

Gurman, A. S., & Kniskern, D. P. (1978a). Deterioration in marital and family therapy: Empirical, clinical and conceptual issues. *Family Process, 17*, 3–20.

Gurman, A. S., & Kniskern, D. P. (1978b). Research on marital and family therapy: Progress, perspective and prospect. In S. L. Garfield & A. E. Bergin (Eds.), *Handbook of psychotherapy and behavior change* (2nd ed., pp. 817–902). New York: Wiley.

Gurman, A. S., & Kniskern, D. P. (1979). Marriage therapy and/or family therapy: What's in a name? *American Association for Marriage and Family Therapy Newsletter, 10,* 1, 5–6, 8.

Gurman, A. S., & Kniskern, D. P. (1981). Family therapy outcome research: Knowns and unknowns. In A. S. Gurman & D. P. Kniskern (Eds.), *Handbook of family therapy* (pp. 742–775). New York: Brunner/Mazel.

Gurman, A. S., & Kniskern, D. P., & Pinsof, W. M. (1986). Research on the process and outcome of marital and family therapy. In S. L. Garfield & A. E. Bergin (Eds.), *Handbook of psychotherapy and behavior change* (3rd ed., pp. 565–626). New York: Wiley.

Gutmann, D. (1977). The cross-cultural perspective: Notes toward a comparative psychology of aging: In J. Birren & K. W. Schaie (Eds.), *Handbook of the psychology of aging* (pp. 302–326). New York: Van Nostrand Reinhold.

Hafner, J. (1986). Marital therapy for agoraphobia. In N. S. Jacobson & A. S. Gurman (Eds.), *Clinical handbook of marital therapy* (pp. 471–494). New York: Guilford Press.

Haley, J. (1973). *Uncommon therapy: The psychiatric techniques of Milton H. Erickson, M.D.* New York: Norton.

Haley, J. (1976). *Problem solving therapy.* San Francisco: Jossey-Bass.

Harkaway, J. E. (Ed.). (1986). *Family therapy collections: Vol. 20. Eating disorders.* Rockville, MD: Aspen.

Hartlaub, G. H., Martin, G. L., & Rhine, M. W. (1986). Recontact with the analyst following termination: A survey of seventy-one cases. *Journal of the American Psychoanalytic Association, 34,* 895–910.

Hatcher, S. L., & Hatcher, R. L. (1983). Set a place for Elijah: Problems of the spouses and parents of psychotherapy patients. *Psychotherapy: Theory, Research, and Practice, 20,* 75–80.

Hauri, P. J., & Sateia, M. J. (1985). Nonpharmacological treatment of sleep disorders. In R. E. Hales & A. J. Frances (Eds.), *Psychiatry update: The American Psychiatric Association annual review* (Vol. 4, pp. 361–378). Washington, DC: American Psychiatric Association.

Hebbel, C. F. (1850/1939). *Freidrich Hebbel's Herodes and Mariamne: A free adaptation* (Clements Dane, Trans.). London: Heinemann.

Henderson, S., Byrne, D. G., & Duncan-Jones, P. (1982). *Neurosis and the social environment.* Sydney: Academic Press.

Henry, W. E., Sims, J. H., & Spray, S. L. (1971). *The fifth profession.* San Francisco: Jossey-Bass.

Hetherington, E. M., Cox, M., & Cox, R. (1977). The aftermath of divorce. In J. J. Stevens, Jr., & M. Matthews (Eds.), *Mother–child, father–child relations* (pp. 149–176). Washington, DC: National Association for the Education of Young Children.

Hilgard, E. R. (1965). *Hypnotic susceptibility.* New York: Harcourt Brace Jovanovich.

Hilgard, E. R. (1974). Toward a neodissociation theory: Multiple cognitive controls in human functioning. *Perspectives in Biology and Medicine, 17,* 301–316.

Hilgard, E. R., & Hilgard, J. R. (1983). *Hypnosis in the relief of pain.* Los Altos, CA: William Kaufman.

Hilgard, J. R. (1970). *Personality and hypnosis: A study of imaginative involvement.* Chicago: University of Chicago Press.

Hilgard, J. R. (1972). Evidence for a developmental–interactive theory of hypnotic susceptibility. In E. Fromm & R. E. Shor (Eds.), *Hypnosis: Research developments and perspectives* (pp. 387–397). Chicago: University of Chicago Press.

Hilgard, J. R. (1974). Imaginative involvement: Some characteristics of the highly hypnotizable and non-hypnotizable. *International Journal of Clinical and Experimental Hypnosis, 22,* 138–156.

Hilgard, J. R. (1979). *Personality and hypnosis* (2nd ed.). Chicago: University of Chicago Press.

Hobbs, N. (1962). Sources of gain in psychotherapy. *American Psychologist, 17*, 741–747.

Holroyd, J. (1980). Hypnosis treatment for smoking. *International Journal of Clinical and Experimental Hypnosis, 28*, 341–357.

Horowitz, M. J., Wilner, N., Marmar, C., & Krupnick, J. (1980). Pathological grief and the activation of latent self images. *American Journal of Psychiatry, 137*, 1137–1162.

Howard, K. I., Kopta, S. M., Krause, M. S., & Orlinsky, D. E. (1986). The dose–effect relationship in psychotherapy. *American Psychologist, 41*, 159–164.

Hoyt, M. F. (1985). Therapist resistances to short-term dynamic psychotherapy. *Journal of the American Academy of Psychoanalysis, 13*, 93–112.

Hugo, V. (1938). *Les miserables* (L. Wraxall, Trans.). New York: Heritage Press. (Original work published 1862)

Humphrey, F. G., & Strong, L. (1976, May). *Treatment of extramarital sexual relationships as reported by clinical members of the American Association of Marriage and Family Counselors.* Paper presented at the conference of the American Association of Marriage and Family Counselors, Hartford, CT.

Hurvitz, N. (1967). Marital problems following psychotherapy with one spouse. *Journal of Consulting and Clinical Psychology, 31*, 38–47.

Ikemi, Y., & Nakagawa, W. (1962). A psychosomatic study of contagious dermatitis. *Kyushmi Journal of Medical Science, 13*, 335–350.

Institute of Medicine. (1979). *Report of a study: Sleeping pills, insomnia, and medical practice.* Washington, DC: National Academy of Sciences.

Jacobson, N. S. (1978). A review of research on the effectiveness of marital therapy. In T. Paolino & B. McCrady (Eds.), *Marriage and marital therapy* (pp. 395–444). New York: Brunner/Mazel.

Jacobson, N. S. (1981). Behavioral marital therapy. In A. S. Gurman & D. P. Kniskern (Eds.), *Handbook of family therapy* (pp. 556–591). New York: Brunner/Mazel.

Jacobson, N. S., & Margolin, G. (1979). *Marital therapy: Strategies based on social learning and behavioral exchange principles.* New York: Brunner/Mazel.

Janoff-Bulman, R. (1985). The aftermath of victimization: Rebuilding shattered assumptions. In C. R. Figley (Ed.), *Trauma and its wake* (pp. 15–35). New York: Brunner/Mazel.

Johnson, D. H., & Gelso, C. J. (1980). The effectiveness of time limits in counseling and psychotherapy: A critical review. *The Counseling Psychologist, 9*, 70–83.

Johnson, S. (1986). Bonds or bargains: Relationship paradigms and their significance for marital therapy. *Journal of Marital and Family Therapy, 12*, 259–267.

Johnson, S. M., & Greenberg, L. S. (1985). Differential effects of experiential and problem-solving interventions in resolving marital conflict. *Journal of Consulting and Clinical Psychology, 53*, 175–184.

Jones, E. (1955). *The life and works of Sigmund Freud* (Vol. 2). New York: Basic Books.

Jung, C. G. (1960). The stages of life. In H. Read, M. Fordham, & G. Adler (Eds.), *The collected works of C. G. Jung: Vol. 8. The structure and dynamics of the psyche* (pp. 384–403). New York: Pantheon. (Original work published 1930–1931)

Kagan, J. (1980). Perspectives on continuity. In O. G. Brim, Jr., & J. Kagan (Eds.), *Constancy and change in human development* (pp. 26–74). Cambridge, MA: Harvard University Press.

Kales, A., Bixler, E. O., Tan, T. L., Scharf, M. B., & Kales, J. D. (1974). Chronic hypnotic-drug use: Ineffectiveness, drug-withdrawal, insomnia, and dependence. *Journal of the American Medical Association, 227*, 513–517.

Kaltreider, N. B., Becker, T., & Horowitz, M. J. (1984). Relationship testing after the loss of a parent. *American Journal of Psychiatry, 141*, 243–246.

Kanfer, F. H., & Saslow, G. (1969). Behavioral diagnosis. In C. Franks (Ed.), *Assessment and status of the behavior therapies* (pp. 417–444). New York: McGraw-Hill.

Kaplan, H. S. (1974). *The new sex therapy.* New York: Brunner/Mazel.

Karacan, I., & Moore, C. A. (1985). Physiology and neurochemistry of sleep disorders. In R. E. Hales & A. J. Frances (Eds.), *Psychiatry update: The American Psychiatric Association annual review* (Vol. 4, pp. 266–293). Washington, DC: American Psychiatric Association.

Karpel, M. A. (1986). *Family resources: The hidden partner in family therapy.* New York: Guilford Press.

Kaslow, F. W. (1981). Divorce and divorce therapy. In A. Gurman & D. Kniskern (Eds.), *Handbook of family therapy* (pp. 662–696). New York: Brunner/Mazel.

Kass, F., Skodol, A. E., Charles, E., Spitzer, R. L., & Williams, J. B. W. (1985). Scaled ratings of DSM-III personality disorders. *American Journal of Psychiatry, 142,* 627–630.

Katz, L., & Stein, S. (1983). Treatment stepfamilies. In B. B. Wolman & G. Stricker (Eds.), *Handbook of family and marital therapy* (pp. 387–420). New York: Plenum.

Katz, N. W. (1979). Comparative efficiency of behavioral training, training plus relaxation, and a sleep/trance hypnotic induction in increasing hypnotic susceptibility. *Journal of Consulting and Clinical Psychology, 47,* 119–127.

Katz, N. W. (1980). Hypnosis and the addictions: A critical review. *Addictive Behaviors, 5,* 41–47.

Keane, T. M., Fairbank, J. A., Caddell, J. M., Zimering, R. T., & Bender, M. E. (1985). A behavioral approach to assessing and treating post-traumatic stress disorder in Vietnam veterans. In C. R. Figley (Ed.), *Trauma and its wake* (pp. 257–294). New York: Brunner/Mazel.

Kegan, R. (1983). *The evolving self.* Cambridge, MA: Harvard University Press.

Kellner, R. (1985). Functional somatic symptoms and hypochondriasis. *Archives of General Psychiatry, 42,* 821–833.

Kernberg, O. (1981, June 20). *Dilemmas in research on long-term psychotherapy.* Paper presented at the meeting of the Society for Psychotherapy Research, Aspen, CO.

Kessler, S. (1975). *The American way of divorce.* Chicago: Nelson-Hall.

Kessler, R. C., & McLeod, J. D. (1985). Social support and mental health in community samples. In S. Cohen & S. L. Syme (Eds.), *Social support and health* (pp. 219–240). New York: Academic Press.

Kiesler, D. J. (1982). Interpersonal theory for personality and psychotherapy. In J. C. Anchin & D. J. Kiesler (Eds.), *Handbook of interpersonal psychotherapy* (pp. 3–24). New York: Springer.

Kihlstrom, J. F. (1985). Hypnosis. *Annual Review of Psychology, 36,* 385–418.

Kinston, W., & Bentovim, A. (1981). Creating a focus for brief marital or family therapy. In S. H. Budman (Ed.), *Forms of brief therapy* (pp. 361–386). New York: Guilford Press.

Kitson, G. C., & Rashke, H. J. (1981). Divorce research: What we need to know. *Journal of Divorce, 4,* 1–37.

Klein, R. H., & Carroll, R. (1986). Patient characteristics and attendance patterns in outpatient group psychotherapy. *International Journal of Group Psychotherapy, 36,* 115–132.

Kleinhauz, M. (1982). Ericksonian techniques in emergency dehypnotization. In J. K. Zeig (Ed.), *Ericksonian approaches to hypnosis and psychotherapy* (pp. 270–278). New York: Brunner/Mazel.

Klerman, G. L., & Clayton, P. (1984). Epidemiologic perspectives on the health consequences of bereavement. In M. Osterweis, F. Solomon, & M. Green (Eds.), *Bereavement: Reactions, consequences, and care* (pp. 15–44). Washington, DC: National Academy Press.

Klerman, G. L., Rounsaville, B., Chevron, E., & Weissman, M. (1984). *Interpersonal psychotherapy of depression.* New York: Basic Books.

Kohl, R. N. (1962). Pathologic reactions of marital partners to improvement of patients. *American Journal of Psychiatry, 118,* 1036–1041.

Kohut, H. (1972). Thoughts on narcissism. *Psychoanalytic Study of the Child, 27*, 360–400.

Kohut, H. (1977). *The restoration of the self.* New York: International Universities Press.

Koss, M. P. (1979). Length of psychotherapy for clients seen in private practice. *Journal of Consulting and Clinical Psychology, 47*, 210–212.

Koss, M. P., & Butcher, J. N. (1986). Research on brief psychotherapy. In S. L. Garfield & A. E. Bergin (Eds.), *Handbook of psychotherapy and behavior change* (3rd ed., pp. 627–670). New York: Wiley.

Kovacs, M., Rush, A. J., Beck, A. J., & Hollon, S. (1981). Depressed outpatients treated with cognitive therapy or pharmacotherapy. *Archives of General Psychiatry, 38*, 33–39.

Kroger, W. S. (1963). *Clinical and experimental hypnosis* (2nd ed.). Philadelphia: J. B. Lippincott.

Kroger, W. S., & Fezler, W. D. (1976). *Hypnosis and modification: Imaginary conditioning.* Philadelphia: J. B. Lippincott.

Kushner, H. (1981). *When bad things happen to good people.* New York: Schocken Books.

Lagner, T. S., & Michael, S. T. (1963). *Life stress and mental health: The Midtown Manhattan Study.* London: Collier/Macmillan.

Lambert, M. J. (1979). Characteristics of patients and their relationship to outcome in brief psychotherapy. *Psychiatric Clinics of North America, 2*, 111–123.

Lambert, M. J., Shapiro, D. A., & Bergin, A. E. (1986). The effectiveness of psychotherapy. In S. L. Garfield & A. E. Bergin (Eds.), *Handbook of psychotherapy and behavior change* (3rd ed., pp. 157–212). New York: Wiley.

Landbook, J. T., & Dawes, R. M. (1982). Psychotherapy outcome: Smith and Glass' conclusions stand up under scrutiny. *American Psychologist, 37*, 504–516.

Lane, T. W. (1986). *A theory of change and a model of psychotherapy research.* Unpublished manuscript, Center for Psychotherapy Research, Department of Psychology, Vanderbilt University.

Langs, R. (1975). Therapeutic misalliances. *International Journal of Psychoanalytic Psychotherapy, 4*, 77–105.

Langsley, D. G. (1978). Comparing clinic and private practice of psychiatry. *American Journal of Psychiatry, 135*, 702–706.

Lankton, S. R., & Lankton, C. H. (1983). *The answer within: A clinical framework of Ericksonian hypnotherapy.* New York: Brunner/Mazel

Lazarus, A. A. (1981). *The practice of multimodal therapy.* New York: McGraw-Hill.

Lazarus, L. W. (1982). Brief psychotherapy of narcissistic disturbances. *Psychotherapy: Theory, Research, and Practice, 19*, 228–236.

Lehrer, P. M., & Woolfolk, R. L. (1984). Are stress reduction techniques interchangeable, or do they have specific effects? A review of the comparative empirical literature. In R. L. Woolfolk & P. M. Lehrer (Eds.), *Principles and practice of stress management* (pp. 404–477). New York: Guilford Press.

Leibovich, M. (1981). Short-term psychotherapy for the borderline personality disorder. *Psychotherapy and Psychosomatics, 35*, 257–264.

Leibovich, M. (1983). Why short-term psychotherapy for borderlines? *Psychotherapy and Psychosomatics, 39*, 1–9.

Leighton, A. H. (1959). *My name is legion: The Stirling County study of psychiatric disorder and sociocultural environment.* New York: Basic Books.

Lerner, M. J. (1970). The desire for justice and reactions to victims: Social psychological studies of some antecedents and consequences. In J. Macaulay & L. Berkowitz (Eds.), *Altruism and helping behavior* (pp. 259–287). New York: Academic Press.

Lerner, M. J. (1980). *The belief in a just world.* New York: Plenum.

Lerner, M. J., & Ellard, J. (1983). *The justice motive: How people define and react to victimization.* Unpublished manuscript, University of Waterloo.

Levin, S. (1962). Indications for analysis and problems of analyzability: Discussion. *Psychoanalytic Quarterly, 31*, 528–531.

Levinson, D., Darrow, C. N., Klein, E. B., Levinson, M. H., & McKee, B. (1978). *The seasons of a man's life.* New York: Knopf.

Lichtenstein, E., & Danaher, B. G. (1976). Modification of smoking behavior: A critical analysis of theory, research and practice. In M. Hersen, R. M. Eisler, & P. M. Miller (Eds.), *Progress in behavior modification* (Vol. 3, pp. 79–132). New York: Academic Press.

Liddle, H. A. (1983). Diagnosis and assessment in family therapy: A comparative analysis of six schools of thought. In B. P. Keeney (Ed.), *Family therapy collections: Vol. 4. Diagnosis and assessment in family therapy* (pp. 1–33). Rockville, MD: Aspen.

Lieberman, M. A., & Borman, L. D. (Eds.) (1979). *Self-help groups for coping with crisis.* San Francisco: Jossey-Bass.

Liebowitz, M. R., Stone, M. H., & Turkat, I.D. (1986). Treatment of personality disorders. In A. J. Frances & R. E. Hales (Eds.), *Psychiatry update: American Psychiatric Association annual review* (Vol. 5, pp. 356–393). Washington, DC: American Psychiatric Association.

Lindemann, E. (1944). Symptomatology and management of acute grief. *American Journal of Psychiatry, 51*, 141–148.

Loewald, H. (1978). *Psychoanalysis and the history of the individual.* New Haven, CT: Yale University Press.

Lopata, H. (1979). *Women as widows: Support systems.* New York: Elsevier/North-Holland.

Lowenthal, M. F., Thurnher, M., & Chiriboga, D. (1975). *Four stages of life.* San Francisco: Jossey-Bass.

Luborsky, L. (1984). *Principles of psychoanalytic psychotherapy: A manual for supportive-expressive treatment.* New York: Basic Books.

Luborsky, L., Chandler, M., Auerbach, A. H., Cohen, J., & Bachrach, H. M. (1971). Factors influencing the outcome of psychotherapy: A review of quantitative research. *Psychological Bulletin, 75*, 145–185.

Luborsky, L., Singer, B., & Luborsky, L. (1975). Comparative studies of psychotherapies. *Archives of General Psychiatry, 32*, 995–1008.

Maas, H., & Kuypers, J. (1974). *From thirty to seventy.* San Francisco: Jossey-Bass.

MacKenzie, K. R., & Livesley, W. T. (1983). A developmental model of brief group therapy. In R. R. Dies & K. R. MacKenzie (Eds.), *Advances in group psychotherapy: Monograph I* (pp. 101–106). New York: International Universities Press.

Madanes, C. (1981). *Strategic family therapy.* San Francisco: Jossey-Bass.

Mahler, M. (1968). *On human symbiosis and the vicissitudes of individuation: Vol. 1. Infantile psychosis.* New York: International Universities Press.

Main, M. (1977). Analysis of a peculiar form of reunion behavior in some day care children: Its history and sequelae in children who are home-reared. In R. Webb (Ed.), *Social development in children: Day care programs and research* (pp. 148–165) Baltimore: Johns Hopkins University Press.

Malan, D. H. (1963). *A study of brief psychotherapy.* New York: Plenum Press.

Malan, D. H. (1976). *The frontiers of brief psychotherapy: An example of the convergence of research and clinical practice.* New York: Plenum.

Mann, J. (1973). *Time-limited psychotherapy.* Cambridge, MA: Harvard University Press.

Mann, J. (1981). The core of time-limited psychotherapy: Time and the central issue. In S. H. Budman (Ed.), *Forms of brief therapy* (pp. 25–44). New York: Guilford Press.

Mann, J., & Goldman, R. (1982). *A casebook in time-limited psychotherapy.* New York: McGraw-Hill.

Marcovitz, F. J., & Smith, J. E. (1983). Patient perceptions of curative factors in short-term group psychotherapy. *International Journal of Group Psychotherapy, 3*, 21–39.

Marmor, J. (1979). Short-term dynamic psychotherapy. *American Journal of Psychiatry, 136,* 149–155.

Marx, J. A., & Gelso, C. J. (1987). Termination of individual counseling in a university counseling center. *Journal of Counseling Psychology, 34,* 3–9.

Mason, A. A. (1952). A case of cogenital ichthyosiform erythrodermia of Brocg treated by hypnosis. *British Medical Journal, 2,* 422–423.

Masters, W. H., & Johnson, V. E. (1970). *Human sexual inadequacy.* Boston, Little, Brown.

Matarazzo, J. (1965). Psychotherapeutic processes. *Annual Review of Psychology, 16,* 181–224.

Mays, D. T., & Franks, C. M. (Eds.). (1985). *Negative outcome in psychotherapy and what to do about it.* New York: Springer.

McCrady, B. S., Noel, N. E., Abrams, D. B., Stout, R. L., Nelson, H. F., & Hay, W. M. (1986). Comparative effectiveness of three types of spouse involvement in outpatient behavioral alcoholism treatment. *Journal of Studies on Alcohol, 47,* 459–467.

McGlashen, T. H. (1986). Schizotypal personality disorder. *Archives of General Psychiatry, 43,* 329–334.

McGoldrick, M., & Carter, E. A. (1980). Forming a remarried family. In E. A. Carter & M. McGoldrick (Eds.), *The family life cycle* (pp. 265–294). New York: Gardner Press.

McGoldrick, M., & Carter, E. A. (1982). The family life cycle. In F. Walsh (Ed.), *Normal family processes* (pp. 167–195). New York: Guilford Press.

McGoldrick, M., Pearce, J. K., & Giordano, J. (Eds.). (1982). *Ethnicity and family therapy.* New York: Guilford Press.

McLean, P. (1982). Behavioral therapy: Theory and research. In A. J. Rush (Ed.), *Short-term psychotherapy for depression.* (pp. 19–49). New York: Guilford Press.

Melges, F. T., & DeMaso, D. R. (1980). Grief resolution therapy: Reliving, revising and revisiting. *American Journal of Psychiatry, 34,* 51–60.

Mellinger, G. D., & Balter, D. (1983). *Prevalence of insomnia and drug treatment.* Paper presented at NIMH Consensus Development Conference on Drugs and Insomnia, Rockville, MD.

Melzack, R., & Wall, P. D. (1982). *The challenge of pain.* New York: Basic Books.

Mendelson, W. B. (1985). Pharmacological treatment of insomnia. In R. E. Hales & A. J. Frances (Eds.), *Psychiatry update: American Psychiatric Association annual review* (Vol. 4, pp. 379–394). Washington, DC: American Psychiatric Association.

Merikangas, K. R., & Weissman, N. M. (1986). Epidemiology of DSM-III Axis II personality disorders. In A. J. Frances & R. EW. Hales (Eds.), *Psychiatry update: American Psychiatric Association annual review* (Vol. 5, pp. 258–278). Washington, DC: American Psychiatric Association.

Messer, S. B. (1986). Behavioral and psychoanalytic perspectives at therapeutic choice points. *American Psychologist, 41,* 1261–1272.

Milton, J. (1962). *Paradise lost* (M. Y. Hughes, Ed.). New York: Odyssey Press. (Original work published 1667).

Minuchin, S. (1974). *Families and family therapy.* Cambridge, MA: Harvard University Press.

Minuchin, S., & Fishman, C. (1981). *Family therapy techniques.* Cambridge, MA: Harvard University Press.

Minuchin, S., Rosman, B., & Baker, L. (1978). *Psychosomatic families.* Cambridge, MA: Harvard University Press.

Mischel, W. (1983). Alternatives in the pursuit of the predictability and consistency of persons: Stable data that yield unstable interpretations. *Journal of Personality, 51,* 578–604.

Morphis, O. L. (1961). Hypnosis and its use in controlling patients with malignancy. *American Journal of Roentgenology, 85,* 897–900.

Mott, T., & Roberts, J. (1979). Obesity and hypnosis: A review of the literature. *American Journal of Clinical Hypnosis, 22,* 3–7.

Murray, H. A. (1938). *Explorations in personality.* New York: Oxford University Press.

Myers, J. K., Lindenthal, J. J., Pepper, A., & Ostrander, D. R. (1972). Life events and mental status: A longitudinal study. *Journal of Health and Social Behavior, 13,* 389–406.

Nadelson, C. M. (1978). Marital therapy from a psychoanalytic perspective. In T. Paolino & B. McCrady (Eds.), *Marriage and marital therapy* (pp. 86–164). New York: Brunner/Mazel.

Neugarten, B. L. (1970). Dynamics of transition from middle age to old age: Adaptation and the life cycle. *Journal of Geriatric Psychiatry, 41,* 71–87.

Neugarten, B. L. (1979). Time, age and the life cycle. *American Journal of Psychiatry, 136,* 149–155.

Nichols, W. C. (1987). *Marital therapy: An integrative approach.* New York: Guilford Press.

Nicholson, R. A., & Berman, J. S. (1983). Is follow-up necessary in evaluating psychotherapy? *Psychological Bulletin, 93,* 261–278

O'Farrell, T. J., Cutter, H. S. G., & Floyd, F. J. (1985). Evaluating behavioral marital therapy for male alcoholics: Effects on marital adjustment and communication from before to after treatment. *Behavior Therapy, 16,* 147–167.

Offer, D. (1969). *The psychological world of the teenager: A study of normal adolescent boys.* New York: Basic Books.

Offer, D. (1984). Preface. In R. Cohen, S. Weissman, & B. J. Cohler (Eds.), *Parenthood as an adult experience.* New York: Guilford Press.

Offer, D., & Offer, J. B. (1975). *From teenage to young manhood: A psychological study.* New York: Basic Books.

Offer, D., Ostrov, E., & Howard, K. I. (1981). *The adolescent: A psychological self-portrait.* New York: Basic Books.

Offer, D., & Sabshin, M. (1984). Patterns of normal development. In D. Offer & M. Sabshin (Eds.), *Normality and the life cycle* (pp. 343–439). New York: Basic Books.

Orlinsky, D. E., & Howard, K. I. (1986). Process and outcome in psychotherapy. In S. L. Garfield & A. E. Bergin (Eds.), *Handbook of psychotherapy and behavior change* (3rd ed., pp. 311–381). New York: Wiley.

Osterweis, M., Solomon, F., & Green, M. (1984). Introduction, In M. Osterweis, F. Solomon, & M. Green (Eds.), *Bereavement: Reactions, consequences, and care* (pp. 3–11). Washington, DC: National Academy Press.

Panel, (1969). Problems of termination in the analysis of adults. (S. K. Firestein, reporter). *Journal of the American Psychanalytic Association, 17,* 222–237.

Panel. (1975). Termination: Problems and techniques (W. S. Robbins, reporter). *Journal of the American Psychoanalytic Association, 23,* 166–176.

Papp, P. (1983). *The process of change.* New York: Guilford Press.

Parad, H. J. (1971). Crisis intervention. In National Association of Social Workers, *Encyclopedia of social work* (pp. 196–202). New York: National Association of Social Workers.

Parad, H. J., & Parad, L. G. (1968). A study of crisis-oriented planned short-term treatment: Part I. *Social Casework, 49,* 346–355.

Parad, L. G., & Parad, H. J. (1968). A study of crisis-oriented planned short-term treatment: Part II. *Social Casework, 49,* 418–426.

Parkes, C. M. (1964). Recent bereavement as a cause of mental illness. *British Journal of Psychiatry, 110,* 198–204.

Parkes, C. M.. & Brown, R. J. (1972). Health after bereavement: A controlled study of young Boston widows and widowers. *Psychosomatic Medicine, 34,* 449–461.

Parkes, C. M., & Stevenson-Hinde, J. (Eds.). (1982). *The place of attachment in human behavior.* New York: Basic Books.

Parloff, M. B., Waskow, I. E., & Wolfe, B. E. (1978). Research on therapist variables in relation to process and outcome. In S. L. Garfield & A. E. Bergin (Eds.), *Handbook of psychotherapy and behavior change* (2nd ed., pp. 233–282). New York: Wiley.

Patterson, G. R., & Hops, H. (1972). Coercion: A game for two: Intervention techniques for marital conflict. In R. Ultich & P. Mountjoy (Eds.), *The experimental analysis of social behavior* (pp. 424–440). New York: Appleton-Century-Crofts.

Patterson, V., Levene, H., & Breger, L. (1977). A one year follow-up study of two forms of brief psychotherapy. *American Journal of Psychotherapy, 31,* 76–82.

Paykel, E. S. (1974). Life stress and psychiatric disorder: Applications of the clinical approach. In B. S. Dohrenwend & B. P. Dohrenwend (Eds.), *Stressful life events: Their nature and effects* (pp. 135–149). New York: Wiley.

Peplau, L. A. (Ed.). (1982). *Loneliness: A sourcebook of current theory, research, and therapy.* New York: Wiley

Perry, C. (1977). Is hypnotizability modifiable? *International Journal of Clinical and Experimental Hypnosis, 25,* 125–146.

Peterson, A. C. (1982). *The early adolescent girl.* Unpublished manuscript.

Pinsof, W. M. (1983). Integrative problem-centered therapy: Toward the synthesis of family and individual psychotherapies. *Journal of Marital and Family Therapy, 9,* 19–35.

Piper, W. E., Debbane, E. G., Garant, J., & Bienvenu, J. (1979). Pretraining for group psychotherapy: A cognitive–experiential approach. *Archives of General Psychiatry, 36,* 1250–1256.

Plakun, E. M., Burkhardt, P., & Muller, J. P. (1984, May). *Fourteen-year follow-up of borderline and schizotypal personality disorders.* Paper presented at the annual meeting of the American Psychiatric Association, Los Angeles.

Platonov, K. (1959). *The word as a psychological and therapeutic factor.* Moscow: foreign Language Publishing House.

Polack, P. R., Egan, D., Vandenbergh, R., & Williams, W. V. (1975). Prevention in mental health. *American Journal of Psychiatry, 132,* 146–149.

Pope, H. (1983). Phenomenology of borderline personality disorder. *Archives of General Psychiatry, 40,* 23–36.

Prochaska, J. O., & DiClemente, C. C. (1982). Transtheoretical therapy: Toward a more integrative model of change. *Psychotherapy: Theory, Research, and Practice, 19,* 276–288.

Rabkin, R. (1977). *Strategic psychotherapy.* New York: Basic Books.

Rahe, R. H., O'Neil, T., Hagan, A., & Arthur, R. J. (1975). Brief group therapy following myocardial infarction: Eighteen months follow-up of a controlled trial. *International Journal of Psychiatry in Medicine, 6,* 349–358.

Rahe, R. H., Tuffli, C. F., Suchor, R. J., & Arthur, R. J. (1973). Group therapy in the outpatient management of post-myocardial infarction patients. *International Journal of Psychiatry in Medicine, 4,* 77–88.

Rahe, R. H., Ward, H. W., & Hayes, V. (1979). Brief group therapy in myocardial infarction rehabilitation: Three to four year follow-up of a controlled trial. *Psychosomatic Medicine, 41,* 229–242.

Reagan, N., & Libby, B. (1980). *Nancy.* New York: Morrow.

Reich, W. (1967). *Reich speaks of Freud* (M. Higgins & C. M. Raphael Eds.). New York: Farrar, Straus & Giroux.

Rice, D. G., & Rice, J. K. (1986). Separation and divorce therapy. In N. S. Jacobson & A. S. Gurman (Eds.), *Clinical handbook of marital therapy* (pp. 279–300). New York: Guilford Press.

Rice, J. K., & Rice, D. G. (1986). *Living through divorce: A developmental approach to divorce therapy.* New York: Guilford Press.

Roazen, P. (1971). *Freud and his followers.* New York: New American Library.

Robin, A., & Foster, S. (in press). *Parent–adolescent conflict: A behavioral–family systems approach to treatment.* New York: Guilford Press.

Robins, L. N. (in press). The epidemiology of antisocial personality. In J. O. Cavenar (Ed.), *Psychiatry*. Philadelphia: J. B. Lippincott.

Roffwarg, H., & Erman, M. (1985). Evaluation and diagnosis of the sleep disorders: Implications for psychiatry and other clinical specialities. In R. E. Hales & A. J. Frances (Eds.), *Psychiatry update: American Psychiatric Association annual review* (Vol. 4, pp. 294–328). Washington, DC: American Psychiatric Association.

Rosenblum, L. A. (1984). Monkeys' responses to separation and loss. In M. Osterweis, F. Solomon, & M. Green (Eds.), *Bereavement: Reactions, consequences and care* (pp. 179–196). Washington, DC: National Academy Press.

Rubenstein, C. M., & Shaver, P. (1982). The experience of loneliness. In A. Peplau & D. Perlman (Eds.), *Loneliness: Theory and research* (pp. 206–223). New York: Wiley.

Rubinstein, E. A., & Lorr, M. (1956). A comparison of terminators and remainers in outpatient psychotherapy. *Journal of Clinical Psychology, 12*, 345–349.

Rutan, J. S., & Stone, W. N. (1984). *Psychodynamic group psychotherapy*. Lexington, MA: Callamore Press.

Sachs, J. S. (1983). Negative factors in brief psychotherapy: An implicit assessment. *Journal of Consulting and Clinical Psychology, 51*, 557–564.

Sager, C. J. (1976). *Marriage contracts and couples therapy*. New York: Brunner/Mazel.

Sager, C. J. (1981). Couples contracts and marital therapy. In A. S. Gurman & D. P. Kniskern (Eds.), *Handbook of family therapy* (pp. 321–344). New York: Brunner/Mazel.

Sager, C. J., Brown, H. S., Crohn, H., Engel, T., Rodstein, E., & Walker, L. (1983). *Treating the remarried family*. New York: Brunner/Mazel.

Salts, C. J. (1985). Divorce stage theory and therapy: Therapeutic implications throughout the divorce process. In D. H. Sprenkle (Ed.), *Divorce therapy* (pp. 13–26). New York: Haworth Press.

Sarbin, T. R., & Coe, W. (1972). *Hypnosis: A social psychological analysis of influence communication*. New York: Holt, Rinehart & Winston.

Scheppele, K. L, & Bart, P. B. (1983). Through women's eyes: Defining danger in the work of sexual assault. *Journal of Social Issues, 39*, 63–81.

Schwartz, R. C., Barrett, M. J., & Saba, G. (1983, October). *Family therapy for bulimia*. Paper presented at the annual conference of the American Association for Marriage and Family Therapy, Washington, DC.

Scott, J. P. (1981). Biological and psychological bases of social attachment. In H. Kellerman (Ed.), *Group cohesion: Theoretical and clinical perspectives* (pp. 207–224). New York: Grune & Stratton.

Seligman, M. E. P. (1975). *Helplessness: On depression, development, and death*. San Francisco: W. H. Freeman.

Seltzer, L. F. (1986). *Paradoxical strategies in psychotherapy: A comprehensive overview and guidebook*. New York: Wiley.

Seltzer, M. (1976). Suggestions for the examination of time-disordered relationships. In J. Gubrium (Ed.), *Time, roles, and self in old age* (pp. 111–125). New York: Human Sciences Press.

Selvini-Palazzoli, M., Boscolo, L., Cecchin, G., & Prata, G. (1978). *Paradox and counterparadox*. New York: Jason Aronson.

Shapiro, D. A., & Shapiro, D. (1982). Meta-analysis of comparative therapy outcome studies: A replication and refinement. *Psychological Bulletin, 92*, 581–604.

Sheehan, P. W. (1979). Hypnosis and the process of imagination. In E. Fromm & R. E. Shor (Eds.), *Hypnosis: Developments in research and new perspectives* (pp. 381–411). Chicago: Aldine.

Sheehy, G. (1976). *Passages: Predictable crises of adult life*. New York: Dutton.

Shutz, W. C. (1966). *The interpersonal underworld*. Palo Alto, CA: Science & Behavior Books.

Siever, L. J., & Klar, H. (1986). A review of DSM-III criteria for the personality disorders. In A. J. Frances & R. E. Hales (Eds.), *Psychiatry update: American Psychiatric Association Annual Review* (Vol. 5, pp. 279–314). Washington, DC: American Psychiatric Association.

Sifneos, P. (1972). *Short-term psychotherapy and emotional crisis.* Cambridge, MA: Harvard University Press.

Sifneos, P.E. (1978a). Evaluation criteria for selection of patients. In H. Davanloo (Ed.), *Basic principles and techniques in short-term dynamic psychotherapy* (pp. 81–84). New York: Spectrum.

Sifneos, P. E. (1978b). Techniques of short-term anxiety provoking therapy. In H. Davanloo (Ed.), *Basic principles and techniques in short-term dynamic psychotherapy* (pp. 433–453). New York: Spectrum.

Sifneos, P. E. (1979). *Short-term dynamic psychotherapy: Evaluation and technique.* New York: Plenum Press.

Silver, R. J. (1982). Brief dynamic psychotherapy: A critical look at the state of the art. *Psychiatric Quarterly, 53,* 275–282.

Silver, R. L., & Wortman, C. B. (1980). Coping with undesirable life events. In J. Garber & M.E.P. Seligman (Eds.), *Human helplessness* (pp. 279–340). New York: Academic Press.

Skynner, A. C. R. (1976). *Systems of family and marital psychotherapy.* New York: Brunner/Mazel.

Skynner, A. C. R. (1981). An open-systems, group analytic approach to family therapy. In A. S. Gurman & D. P. Kniskern (Eds.), *Handbook of family therapy* (pp. 39–84). New York: Brunner/Mazel.

Small, L. (1979). *The briefer psychotherapies.* New York: Brunner/Mazel.

Smith, M. L., Glass, G. V., & Miller, T. I. (1980). *The benefits of psychotherapy.* Baltimore: Johns Hopkins University Press.

Sobel, D. (1982, November 21). A new and controversial short-term psychotherapy. *New York Times Magazine,* p. 58.

Solsberry, V., & Krupnick, J. (1984). Adults reactions to bereavement. In M. Osterweis, F. Solomon, & M. Green (Eds.), *Bereavement: Reactions, consequences, and care* (pp. 47–68). Washington, DC: National Academy Press.

Sophocles, (1949). Oedipus the King (D. Grene, Trans.). In C. A. Robinson (Ed.), *An anthology of Greek drama, first series* (pp. 51–100). New York: Holt, Rinehart & Winston. (Original work produced ca. 429 B.C.)

Spanos, N. P., & Barber, T. X. (1976). Behavior modification and hypnosis. In M. Hersen, R. M. Eisler, & P. M. Miller (Eds.), *Progress in behavior modification* (Vol. 3, pp. 110–142). New York: Academic Press.

Spanos, N. P., Valois, R., Ham, M. W., & Ham, M. L. (1973). Suggestibility and vividness and control of imagery. *International Journal of Clinical and Experimental Hypnosis, 21,* 305–311.

Spiegel, H. (1974). *Manual for hypnotic induction profile.* New York: Soni Medica.

Spiegel, H., & Linn, L. (1969). The "ripple effect" following adjunct hypnosis in analytic psychotherapy. *American Journal of Psychiatry, 126,* 53–58.

Spiegel, H., & Spiegel, D. (1978). *Trance and treatment: Clinical uses of hypnosis.* New York: Basic Books.

Spielman, A. J. (1986). Assessment of insomnia. *Clinical Psychology Review, 6,* 11–25.

Sprenkle, D. H., & Weis, D. L. (1978). Extramarital sexuality: Implications for marital therapists. *Journal of Sex and Marital Therapy, 4,* 279–291.

Stangl, D., Pfohl, B., Zimmerman, M., Bowers, W., & Corenthal, C. (1985). A structured interview for the DSM-III personality disorders. *Archives of General Psychiatry, 42,* 591–596.

Stanton, M. D. (1981). Strategic approaches to family therapy. In A. S. Gurman & D. P. Kniskern (Eds.), *Handbook of family therapy* (pp. 361–402). New York: Brunner/Mazel.

Stanton, M. D., Todd, T., & Associates, (1982). *The family therapy of drug addiction.* New York: Guilford Press.

Stern, J. A., Brown, M., Ulett, G. A., & Sletten, I. (1977). A Comparison of hypnosis, morphine, Valium, aspirin, and placebo in the management of experimentally induced pain. *Annals of the New York Academy of Sciences, 296,* 175–193.

Stinchcombe, A. L., Adams, R., Heimer, C. A., Scheppele K. L., Smith, T. W., & Taylor, D. G. (1980). *Crime and punishment: Changing attitudes in America.* San Francisco: Jossey-Bass.

Stone, W. N., & Rutan, J. S. (1984). Duration of group psychotherapy. *International Journal of Group Psychotherapy, 32,* 29–47.

Storm, C. L., & Sprenkle, D. H. (1982). Individual treatment in divorce therapy: A critique of an assumption. *Journal of Divorce, 5,* 87–97.

Strauss, M. A., Gelles, R. J., & Steinmetz, S. K. (1980). *Behind closed doors: Violence in the American family.* Garden City, NY: Doubleday.

Strupp, H. H. (1980a). Success and failure in time-limited psychotherapy: A systematic comparison of two cases (Comparison 1). *Archives of General Psychiatry, 37,* 595–603.

Strupp, H. H. (1980b). Success and failure in time-limited psychotherapy: A systematic comparison of two cases (Comparison 2). *Archives of General Psychiatry, 37,* 708–716.

Strupp, H. H. (1980c). Success and failure in time-limited psychotherapy: With special reference to the performance of a lay counselor (Comparison 3). *Archives of General Psychiatry, 37,* 831–841.

Strupp, H. H. (1980d). Success and failure in time-limited psychotherapy: Further evidence (Comparison 4). *Archives of General Psychiatry, 37,* 947–954.

Strupp, H. H., & Binder, J. L. (1984). *Psychotherapy in a new key: A guide to time-limited dynamic psychotherapy.* New York: Basic Books.

Stuart, R. B. (1978). *Act thin, stay thin.* New York: Norton.

Stuart, R. B. (1980). *Helping couples change: A social learning approach to marital therapy.* New York: Guilford Press.

Stunkard, A. J. (1985). Obesity. In R. E. Hales & A. J. Frances (Eds.), *Psychiatry update: American Psychiatric Association annual review* (Vol. 4, pp. 419–437). Washington, DC: American Psychiatric Association.

Stunkard, A. J., & Mendelson, M. (1967). Obesity and the body image: I. Characteristics of disturbance in the body image of some obsese persons. *American Journal of Psychiatry, 123,* 1296–1300.

Sullivan, H. S. (1953). *The interpersonal theory of psychiatry.* New York: Norton.

Surman, O.S., Gottlieb, S. K., Hackett, T. P., & Silverberg, E. L. (1973). Hypnosis in the treatment of warts. *Archives of General Psychiatry, 28,* 439–441.

Sutcliffe, J. P., Perry, G. W., & Sheehan, P. W. (1970). The relation of some aspects of imagery and fantasy to hypnotizability. *Journal of Abnormal Psychology, 76,* 279–287.

Taylor, S. (1983). Adjustment to threatening life events: A theory of cognitive adapation. *American Psychologist, 38,* 1161–1173.

Tellegen, A., & Atkinson, G. (1974). Openness to absorbing and self-altering experiences ("absorption"), a trait related to hypnotic susceptibility. *Journal of Abnormal Psychology, 83,* 268–277.

Tennyson, A. (1979). In memoriam A. H. H. In M. H. Abrams (General Ed.), *The Norton anthology of English literature* (4th ed., Vol. 2, pp. 1127–1174). New York: Norton. (Original work published 1850)

Thibaut, J., & Kelley, H. (1959). *The social psychology of groups.* New York: Wiley.

Thoits, P. (1985). Negative outcome: The influence of factors outside therapy. In D. T. Mays & C. M. Franks (Eds.), *Negative outcome in psychotherapy and what to do about it* (pp. 249–263). New York: Springer.

Ticho, E. (1972). Termination of psychoanalysis: Treatment goals, life goals. *Psychoanalytic Quarterly, 41,* 315–333.

Tolstoy, L. (1965). *Anna Karenina* (C. Garnett, Trans.; L. J. Kent & N. Berberova, Eds.). New York: Modern Library. (Original work published 1878)

Toomin, M. K. (1972). Structured separation with counseling: A therapeutic approach for couples in conflict. *Family Process, 11,* 299–310.

Troll, L. (1975). *Early and middle adulthood.* Monterey, CA: Brooks/Cole.

Tuckman, B. W. (1965). Developmental sequence in small groups. *Psychological Bulletin, 63,* 383–399.

Turner, R. J. (1983). Direct, indirect, and moderating effects of social support on psychological distress and associated conditions. In H. B. Kaplan (Ed.), *Psychosocial stress: Trends in theory and research* (pp. 105–155). New York: Academic Press.

Turner, R. M. (1986). Behavioral self control procedures for disorders of initiating and maintaining sleep (DIMS). *Clinical Psychology Review, 6,* 27–38.

U.S. Bureau of the Census, (1977). *Marital status and living arrangements: March 1976.* (Current Population Reports, Series P-20, No. 306). Washington, DC: U.S. Government Printing Office.

Vaillant, G. (1977). *Adaptation to life.* Boston: Little, Brown.

Vaillant, G., & McArthur, C. (1972). National history of psychological health: I. The adult life cycle from 18–50. *Seminars in Psychiatry, 4,* 415–427.

Van Dyck, R. (1982). How to use Ericksonian approaches when you are not Milton H. Erickson. In J. K. Zeig (Ed.), *Ericksonian approaches to hypnosis and psychotherapy* (pp. 37–47). New York: Brunner/Mazel.

Visher, E. B., & Visher, J. S. (1979). *Stepfamilies: A guide to working with stepparents and stepchildren.* New York: Brunner/Mazel.

Visher, J. S., & Visher, E. B. (1982). Stepfamilies and stepparenting. In F. Walsh (Ed.), *Normal family processes* (pp. 331–353). New York: Guilford Press.

Wachtel, P. L. (1977). *Psychoanalysis and behavior therapy: Toward an integration.* New York: Basic Books.

Wachtel, P. L. (1982). Interpersonal therapy and active intervention. In J. C. Anchin & D. J. Kiesler (Eds.), *Handbook of interpersonal psychotherapy* (pp. 46–63). New York: Pergamon Press.

Wadden, T. A., & Anderton, C. H. (1982). The clinical use of hypnosis. *Psychological Bulletin, 91,* 215–243.

Wallerstein, J., & Kelly, J. (1980). *Surviving the breakup.* New York: Basic Books.

Watkins, P., & Soledad, G. (1979). *My life with Charles Manson.* New York: Bantam Books.

Watzlawick, P., Fisch, R., & Segal, L. (1982). *The tactics of change.* San Francisco: Jossey-Bass.

Weakland, J. H., Fisch, R., Watzlawick, P., & Bodin, A. (1974). Brief therapy: Focused problem resolution. *Family Process, 13,* 141–168.

Weiner-Davis, M. (1987). Confessions of an unabashed marriage saver. *The Family Therapy Networker, 11*(1), 53–56.

Weinstein, N. D. (1980). Unrealistic optimism about future events. *Journal of Personality and Social Psychology, 39,* 806–820.

Weiss, R. S. (1974). The provisions of social relationships. In Z. Rubin (Ed.), *Doing unto others* (pp. 17–26). Englewood Cliffs, NJ: Prentice-Hall.

Weiss, R. S. (1975). *Marital separation.* New York: Basic Books.

Weiss, R. S. (1982). Attachment in adult life. In C. M. Parkes & J. Stevenson-Hinde (Eds.), *The place of attachment in human behavior* (pp. 171–184). New York: Basic Books.

Weissman, M. M., Klerman, G. L., Prusoff, B. A., Sholomskas, D., and Padian, N. (1981). Depressed outpatients: Results one year after treatment with drugs and/or interpersonal psychotherapy. *Archives of General Psychiatry, 36,* 51–55.

Weitzenhoffer, A. M. (1972). Behavior therapeutic techniques and hypnotic models. *American Journal of Clinical Hypnosis, 15,* 71–82.

Werner, E. E., & Smith, R. S. (1982). *Vulnerability and invincibility.* New York: McGraw-Hill.

Wile, D. E. (1981). *Couples therapy: A non-traditional approach.* New York: Wiley.

Willard, R. D. (1977). Breast enlargement through visual imagery and hypnosis. *American Journal of Clinical Hypnosis, 19,* 195–200.

Williamson, D. S. (1977). Extramarital involvements in couple interaction. In R. F. Stahmann & W. J. Heibert (Eds.), *Klemer's counseling in marital and sexual problems* (2nd ed.). Baltimore: Williams & Wilkins.

Williamson, D. S. (1981). New life at the graveyard. *Journal of Marriage and Family Counseling, 4,* 93–101.

Wilson, G. T. (1981). Behavior therapy as a short-term therapeutic approach. In S. H. Budman (Ed.), *Forms of brief therapy* (pp. 131–166). New York: Guilford Press.

Wilson, J. P., Smith, W. K., & Johnson, S. K. (1985). A comparative analysis of PTSD among various survivor groups. In C. R. Figley (Ed.), *Trauma and its wake* (pp. 142–172). New York: Brunner/Mazel.

Wilson, S. C., & Barber, T. X. (1978). The Creative Imagination Scale as a measure of hypnotic responsiveness: Applications to experimental and clinical hypnosis. *American Journal of Clinical Hypnosis, 20,* 235–249.

Wilson, S. C., & Barber, T. X. (1981). Vivid fantasy and hallucinatory abilities in the life histories of excellent hypnotic subjects ("somnambules"): Preliminary report with female subjects. In E. Klinger (Ed.), *Imagery: Vol. 2. Concepts, results, and applications* (pp. 133–149). New York: Plenum.

Wilson, S. C., & Barber, T. X. (1983). The fantasy-prone personality: Implications for understanding imagery, hypnosis and parapsychological phenomena. In A. A. Sheikh (Ed.), *Imagery: Current theory, research, and application* (pp. 340–387). New York: Wiley.

Windholz, M. J., Marmar, C. R., & Horowitz, M. J. (1985). A review of the research on conjugal bereavement: Impact on health and efficacy of intervention. *Comprehensive Psychiatry, 26,* 433–447.

Wolberg, L. R. (1965). The techniques of short-term psychotherapy. In L. R. Wolberg (Ed.), *Short-term psychotherapy* (pp. 127–200). New York: Grune & Stratton.

Wolberg, L. R. (1980). *Handbooks of short-term psychotherapy.* New York: Grune & Stratton.

Wolberg, L. R. (1982). *Hypnosis: It is for you?* New York: Dembner Books.

Wolff, S., & Chick, J. (1980). Schizoid personality in childhood: A controlled follow-up study. *Psychological Medicine, 10,* 85–100.

Woody, G. E., Luborsky, L., McLellan, T., O'Brien, C. P., Beck, A. T., Blaine, J., Herman, J., & Hole, A. (1983). Psychotherapy for opiate addicts: Does it help? *Archives of General Psychiatry, 40,* 639–645.

Worden, J. W. (1982). *Grief counseling and grief therapy: A handbook for the mental health practitioner.* New York: Springer.

Yalom, I. D. (1975). *The theory and practice of group psychotherapy* (2nd ed.). New York: Basic Books.

Yalom, I. D. (1980). *Existential psychotherapy.* New York: Basic Books.

Yalom, I. D. (1985). *The theory and practice of group psychotherapy* (3rd ed.). New York: Basic Books.

Zeig, J. F. (1980). *Teaching seminar with Milton H. Erickson, M.D.* New York: Brunner/ Mazel.

Zetzel, E. (1968). *The capacity of emotional growth.* New York: International Universities Press.

Zola, I. K. (1973). Pathways to the doctor—from person to patient. *Social Science and Medicine, 7,* 677–689.

Zusne, L. (1986). Some factors affecting the birthday and death day phenomenon. *Omega, 17,* 9–22.

Index

Accessibility, attachment and, 156
Acknowledgment, of group crisis, 277
Addiction to psychotherapy, 43, 44
Addressing group crisis, 277
Adjustment to personal catastrophe, 81, 82
Adult, unattached young, predictable tasks of, 155
Adult development
  chance encounters and, 70–72, 99
  considerations in I-D-E focus, 38, 39
  effect of childhood development, 97
  ordered-change account perspective, 106
  perspective
    of brief therapist, 14, 31; emotions and, 97, 98; personal narrative, 101, 102
  phenomenological position, 100
Affection, in family, 155, 156
Age, patient
  limitations on one's life, acceptance of, 113
  relationship to loneliness, 75
  significance of birthday, 38, 39
Aggression, inhibition of, 330
Agoraphobia, case example, 145–148
Alcoholics Anonymous, 41, 42
Alcoholism
  in divorce decision, case example of, 174–176
  initiation of therapy and, 41, 42
  treatment focus and, 65, 66
Alexander, F., 2, 3, 224, 225, 283, 284
Analytic therapy, regrieving for loss, 87–89
Anniversaries, patient, 39, 40
Antisocial disorders
  classification of, 217
  treatment of, 234–238
Anxiety
  anticipatory, 77, 78
  hypnosis for, 209–211
"Anxious cluster" disorders
  classification of, 217, 218
  treatment of, 239–242
Assets, individual and family/couple, 152
Attachment
  accessibility and, 156
  family, 155, 156
  research background, 74, 75
  types of, 75, 76
Attitudinal factors, 10–16
Attribution-oriented reframing, 128–138
Avoidant disorders
  classification of, 217, 218
  treatment of, 239–242

Bandura, A., 69–71, 99
Behavior
  change, in developmental dysynchrony therapy, 110–112
  functional analysis of, 131
Behavioral therapy, regrieving for loss, 87–89
Bereavement (see also Interpersonal loss)
  impact on health, 77
Binder, J. L., 287
Binuclear family, 164, 181
"Birthday–death day" phenomenon, 38, 39
Bonds, stepfamilies and, 185, 186
Borderline character disorders
  classification of, 217
  severe, interminable brief therapy for, 242–244
  treatment of, 234–238
Boundaries
  of family and couple, 154
  stepfamilies and, 186
Boxer, A. M., 100, 101
Braid, James, 191
Brief therapy (see specific aspects or applications of)
Business aspects, of long-term therapy, 13

Cancer
  emotional recovery from mastectomy, 86, 87
  psychological adjustment to, 81, 82
Carter, E. A., 185, 186
Case transcript, David, 303–371
Chance encounters
  effect on patient's life course, 70–72
  life paths and, 99
Change
  character
    in brief therapy, 14; in long-term therapy, 11, 12
  in developmental dysynchrony therapy, 110–112
  predictability of, 218
  realistic timetable for, 367
  vs. cure, 371
Character disorders (see Personality disorders)
Childhood
  development
    of attachment, 74, 75; emotional, effect on adult personality, 97; faulty learning during, 68, 69
  learning to inhibit aggression during, 330
  punishment, hypnotic susceptibility and, 192, 193
Children
  inclusion in marital therapy, 167
  launching, predictable tasks of, 155